Cholestatic Liver Diseases: Therapeutic Options and Perspectives

FALK SYMPOSIUM 136

Cholestatic Liver Diseases: Therapeutic Options and Perspectives

In honour of Hans Popper's 100th birthday

Edited by

U. Leuschner
Innere Medizin II
Klinikum der Johann Wolfgang
Goethe-Universität Frankfurt
Frankfurt
Germany

U. Broomé
Department of Gastroenterology
and Hepatology, K63
Huddinge University Hospital
Huddinge
Sweden

A. Stiehl
Medizinische Universitätsklinik
Heidelberg
Germany

Proceedings of Falk Symposium 136 (Part I of the XII Falk Liver Week)
held in Freiburg, Germany, October 15–16, 2003

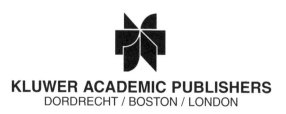

KLUWER ACADEMIC PUBLISHERS
DORDRECHT / BOSTON / LONDON

Library of Congress Cataloging-in-Publication Data is available.

ISBN 0-7923-8793-7

Published by Kluwer Academic Publishers, BV
P.O. Box 17, 3300 AA Dordrecht, The Netherlands.

Sold and distributed in North, Central and South America
by Kluwer Academic Publishers,
101 Philip Drive, Norwell, MA 02061, USA.

In all other countries, sold and distributed
by Kluwer Academic Publishers, Distribution Center,
P.O. Box 322, 3300 AH Dordrecht, The Netherlands.

Printed on acid-free paper

Printed and bound in Great Britain by MPG Books, Bodmin, Cornwall.

Contents

CONTENTS

SECTION III: CLINICS OF PRIMARY BILIARY CIRRHOSIS

SECTION IV: OVERLAP SYNDROMES

SECTION V: TREATMENT OF PRIMARY BILIARY CIRRHOSIS

List of Principal Contributors

DH Adams
Liver Research Group
5th Floor, Institute of Biomedical
  Research
Wolfson Drive
The University of Birmingham Medical
  School
Edgbaston
Birmingham, B15 2TT
UK

NV Bergasa
Columbia University
College of Physicians and
  Surgeons
Digestive and Liver Diseases
630 West 168th Street
New York, NY 10032
USA

A Bergquist
Department of Gastroenterology and
  Hepatology, K63
Huddinge University Hospital
141 86 Stockholm
Sweden

U Beuers
Medizinische Klinik II –
Grosshadern
Ludwig-Maximilians-Universität
  München
Marchioninistr. 15
D-81377 München
Germany

KM Boberg
Medical Department
Rikshospitalet
0027 Oslo
Norway

CE Broelsch
Department of General Surgery and
  Transplantation
University Hospital Essen
Hufelandstr. 55
D-45122 Essen
Germany

U Broomé
Department of Gastroenterology and
  Hepatology, K63
Huddinge University Hospital
141 86 Huddinge
Sweden

RW Chapman
John Radcliffe Hospital
University of Oxford
Department of Gastroenterology
Headley Way, Headington
Oxford, OX3 9DU
UK

E Christensen
Clinic of Internal Medicine I
Bispebjerg University Hospital
Bispebjerg Bakke 23
DK 2400 Copenhagen NV
Denmark

AJ Czaja
Mayo Clinic
Division of
  Gastroenterology and Hepatology
200 First Street SW
Rochester, MN 55905
USA

VJ Desmet
Catholic University of Leuven
University Hospital St. Rafael
Department of Morphology and
  Molecular Pathology
Minderbroederstraat 12
B-3000 Leuven
Belgium

HP Dienes
Pathologie
Klinikum der Universität
Joseph-Stelzmann-Str. 9
D-50931 Köln
Germany

PT Donaldson
Centre for Liver Research
University of Newcastle
The Medical School
Framlington Place
Newcastle upon Tyne, NE2 4HH
UK

KA Fleming
University of Oxford
Medical Sciences Office
Level 3, John Radcliffe Hospital
Headington
Oxford OX3 9DU
UK

ME Gershwin
Division of Rheumatology,
  Allergy and Clinical
  Immunology
University of California at
  Davis School of Medicine
TB 192
Davis, CA 95616
USA

J Heathcote
University of Toronto
Toronto Western Hospital
Fell Pavilion 6B-170
399 Bathurst Street
Toronto, Ontario
M5T 2S8
Canada

OFW James
Centre for Liver Research
University of Newcastle
The Medical School
Framlington Place
Newcastle upon Tyne, NE2 4HH
UK

DEJ Jones
Centre for Liver Research
University of Newcastle
The Medical School
Floor 4, William Leech Building
Framlington Place
Newcastle upon Tyne, NE2 4HH
UK

R Joplin
Liver Research Laboratories
University Hospital Birmingham
Birmingham
B15 2TH
UK

KV Kowdley
University of Washington,
  Medical Center
Gastroenterology and Hepatology
Box 356174
1959 NE Pacific Street
Seattle, WA 98195
USA

U Leuschner
Innere Medizin II
Klinikum der Johann Wolfgang
  Goethe-Universität Frankfurt
Theodor-Stern-Kai 7
D-60596 Frankfurt
Germany

AW Lohse
I Medizinische Klinik und Poliklinik
Johannes-Gutenberg-Universität
  Mainz
Langenbeckstr. 1
D-55131 Mainz
Germany

IG McFarlane
King's College Hospital
Institute of Liver Studies
Denmark Hill
London
SE5 9RS
UK

G Mieli-Vergani
Paediatric Liver Service
King's College Hospital
Denmark Hill
London, SE5 9RS
UK

J Neuberger
Queen Elizabeth Hospital
The Liver and Hepatobiliary Unit
3rd Floor, Nuffield House
Birmingham
B15 2TH
UK

JL Newton
Institute for Ageing and Health
School of Clinical Medical
  Sciences
Care of the Elderly Offices
Royal Victoria Infirmary
Newcastle upon Tyne
NE1 4LP
UK

R Olsson
Department of Medicine
Sahlgrenska University Hospital
41345 Goteborg
Sweden

CY Ponsioen
Hilversum Hospital
Department of Internal Medicine
PO Box 10016
1201 DA Hilversum
The Netherlands

R Poupon
Hôpital Saint-Antoine
Service d'Hepato-Gastro-
  Enterologie
184, rue du Faubourg St. Antoine
F-75571 Paris
France

SM Riordan
Prince of Wales Hospital
Gastrointestinal and Liver Unit
Barker Street
Randwick
NSW 2031
Australia

E Schrumpf
University of Oslo, Medical
  Department
Rikshospitalet
Section of Gastroenterology and
  Hepatology
0027 Oslo
Norway

D Schuppan
Department of Medicine I
Department of Gastroenterology and
  Hepatology
University of Erlangen-Nürnberg
Ulmenweg 18
D-91054 Erlangen
Germany

A Stiehl
Medizinische Universitätsklinik
Bergheimer Str. 58
D-69115 Heidelberg
Germany

CP Strassburg
Department of Gastroenterology,
 Hepatology and Endocrinology, and
 Heisenberg Scholar of the Deutsche
 Forschungsgemeinschaft
Hannover Medical School
Carl-Neuberg-Str. 1
D-30625 Hannover
Germany

MG Swain
University of Calgary
Health Sciences Center
3330 Hospital Drive NW
Calgary, Alberta
T2N 4N1
Canada

GP van Berge Henegouwen
Department of Gastroenterology and
 Hepatology
University Medical Centre Utrecht,
 F02.618
PO Box 85500
3508 GA Utrecht
The Netherlands

HR van Buuren
Department of Gastroenterology
Erasmus Medical Centre
 Rotterdam
PO Box 2040
3000 CA Rotterdam
The Netherlands

JM Vierling
Cedars-Sinai Medical
 Center – UCLA
Hepatology and Liver Transplantation
 Programs
8635 West Third Street
Los Angeles
CA 90048
USA

Preface

This book comprises the scientific contributions to the Falk Symposium No. 136 "Cholestatic Liver Diseases: Therapeutic Options and Perspectives", held in Freiburg, Germany, in October 2003.

During the last two decades, knowledge about cholestatic liver diseases and concomitant diseases, such as ulcerative colitis, cholangio- and hepatocellular carcinoma, pancreas and colon cancer, has increased considerably. Studies on ursodeoxycholic acid therapy alone or in combination with immunosuppressive compounds, and their positive effects on biliary liver diseases as well as on so-called overlap syndromes or intestinal tumours, are published in increasing numbers and stimulate the discussion whether or not ursodeoxycholic acid is able to improve the general condition and/or life expectancy of our patients.

On the other hand, genetics, aetiological and pathogenetic aspects are still difficult to comprehend, but are the absolute prerequisite for the development of better treatment options. In this book, both progress in basic research and especially in clinical application of recent data to medical treatment are presented.

The Falk Symposium No. 136, part of the XII Falk Liver Week, was an international and interdisciplinary symposium at the highest scientific level. The editors are grateful to the contributors, but especially extend their thanks to Dr. Herbert Falk and Ursula Falk and the staff of the Falk Foundation e.V. for the generous support. They also thank Lancaster Publishing Services Ltd., Lancaster, U.K., for their excellent cooperation in producing this book.

Prof. Dr. Ulrich Leuschner
Prof. Dr. Ulrika Broomé
Prof. Dr. Adolf Stiehl

Section I
Epidemiology and aetiology of primary biliary cirrhosis

1
Epidemiology of primary biliary cirrhosis

O. F. W. JAMES

INTRODUCTION

Modern epidemiology may be valuable in giving clues as to the cause of a disease – for example in the case of the Broad Street pump and typhoid. High-quality epidemiological studies of primary biliary cirrhosis (PBC) are increasingly bringing this disease to the attention of health-service planners (for example in provision of liver transplantation services), as well as informing patients and patient support groups. We have recently carried out a systematic review of studies of PBC epidemiology, and this summary is drawn from the systematic review[1].

METHODS

Studies were identified from systematic searches of the electronic forms of the Medline and Embase databases. Both databases were searched from their date of inception (1966 for Medline and 1980 for Embase) using search strings designed to be as comprehensive as possible. In addition, abstracts from relevant hepatology meetings were hand-searched. The reference lists of all relevant studies were examined to identify further studies. Inclusion and exclusion criteria were adapted from Jacobson et al.[2]. Papers were included if they reported the incidence or prevalence of PBC in a population of defined size; any clinical definition of PBC was allowed. Papers were excluded if they: (a) consisted of case reports of case series in which the size of the catchment population was not given or was not calculable (i.e. missing denominator data); (b) reported only the frequency of PBC within a subgroup of patients with another condition (for example patients with other autoimmune disease or coeliac disease); (c) only reported the frequency of another medical condition among patients with PBC; or (d) comprised a review article containing no original data.

POPULATION SCREENING STUDIES

No study has until now screened an unselected population for PBC. Matallia et al. studied the incidence of antimitochondrial antibodies (AMA) in Italy using 1530 blood samples (975 from women) acquired from blood donors or adults undergoing endoscopy[3]. Nine individuals were positive for AMA by ELISA. There was no follow-up to determine which patients had PBC.

Perhaps the most interesting screening study was that in which 17 899 survivors of the Nagasaki atomic bomb explosion were screened for PBC[4]. A total of 870 (653 female) serum specimens revealed raised serum alkaline phosphatase, and 484 survivors agreed to further investigation; 28 were AMA-positive. The frequency of PBC (defined as AMA-positive and raised alkaline phosphatase) – 1565 cases per million – varied with distance from the explosion. The importance of this finding is quite unclear, but intriguing.

EPIDEMIOLOGICAL STUDIES OF THE FREQUENCY OF PBC

Eight epidemiological studies were published before 1986. Generally these were of relatively low quality and all were in populations which were subsequently restudied using better methodology. They are of limited use for our current understanding of the epidemiology of PBC and will be discussed further only in the context of studies of the same area repeated at a later date. Later studies of PBC epidemiology are summarized in Table 1.

European studies

United Kingdom

Nine groups have reported the prevalence of PBC in the United Kingdom. Three of these have only been published in abstract form, or in correspondence. In Sheffield a recent study by Ray-Chadhuri et al. presented updated incidence and prevalence data using the methods of James et al.[5,6]. The prevalence of PBC increased during the study period from 57 cases per million in 1987 to 238 in 1999. Mean annual incidence was around 20 per million per year. In Tayside, Scotland, a recent study reviewing earlier surveys demonstrated a rise in prevalence from 186 per million in 1986 to 379 per million in 1996. The latter figure was due to comprehensive case finding with clear diagnostic criteria, and a well-defined population at risk. This may have contributed to the high prevalence found.

A series of studies of PBC epidemiology have been carried out by our own group over more than 20 years. Results were summarized by James et al. in 1999[5]. This most recent study used multiple case-finding strategies to identify a comprehensive cohort of patients with PBC, including those under primary care and those in whom the diagnosis was possible based upon the results of prior investigations, but not made by the clinician caring for the patient at this time. Cases were identified by questionnaires to all relevant physicians in the study area, follow-up of all positive AMA results from immunology laboratories, examination of the case records of patients with PBC recorded on their death

Table 1 Summary results of epidemiological studies of PBC published since 1986

Year of publication	Area of study	Period of survey	No. of PBC cases	Population at risk	Mean incidence (per million per year)	Final point prevalence (per million)
1986	Nottingham, England	1970–1984	38	573 000	4.4	42
1986	Picardy, France	1975–1984	31	2 380 000	2.6	13
1987	West of Scotland	1965–1980	195	3 000 000	13.3	93
1987	Asturias, Spain	1973–1985	29	1 131 000	2.0	21
1988	Midi-Pyrenees, France	1984–1985	66	2 330 000	8.5	
1989	Navarra, Spain	1974–1987	39	523 000	9.5	62
1990	Northern Sweden	1973–1982	111	570 000	13.3	151
1990	Madrid, Spain	1974–1988	45	747 000	4.6	46
1990	Northeast England	1965–1987	411	1 920 000	15.0	129
1990	Ontario, Canada	1987	189	8 900 000	3.3	22
1991	Denmark	1981–1985	233	5 110 000	9.0	
1991	Quebec, Canada	1980–1986	228	8 970 000	3.9	25
1991	Granada, Spain	1976–1989	25	443 000	4.0	36
1992	Israel	1980–1990	30	4 500 000	0.7	6.7
1995	Estonia	1973–1992	69	1 530 000	2.3	27
1995	Victoria, Australia	1990–1991	84	4 390 000		19
1996	Birmingham, England	1982–1994	4	277 000		14
1996	Winnipeg, Canada	1987–1994	52	650 000	12.3	
1996	Netherlands	1979–1992	596	15 000 000	2.8	
1998	Akershus, Norway	1985–1994	21	180 000	12.0	120
1998	Oslo, Norway	1986–1995	21	130 000	16.2	146
1998	Swansea, Wales	1984–1996	67	251 000		203
1999	Northeast England	1987–1994	770	2 040 000	26.6	251
1999	Hiroshima, Japan	1988–1997	156	2 870 000		54
2000	Olmstead County, USA	1975–1995	46	107 000	27.0	402
2001	Sheffield, England	1987–1999	172	529 000	20.5	238
2001	Dundee, Scotland	1986–1996	294	560 000	49.0	379
2002	Alaska, USA	1984–2000	18	100 000		289
2002	Japan	1968–1998	4361	125 000 000	2.3	27

5

certificates and a review of centrally maintained discharge diagnosis databases. The denominator population (approximately 2.05 million) was clearly defined by health authority boundaries and calculated from annually updated census estimates. Case definition remained unchanged; 770 cases (694 female, 469 asymptomatic at diagnosis) of PBC prevalent or incident between 1987 and 1994 were identified. The incidence of PBC rose from 23 per million in 1987 to 32.3 per million in 1994 (91 per million in women aged over 40). Overall prevalence rose from 149 to 251 per million during this time (541–940 per million in women aged over 40). This frequency is among the three highest recorded in unselected populations worldwide; it may reflect the use of highly comprehensive case-finding methods or may reflect local excesses of disease due to environmental or genetic factors. While the prevalence of PBC rose in northeast England from 18 per million in 1976 to 251 per million in 1994, and the annual incidence rose from 11.3 cases per million in 1976 to a median 30 per million between 1987 and 1994, it is still unclear as to whether this extraordinary increase is due to improved PBC case identification methods and general awareness among doctors, or whether it represents a true increase. The same may be said of other studies from around the world which have also reported steadily increasing prevalence and incidence. It is fair to say that in the good Tayside, Scotland, study and our own studies, where consistent case-finding methods have been adopted over a 4- or 5-year period in more recent times, no statistically significant increase in annual incidence has now been observed.

Two other UK studies are worth mentioning. First, Anand et al. identified cases of PBC in UK resident patients of non-European origin treated at the Queen Elizabeth Hospital, Birmingham, between 1982 and 1994[8]. Six cases occurred in Asian patients (three of Indian origin, two Pakistani, one Malaysian – all female), four of these lived in Birmingham. The period prevalence of PBC was 14 per million in the regional Asian population (100 per million in Asian women aged over 35). While this was a methodologically incomplete study, its interest lies in the fact that, as the authors remark, this incidence contrasts with the extremely low frequency of PBC reported in Asia (see below), and suggests evidence for an acquired environmental risk for the disease.

Kingham and Parker estimated the prevalence of PBC in Swansea, Wales, from a meticulous case register maintained between 1984 and 1996, and from a review of hospital records of any patient with positive AMA or liver biopsy suggestive of PBC in this period[9]. Within a defined study population ($n = 251\,000$), 67 cases of PBC were identified, giving a period prevalence of 251 cases per million and a final point prevalence of 203 cases per million. In summary of these UK studies from four distinct locations (excluding the Birmingham study) prevalence of above 200 per million and, allowing for methodological imperfections, more probably up to 300 per million, looks very plausible. Extrapolation of this figure to the overall UK population would suggest that there may be around 18 000 patients with this disease in the UK.

France

Two studies have reported the frequency of PBC in France; however, neither of these used modern epidemiological methods and in both studies other flaws suggested many missed cases. Accordingly it is very difficult to give an authoritative up-to-date estimation of prevalence in France[10,11].

Spain

Five case series reporting the frequency of PBC in different regions of Spain were published between 1984 and 1991. In none of these were rigorous case finding or epidemiological methods used. However, it is of interest that in the most thorough of these[12] Borda et al. found an increasing incidence of PBC from 4.1 per million in 1974 to 25.2 in 1987 (78 cases per million in women over age 25). The prevalence of PBC was 62 per million (186 in women over age 25). Given the incompleteness of the methods used, these figures are broadly comparable to those found in the UK.

Sweden

Three groups have reviewed the frequency of PBC in Sweden. The most recent of these was a rigorous study in northern Sweden carried out between 1973 and 1982 by Danielsson et al.[13]. Cases of PBC were identified from case registers and a survey of physicians in all hospitals in a study area, and by retrospective examination of all positive AMA from the laboratories serving the areas. A total of 111 cases (72 initially asymptomatic) were identified in a population of 570 000. Average incidence of PBC was 13.3 per million over the study period with no secular trend. Point prevalence in 1982 was 151 cases per million. This was a well-designed study in which cases were identified from multiple sources to obtain as complete a case register as possible. The size of the population and the cohort of patients mean that confidence limits for estimates of frequency are relatively tight.

Norway

Boberg et al. reviewed the frequency of autoimmune liver disease, including PBC, treated at one hospital in Oslo between 1986 and 1995[14]. The hospital is one of four in Oslo, and has a catchment area of 130 000. Patients were identified from coding of admission and discharge diagnosis. Twenty-one cases of PBC were treated during the study. The mean annual incidence was 16 per million. Prevalence rose from 78 to 146 per million between 1986 and 1995. The authors agree that the study may have underestimated prevalence and incidence; however, since the study only included patients seen in the single tertiary case centre, it did not attempt to ascertain patient flows between hospitals. Two other smaller studies with very small numbers of patients in limited populations came to not-dissimilar findings, but estimates of incidence and prevalence have very wide confidence limits.

The Netherlands and Denmark

In each of these countries an overall estimate of the frequency of PBC has been carried out for the country as a whole, using national statistics of death certification or hospital admissions. Because, in both studies, routinely collected data were used, no standardized diagnostic criteria could be applied, and case definition could not be verified. In the Dutch study a very severe underestimate of PBC frequency must have occurred, since those patients with PBC whose death was due to non-liver-related disease were not included[15]. In Denmark the study may have missed significant numbers of patients since only in-patient episodes were recorded[16].

Other European countries

No formal epidemiological evaluations of PBC are reported from several European countries. A number of large single-centre case series have been published from Italy[17,18] and Greece[19], indicating that PBC in these countries may well occur at a similar frequency to that reported elsewhere.

In summarizing European studies outside the UK, apart from the Swedish study reported, there are such significant methodological and statistical problems that comparison between countries is really impossible beyond saying that PBC probably has a not-dissimilar incidence and prevalence in major European countries – both northern and southern. More comprehensive studies are eagerly awaited.

North American studies

Canada. Two epidemiological studies were carried out about 15 years ago in Ontario[20] and Quebec[21]. Both studies had incomplete case-finding methods but each showed prevalence around 25 per million and incidence about 3.5 per million. Each series probably grossly underestimates asymptomatic patients.

The United States. Two studies have reported the frequency of PBC in the USA. Kim et al.[22] recently reported the frequency of PBC in Olmstead County, Rochester (population 106 500). The main data source was the Rochester Epidemiology Project. This extremely thorough study suggested the age- and sex-standardized prevalence in December 1995 was 402 cases per million (654 cases per million in women). The average annual incidence was 27 cases per million. There were no secular trends reported.

In Alaskan natives Hurlburt et al.[23] identified PBC through review of outpatient records in all clinics in the State of Alaska, together with other case-finding methods. Point prevalence in 2000 was 289 per million. These data contradict the widely held belief that PBC is largely restricted to populations of European ethnic origin. Because both of the American studies were carried out on small populations, confidence limits must be wide.

Africa

No studies of the frequency of PBC in Africa have been published. One case series from Cape Town reported eight cases ever diagnosed. Two of these had originated from northeast England[24].

Australasian studies

Watson et al.[25] identified cases of PBC in the State of Victoria using incomplete case-finding methods; the prevalence of PBC was low at 19.1 per million. The disease was less frequent in patients born in Australia, and prevalence was

47.8 per million among first-generation European migrants. This might suggest an environmental risk factor. The group is currently undertaking a new study using more complete methods for case identification. Preliminary results suggest that the true incidence is now 50% higher than previously reported (Angus, personal communication, 2003).

Japan

The Japanese government has undertaken biannual surveys of the frequency of PBC in Japan (population 125 million) since 1980 through the Intractable Liver Disease Research Project team. Results were published most recently in 1997[26]. The annual incidence of PBC has been between 1.9 and 3.2 new cases per million, and point prevalence has risen to 54.3 per million in Japan[27]. Although this programme, and its accompanying spin-off studies, is by far the largest reported survey of PBC, the investigators agree that they may have missed a large proportion of cases since only a single case-finding method was used. Taking this into account it is clear that the prevalence of PBC in Japan is probably comparable to that in parts of Europe.

Other Asian countries

We have found no studies of the prevalence of PBC elsewhere in Australasia, although case series indicate that there is possibly a low to intermediate prevalence in Taiwan and Singapore[1]. In India only one case of PBC was identified among almost 28 000 new referrals with chronic liver disease to the major liver referral centre in India[8]. The total number of patients reported from Indian centres is 16.

GEOGRAPHICAL VARIATION IN THE FREQUENCY OF PBC

The above worldwide studies vary in their estimates of the frequency of PBC. It is very difficult to know to what extent differences in study methods or true geographical variation may have contributed to differences between Asia and Africa on the one hand and Europe and North America on the other. Eleven studies have used aggregated data to compare the frequency of PBC in subregions of their study areas; these are summarized in ref. 1. While the majority of these are of poor methodological quality, three interesting findings have emerged, one of which has subsequently been retracted.

In an early study Triger found that in Sheffield, UK, 30 (88%) of 34 cases of PBC extracted their home drinking water from a single reservoir[28]. This reservoir, however, served only 40% of the population living in the study area. Recent re-evaluation of these data in a much larger cohort has not confirmed this finding (odds ratio 0.88; 95% CI 0.57–1.31), suggesting that the original result probably occurred from a type I error[6].

The second finding emerging from studies of geographical variation in the frequency of PBC, arising from several of these in Europe, suggests that PBC may be less common in rural areas; however, methods used were incomplete and numbers were small.

We have recently performed a large study to examine spatial variation in risk for PBC on a cohort of 770 patients using point process analysis[29]. There were very substantial, statistically significant, anomalies in the spatial distribution of patients. These appeared to arise both from large-scale variation in the risk of disease and from local clustering of cases. Extraordinary clusters of disease were noticed in several urban areas (up to 13 cases per km^2). No obvious demographic or geographical features were found to explain this variation, although they do suggest the presence of one or more unidentified environmental risk factors. These studies are at present being repeated with a fresh cohort of patients.

CASE–CONTROL STUDIES OF RISK FACTORS FOR PBC

Two case–control studies have examined a variety of putative environmental risk factors for PBC. Parikh-Patel et al. identified 241 patients with PBC from an internet mail list server. These were compared with age-matched controls selected from the siblings and friends of these patients, and chosen by the patients themselves[30]. Increased frequency of smoking (OR 2.0; CI 1.1–3.8), urinary tract infection (2.1; 1.1–3.4), tonsillectomy (1.9; 1.0–3.4) and shingles were found in cases. However, methods of selection for both cases and controls were unconventional and were certainly susceptible to marked selection bias. An earlier smaller case–control study from our own group[31] also identified smoking as a powerful risk factor for PBC (2.4; 1.4–4.1) as well as finding an unexpected association with psoriasis (4.6;1.2–17.3) and a negative association with eczema (0.13; 0.02–1.0).

SUMMARY

Substantial increases in prevalence of PBC have been detected wherever studies have been carried out over 10 or more years. Together these data strongly suggest that in many countries the frequency with which PBC is diagnosed has increased very considerably between 1980 and the present time. Unfortunately the reasons for this change may be complex. There may have been a true increase in the incidence of PBC, reflecting either increased exposure to a currently unknown environmental agent, or demographic changes with an increased elderly at-risk population. The prevalence may also have increased due to increased survival of patients either due to improved care or earlier diagnosis.

To complicate matters further, it is likely that some of the apparent increase in PBC frequency may have resulted from increased use of diagnostic tests, increased clinician or patient awareness of the disease, and increased use of well-person screening or investigation of ill-defined symptoms.

We suggest that, as with other diseases, modern epidemiological instruments used in well-designed studies may both provide important clues to the cause or causes of the disease and guide future provision of services for PBC sufferers.

References

1. Prince MI, James OFW. The epidemiology of primary biliary cirrhosis. Clin Liver Dis. 2003;7:795–819.
2. Jacobson DL, Grange SJ, Rose NR, Graham NM. Epidemiology and estimated population burden of selected autoimmune diseases in the United States. Clin Immunol Immunopathol. 1997;84:223–43.
3. Mattalia A, Quaranta S, Leung PS et al. Characterization of antimitochondrial antibodies in healthy adults. Hepatology. 1998;27:656–61.
4. Ohba K, Omagari K, Kinoshita H et al. Primary biliary cirrhosis among atomic bomb survivors in Nagasaki, Japan. J Clin Epidemiol. 2001;54:845–50.
5. James OFW, Bhopal R, Howel D, Gray J, Burt AD, Metcalf JV. Primary biliary cirrhosis once rare, now common in the United Kingdom? Hepatology. 1999;30:390–4.
6. Ray-Chadhuri D, Rigney E, McCormack K et al. Epidemiology of PBC in Sheffield updates: demographic and relation to water supply. London: British Association for the Study of the Liver. 2001:42.
7. Steinke D, Weston T, Morris A, Macdonald T, Dillon J. Incidence, prevalence and resource use of primary biliary cirrhosis in Tayside, Scotland. J Hepatol. 2001;31:532A.
8. Anand AC, Elias E, Neuberger JM. End-stage primary biliary cirrhosis in a first generation migrant South Asian population. Eur J Gastroenterol Hepatol. 1996;8:663–6.
9. Kingham JG, Parker DR. The association between primary biliary cirrhosis and coeliac disease: a study of relative prevalence. Gut. 1998;42:120–2.
10. Cales P, Cales V, Oksman F, Vinel JP, Pascal JP. Significance of antimitochondrial antibodies, in a population of 111 patients from the Midi-Pyrenees region. Presses Med. 1988;17:742–5.
11. Sevenet F, Capron JP. [Asymptomatic forms of primary biliary cirrhosis seen in 10 years in Picardie]. Presse Med. 1986;15:1957–60.
12. Borda F, Huarte MP, Zosaya JM et al. Primary biliary cirrhosis in Navarra. Med Interna. 1989;6:63–6.
13. Danielsson A, Boqvist L, Uddenfeldt P. Epidemiology of primary biliary cirrhosis in a defined rural population in the northern part of Sweden. Hepatology. 1990;11:458–64.
14. Boberg KM, Aadland E, Jahnsen J, Raknerud N, Stiris M, Bell H. Incidence and prevalence of primary biliary cirrhosis, primary sclerosing cholangitis and autoimmune hepatitis in a Norwegian population. Scand J Gastroenterol. 1998;33:99–103.
15. Van Dam G, Gips C. Primary biliary cirrhosis (PBC) in a European country – a description of death rates in The Netherlands (1979–1992). Hepatogastroenterology. 1996;43:906–13.
16. Sorensen HT, Thulstrup AM, Blomqvist P, Norgaard B, Fonger K, Ekbom A. Risk of primary biliary liver cirrhosis in patients with coeliac disease: Danish and Swedish cohort data. Gut. 1999;44:736–8.
17. Floreani A, Baragiotta A, Baldo V, Menegon T, Farinati F, Naccarato R. Hepatic and extrahepatic malignancies in primary biliary cirrhosis. Hepatology. 1999;29:1425–8.
18. Vogel A, Strassburg C, Manns M. Genetic association of vitamin D receptor polymorphisms with primary biliary cirrhosis and autoimmune hepatitis. Hepatology. 2002;35:126–31.
19. Hadziyannis S, Hadziyannis E. A randomised controlled trial of ursodeoxycholic acid (UDCA) in primary biliary cirrhosis (PBC). Hepatology. 1988;8:1421.
20. Witt-Sullivan H, Heathcote J, Cauch K et al. The demography of primary biliary cirrhosis in Ontario, Canada. Hepatology. 1990;12:98–105.
21. Villeneuve JP, Fenyves D, Infante-Rivard C. Descriptive epidemiology of primary biliary cirrhosis in the province of Quebec. Can J Gastroenterol. 1991;5:174–8.
22. Kim WR, Lindor KD, Locke GR 3rd et al. Epidemiology and natural history of primary biliary cirrhosis in a US community. Gastroenterology. 2000;119:1631–6.
23. Hulburt K, McMahon B, Deubner H, Hsu-Trawinski B, Williams J, Kowdley K. Prevalence of autoimmune liver disease in Alaska natives. Am J Gastroenterol. 2002;97:2402–7.
24. Robson S, Hift R, Kirsch R. Primary biliary cirrhosis. A retrospective survey at Groote Schuur Hospital, Cape Town. S Afr Med J. 1990;78:19–22.
25. Watson R, Angus P, Dewar M, Goss B, Sewell R, Smallwood R. Low prevalence of primary biliary cirrhosis in Victoria, Australia. Gut. 1995;36:927–30.

26. Mori M, Tamakoshi A, Kojima M et al. Nationwide survey of intractable hepatic disorders in Japan. In: Ohio Y, editor. Annual Report of Research Committee On Epidemiology of Intractable Disease. Tokyo: Ministry of Health and Welfare, Japan; 1997:23–7.
27. Tsuji K, Watanabe Y, Van De Water J et al. Familial primary biliary cirrhosis in Hiroshima. J Autoimmun. 1999;13:171–8.
28. Triger D. Primary biliary cirrhosis: an epidemiological study. Br Med J. 1980;281:772–5.
29. Prince M, Chetwynd A, Diggle P, Jarner M, Metcalfe J, James O. The geographical distribution of primary biliary cirrhosis in a well defined cohort. Hepatology. 2001;34:1083–8.
30. Parikh-Patel A, Gold EB, Worman H, Krivy KE, Gershwin ME. Risk factors for primary biliary cirrhosis in a cohort of patients from the United States. Hepatology. 2001;33:16–21.
31. Howel D, Fischbacher C, Bhopal R, Gray J, James O. An exploratory population-based case–control study of primary biliary cirrhosis. Hepatology. 2000;31:1055–60.

2
Genetic components of primary biliary cirrhosis

T. K. MAO, A. A. ANSARI, U. BEUERS and
M. E. GERSHWIN

INTRODUCTION

Autoimmune diseases, including primary biliary cirrhosis (PBC), are thought to arise from chronic immune activation in genetically susceptible individuals[1,2]. Primary biliary cirrhosis (PBC) is a chronic and progressive inflammatory liver disease characterized by the destruction of small biliary epithelial cells (BECs)[3-5]. It is generally believed that the targeted attack on the biliary epithelium is autoimmune-mediated, yet mechanisms of pathogenesis of PBC remain undefined. Serological investigations show high titres of antimitochondrial antibodies in 90–95% of PBC cases[6], while histological examination of PBC livers demonstrated marked infiltration of lymphocytes in the portal area, adjacent to the intrahepatic biliary epithelium[7]. The apparent paradox in PBC is that mitochondrial autoantigens are ubiquitous, present in most metabolically active cells, yet pathogenesis specifically targets BECs. However, a line of evidence, including epidemiological studies, case findings and twin concordance studies, has clearly demonstrated that genetic predisposition is a major factor in disease susceptibility. Data from such studies are reviewed and highlighted; in particular the genetic associations in PBC.

FAMILIAL PREVALENCE OF PBC

Since the early 1970s numerous case reports identifying family members with PBC have suggested that disease prevalence is increased within first-degree relatives (summarized in refs 8 and 9). Such isolated studies, which have hinted at a genetic component in the development of PBC, have subsequently been confirmed in comprehensive, geo-epidemiological studies of familial PBC. A summary of the available data is presented in Table 1.

Table 1 Summary of epidemiological studies of familial PBC

Country	Year	Researchers	No. of indexed patients	Familial prevalence	Affected family members
US	1994	Bach and Schaffner[10]	396	4.3%	16/18 first-degree relations: 7 M/D, 5S/S, 1B/B, 1S/S/D, 1S/S/S/B 2/18 second-degree relation: 1S/S/C, 1A/N
England	1983	Hamlyn et al.[14]	117	1%	Not specified
England	1990	Myszor et al.[15]	347	2.4%*	4/4 first-degree relations: 2M/D, 1S/S, 1S/B
England	1995	Brind et al.[16]	736	1.33%	10/10 first-degree relations: all M/D
England	1999	Jones et al.[17]	157	6.4%	8/10 first-degree relations (not specified) 2/10 second-degree relations (not specified)
Sweden	1990	Danielsson et al.[18]	111	4.5%	Not specified
Italy	1997	Floreani et al.[19]	156	3.8%	5/6 first-degree relations: 2M/D, 2S/B, 1S/S 1/6 second-degree relation: 1C/C
Japan	1999	Tsuji et al.[8]	156	5.1%	8/8 first-degree relations: 4M/D, 1M/D/D, 2B/S, 1S/S

* Included indexed PBC patients in their calculation (please refer to text).
Abbreviations used: M, mother; D, daughter; S, sister; B, brother; C, cousin; A, aunt; N, niece.

In North America Bach and Schaffner[10] performed a retrospective review of charts and a prospective mail survey to estimate the prevalence of PBC in family members with this disease. Of the 396 indexed patients with PBC in the New York area, 17 families were shown to have more than one family member diagnosed with PBC, translating to a familial prevalence of 42 820 per million or 4.3%. At the time, a lack of epidemiological data on the occurrence of PBC in the general population of the United States compelled Bach and Schaffner to compare their findings to data from various regions of Europe, which had indicated the prevalence of PBC between 7 and 75 per million. Although the apparent prevalence of disease seen within families is much greater (approximately 1000-fold) than the European population, the authors still regarded the value as 'conservative' as the figure rises significantly to 14.9% if family members with liver disease suggestive of PBC are included. In the first and only population-based epidemiological study conducted in the United States, in 2000, it was discovered that Olmsted County (Minnesota) displayed the highest prevalence of PBC to date at 402 per million or 0.04%[11]. This figure nearly doubled the previous hot spot of Newcastle-upon-Tyne, England, where the prevalence was reported to be 240 per million[12]. Even with the recent epidemiological data in the United States, the familial prevalence from the Bach and Schaffner study is still 100-fold greater than the geographically matched population, and therefore does not diminish the suggestion that family history of PBC is a predisposing factor for the development of disease.

In England, where population-based epidemiological studies have been thoroughly investigated[13], there have been four studies based on two research groups examining the clustering of PBC among family members[14–17]. The first, which was documented in 1983 by Hamlyn et al.[14], reported that 1% of the 117 cases studied in the Newcastle-upon-Tyne area had a family member with the disease. At the time the prevalence in the general population varied within the region from 37 per million (0.0037%) in rural areas to 144 per million (0.014%) in industrial urban areas. In 1990 the same group of investigators expanded their study to include most of northern Europe[15]. They examined the records of 347 patients to identify four families with affected first-degree family members (two sibling pairs and two mother/daughter pairs), and believed that translated into a familial prevalence of 2.4%. However, this percentage is misleading since they included indexed PBC patients into their calculation (8/347), which led to a doubling of the true percentage of familial prevalence ($(4/347) \times 100\% = 1.2\%$). As a result the susceptibility of family members of patients developing PBC is relatively similar to their previous study, despite their claim that prevalence of the general population in England was steadily increasing from 18 to 128.5 per million in a 10-year span. The same group has recently reassessed the prevalence of familial PBC in Newcastle-upon-Tyne and surrounding districts[17]. Of the 157 indexed patients, Jones et al. identified 10 patients with family members diagnosed with the disease for a familial prevalence of 64 000 per million or 6.4%. Several factors may have accounted for the marked increase of prevalence among affected family members: (1) probable diagnosis of PBC was included in their investigation (i.e. patients met two of three criteria that included cholestatic liver function tests, serum AMA titres of $\geq 1{:}40$ and compatible/diagnostic liver histology) while only definite cases were examined in prior studies. (2) Two of 10 identified families were of second-degree relatives, while in the 1990 study all were first-degree relatives. However, it was not mentioned whether or not, in the 1990 study, they omitted second-degree relatives, or simply that such cases were not discovered. Additionally, Jones et al. stated that, due to large numbers of first-degree relatives among the PBC patients (total of 1118), the prevalence of PBC in first-degree relatives was <1%. In a study conducted by a separate group in England it was demonstrated that 10 of the 736 PBC patients were discovered to have a history of PBC in a family member, resulting in a familial prevalence of 1.33% (13 300 per million).

Studies of frequency of familial PBC were also examined in other parts of Europe, as well as Asia. In 1990 Danielsson et al. conducted a study in northern Sweden where a familial prevalence of 4.5% (45 000 per million) was discovered from a group of 111 PBC patients[18]. In Italy, Floreani et al.[19] reviewed the charts of 156 patients and observed six families (3.8% or 38 000 per million) with a definite diagnosis of PBC in a blood relative. Most recently in Hiroshima, Japan, where PBC is a reportable disease with comprehensive enrollment of patients,

Tsuji et al.[8] reported 156 new patients with PBC in a population of 2 873 000 during the period 1988–1997; thus, the prevalence of PBC in this general population was 54 cases per million (0.0054%). Eight of the indexed patients were identified with at least one family member with diagnosis compatible with PBC, reflecting a familial prevalence of 5.1% (51 280 per million); that is nearly 1000-fold higher than the general population.

Cumulatively, the data from these studies displayed a familial prevalence of PBC in the range 1–6%, suggesting that family members of PBC patients are much more likely to develop the disease than are the general population, which is reported to be in the neighbourhood of 5–402 per million[11,13]. Although familial prevalence is strikingly higher than the frequency detected in the general population, we cannot hastily assume that PBC is purely a genetic disease, for such pronounced discrepancy may simply be due to shared environmental factors (i.e. food and water supply) by family members. Ultimately, environmental factors such as infectious agents, commonly exposed-to chemicals, or hormonal stimulation may be discovered to play a major role in the susceptibility of this complex disease.

TWINS STUDIES

The classical epidemiological strategy to delineate any genetic influences in the development of multifactorial diseases is through the study of concordance rates in twins. In most human autoimmune diseases the concordance rates in monozygotic twins (i.e. genetically identical) are generally less than 50%[20]. Until recently there have been only two reported studies of twins with regard to PBC. A case study in 1973 identified a set of twin sisters, both diagnosed with PBC, yet their zygosity was undetermined[21]. In 1994 Kaplan et al.[22] described a pair of identical twins discordant for the disease, although the monozygosity of the set has been challenged[23]. Most recently our laboratory has been able to identify 15 sets of twins, seven of which were confirmed to be monozygotes. Upon subsequent re-evaluation of patient charts the concordance rate in the monozygotic twins was 0.57, i.e. in four sets both individuals were diagnosed with PBC, while none of the dizygotic sets was found concordant for PBC. Hence, the concordance rate for PBC in identical twins is among the highest reported in autoimmune diseases. The dramatic discrepancy in the concordance rate of dizygotic twins compared with that of monozygotic twins supports the presence of multiple genes contributing to the genetic disposition of PBC.

MHC GENES ASSOCIATED WITH PBC

The structure of the major histocompatibility complex (MHC) consists of three regions located on chromosome 6 that are termed MHC class I, II, and III. In humans the class I region contains three main genes called human leucocyte antigen (HLA)-A, -B, and -C, which encodes for the polymorphic heavy chain (α-chain) of the class I heterodimer, whereas the invariant β_2-microglobulin is located on a different chromosome 15. The class II region includes genes encoding HLA-DR, -DP, and -DQ molecules, as well as transporter proteins (TAP1 and

TAP2) and LMP genes encoding for proteasome subunits involved in antigen processing. Unlike HLA class I heterodimers, both the α- and β-polypeptides for DR, DP, and DQ molecules are encoded on chromosome 6: the α-chain by an A gene and the β-chain by a B gene. While the DRA gene is invariable the DRB, DQA, DQB, DPA, and DPB genes are all polymorphic. The class III region is composed of genes for complement factors C4 and proinflammatory cytokines such as tumour necrosis factor (TNF)-α and TNF-β. Moreover, the genes contained within the MHC region are extremely polymorphic and polygenic, especially the HLA class I and II heterodimers. Although the precise mechanism by which MHC genes predispose an individual to autoimmunity is still not clear, it is generally believed that a particular polymorphic variant of the MHC influences immune responses by enhancing the binding to a self-peptide, thereby increasing its antigenicity when interacting with T cell receptors[1]. Consequently, polymorphisms in histocompatibility genes can alter the expressed repertoire of T cells, skewing the immune system to favour autoimmune reactions.

There have been extensive studies associating certain HLA polymorphisms and haplotypes with the susceptibility and progression of PBC (data are summarized in Table 2). Although many studies have addressed the potential association of HLA class I molecules with PBC in different ethnic populations (Spain[24], Japan[25,26], England[27,28], US[29,30], Germany[31], and Denmark[32]), the results were essentially unanimous. Thus no associations have been found in class I molecules with the predisposition of PBC across various ethnic groups. However, most recently a group in Italy reported that PBC in Italian patients is associated with various HLA-B alleles, including B*15, B*41, B*55, and B*58[33].

On the contrary, there have been several putative MHC class II molecules that are associated with PBC in both the Caucasian and Asian populations. In Caucasians, HLA-DR8 (DRB1*08) was identified as a risk factor by several groups[31,34–38]. Interestingly, the HLA-DR8 allele is known to be in linkage disequilibrium with DQB1*0402 in the Caucasian population[39] and this non-random association between these two alleles represents the strongest immunogenic association with PBC of European descent[35,38]. Moreover, Donaldson et al.[40] recently suggested that the linkage of the DQA1*0401 allele to the DR8-DQB1*0402 haplotype appears to be principally associated with disease progression, rather than disease susceptibility, as the combination was detected only in later stages of disease. However, several other investigators have disputed the relative importance of DR8 molecules[27,32,33,41,42], and felt that PBC in Europeans is associated with other MHC class II molecules such as DR3[24,32] and DPB1*0301[43]. Results from some of the studies have suggested that certain class II variants reduce the risk of developing PBC in Americans, which included DR5[34], DQw3[30], DQA1*0102 and DQB1*0602[37]. In 2003 Invernizzi et al. suggested that Italian patients with the DRB1*11 allele were protected from disease onset[33]. Nevertheless, some groups were unable to detect associations with any HLA-DR[27–29,41,42] or -DPB antigens[44]. In the Asian population, particularly the Japanese, MHC class II association studies have also been conducted, yet the results are also conflicting. However, DR2[25], DPB1*0501[45] and DRB1*0803[26] have all been reported to be implicated with the predisposition of PBC. In contrast, two purported alleles have been documented to confer resistance to PBC in Japanese patients: DR52[45] and DQA1*0102[26]. Overall,

Table 2 Summary of the association of HLA molecules with susceptibility of PBC

Year	Country	HLA investigated	Significant association with	PBC	Controls	p (corrected)	RR	Refs.
1979	Spain	A, B, C, DRw	DRw3	57.1% (12/21)	14.8% (11/74)	<0.004	7.6	24
1983	Japan	A, B, DR	DR2	68% (15/22)	30% (15/50)	<0.042	5.00	25
1985	England	A, B, DR	No associations					27
1987	England	A, B, DR, C4A, C4B, Bf, C3	C4B2	45% (15/33)	17% (53/307)	0.014		28
1987	US	DR, DQ	DR8 DR5 decreased in PBC	30.1% (35/114) 9.6% (11/114)	4.7% (8/171) 25.2% (43/171)	<0.0001 0.0118		34
1987	US	A, B, DR(1–7)	No associations (DR8 not tested)					29
1990	US	A, B, C, DR7, DRw8, DRw17, DQw2, DQw3	DRw8 DQw3 decreased in PBC	18.4% (6/35) 26.3% (9/35)	4.7% (73/1546) 53.5% (827/1546)	0.02 <0.001	3.1 0.3	30
1991	Germany	A, B, C, DR, C4A, C4B, Bf	DRw8 C4A-Q0 DRw8/C4A-Q0	36% (9/25) 72% (18/25) 20% (5/25)	3.6% (6/169) 34.5% (51/148) 0.7% (1/148)	0.00013 0.0056 9.7 E-7*	15.28 4.89 183.75	31
1992	England	DRB, DQB	DR8 DR8/ DQB1*0402	11% (18/159) 11% (10/89)	4% (6/162) 2.2% (4/181)	<0.01 <0.001	3.3 5.4	35
1992	Denmark	A, B, C, DRB, DQA, DQB, DPA, DPB	DR3	52.2% (12/23)	24.6% (296/1204)	<0.05	3.4	32
1993	Japan	DR, DQ, DPB1	DQ3 DPB1*0501 DPB1*0402 decreased in PBC DR52 (DRB3) decreased in PBC	80.9% (38/47) 85.1% (40/47) 2.2% (1/47) 34% (16/47)	51.3% (77/150) 55.3% (83/150) 23.3% (35/150) 54% (81/150)	<0.05 <0.01 <0.05 <0.05	1.5	45
1993	England	DRB1, DRB3, DQA, DQB	DR8	18.5% (24/130)	9.1% (33/363)	<0.005**	2.0	36

18

Year	Country	Genes studied	Association	Cases	Controls	p value	OR	Ref
1994	Japan	A, B, C DRB1, B3, B5 DQA1, B1	DRB1*0803 DQA1*0103 DQB1*0601 DQA1*0102 decreased in PBC	35.5% (22/62) 43.5% (27/62) 43.5% (27/62) 3.2% (2/62)	7.4% (32/430) 18.4% (79/430) 17.9% (77/430) 16.3% (70/430)	<0.0001 <0.0001 <0.0001 0.0288	6.84 3.43 3.54	26
1994	England	DRB1, DQB1, DPB1	No association					41
1994	US	DRB1, DQA1, DQB1	DRB1*0801 DRB1*0901 DQA1*0401/0601 DQA1*0102 decreased in PBC DQB1*0602 decreased in PBC	7.8% (8/102) 3.9% (4/102) 9.8% (10/102) 5.9% (6/102) 2.9% (3/102)	1.9% (9/480) 0.8% (4/480) 2.7% (13/480) 18.8% (90/480) 12.1% (58/478)	<0.05 <0.05 <0.001 <0.001 <0.025	4.5*** 4.9*** 8.3*** 0.3*** 0.2***	37
1995	Germany	DPB1	DPB1*0301	50% (16/32)	12.8% (6/47)	<0.015	6.8	43
1995	England	DPB1	No association					44
2001	England	DRB, DQA, DQB	DRB1*0801 DRB1*0801/ DQA1*0401/ DQB1*0402 (late stage)	15% (25/164) 23% (21/88)	2.9% (3/102) 2.9% (3/102)	0.0014 4.4 E−6	5.9*** 15.5***	40
2002	Sweden	DRB1, DQB1, DPB1	DRB1*08 DQB1*0402	29.3% (29/99) 28.6% (28/98)	11.4% (18/158) 10.8% (17/158)	0.001 0.001	3.22 3.32	38
2003	Italy	A, B, DRB1	B*15 B*41 B*55 B*58 DRB1*11	8% (9/112) 3.1% 3.6% (4/112) 1.8% (2/112) 10.7% (16/149)	3.4% (19/558) 0.3% 1.3% 0.3% 27.6% (154/558)	0.0039 8.8 E−15 0.034 0.00042 1.6 E−6	2.5*** 12.0*** 2.9*** 6.8*** 0.3***	33
2003	Brazil	DR, DQ	No associations					42

* Fisher's p value, ** Uncorrected p value, *** Odds ratio.

the association of MHC class II molecules with the susceptibility of PBC is still debatable and significantly weaker than what has been reported for other autoimmune diseases[46,47].

Other genes within the MHC class II regions have also been analysed for possible genetic influences on the development of PBC. Although TAP genes are not as polymorphic as their neighbouring class II genes, they function to transport antigenic peptides across the endoplasmic reticulum prior to being loaded onto MHC molecules. Hence, certain variants of the TAP genes can skew the type of peptides that are readily available for antigen presentation. There has been only one attempt to reveal any polymorphisms of TAP genes that influences the development of PBC; however, no associations were found[48].

Several laboratories have also scrutinized genes encoded within the MHC class III region for disease association. Strong correlations with PBC have been described for complement factors, including C4B 2 allotype[28] in British patients and C4A*Q0 allele[31] in Germans. Furthermore, several groups have also investigated the association of polymorphisms within the TNF-α promotor with PBC. It is well established that TNF-α is an important mediator of inflammation, and biallelic polymorphism has been discovered at position −308 within the TNF-α promoter region, including a common variant with a G (TNF1), and an uncommon variant with an A (TNF2)[49]. Several studies have demonstrated that the transcription at position −308 from G to A (TNF2) augments production of TNF-α[50–52]. An investigation conducted in the UK by Gordon and colleagues reported that PBC patients are associated with reduced carriage of TNF2[53]. In contrast, two other studies were unable to detect a difference in TNF1/TNF2 carriage between patients and controls, thereby suggesting that neither TNF1 nor TNF2 represented a risk factor for PBC[54,55]. However, Tanaka et al.[54] observed a significantly higher Mayo score for disease severity in patients who were heterozygotes compared to those with the homozygous TNF1/TNF1 genotype. Therefore, Tanaka et al. propose that TNF2 may play a role in progression, rather than induction, of disease, due to the association of TNF2 with more advanced disease. However, this hypothesis was still contested, since Jones et al.[55] reported that the TNF1/TNF1 genotype was present more frequently in advanced-stage PBC patients than in patients with less severe disease. Most recently, in 2003, Bittencourt et al. argued that TNF-α alleles were not associated with susceptibility or progression of PBC in Brazilian patients[42]. Clearly, additional studies are needed with a larger number of patients to clarify the discrepancies in these studies.

OTHER PURPORTED SUSCEPTIBILITY GENES

With the recent advances in molecular technology, single-nucleotide polymorphisms (SNPs) are being uncovered at an explosive rate. This has allowed many investigators to venture into non-MHC genes to discover any variants that confer susceptibility to PBC. A summary of purported susceptibility gene studies is provided in Table 3.

Cytotoxic T lymphocyte antigen-4 (CTLA-4) is a molecule expressed on the surface of activated T cells and serves a critical role in regulating and/or

Table 3 Summary of association of non-MHC genes with susceptibility of PBC

Purported gene	Country	# PBC patients	# Controls	Strength of association: odds ratio	p-Value	Reference
CTLA-4	England, Brazil	200, 50	200, 67	2.45	0.000063 NS	Agarwal et al.[56] Bittencourt et al.[42]
IL-1β	England	164	101	2.37	0.00078	Donaldson et al.[40]
MBL	Japan	65	218	2.51	0.003	Matsushita et al.[63]
NRAMP1	England	53	78		<0.024	Graham et al.[68]
IL-10	England, Italy, Japan	171, 94, 65	141, 72, 71	1.2, 2.44	0.49 (NS) <0.041 NS	Zapalla et al.[70] Matsushita et al.[69]
Eta-1/osteopontin	Japan	50	34		0.16–0.72 (NS)	Kikuchi et al.[74]
CD14	France	30	27		NS	Corpechot et al.[72]
CD40 ligand	Japan	No gene mutations detected in 24 patients				Higuchi et al.[71]
eNOS	Italy	109	242		NS	Selmi et al.[73]

NS: no significance.

terminating peripheral T cell responses by competing with the co-stimulatory molecule CD28 for their natural ligands (CD80/86) present on mature antigen-presenting cells. The CTLA-4 gene contains a SNP in exon 1, where an adenine is substituted for a guanine in position 49, and hence a threonine in lieu of alanine in the protein. In a study conducted in northern England Agarwal et al. demonstrated a significant difference in allele frequencies among 200 PBC patients versus 200 controls[56]. However, no particular CTLA-4 genotypes were found to be associated with PBC in Brazilian patients[42].

An early report indicating abnormal production of interleukin (IL)-1 by monocytes in PBC[57] sparked a subsequent investigation on IL-1 gene polymorphisms in this chronic progressive inflammatory disease. In 2001 an English group reported a significantly higher frequency of the IL-1B*1,1 genotype in PBC patients with early-stage disease compared to late-stage disease, suggesting that the IL-1 gene is associated with disease susceptibility[40].

The proposal that mucosal immune response against pathogens may be involved in the induction of PBC[58] has directed several studies towards the mucosal immune system in PBC patients[59,60]. Interestingly, mannose-binding lectin (MBL) is secreted into luminal fluid[61,62], suggesting that MBL plays an important role in innate mucosal responses. Additionally, several SNPs identified in the MBL gene prompted Matsushita et al. to characterize the MBL genotype in PBC patients. The results revealed a significant increase in HYPA/HYPA genotype, which is linked to hyper-production of MBL[63]. The author proposes that this genotype is reflective of the significant increase of serum MBL in PBC patients, and possibly increasing luminal secretion of MBL to a level where the complement cascade is inappropriately activated on the surface of biliary epithelial cells.

Natural resistance-associated macrophage protein1 (NRAMP1) is a membrane protein expressed by mononuclear phagocytes, and is shown to be involved in macrophage activation by up-regulating MHC class II genes, as well as secretion of TNF-α and IL-1β. At least 10 polymorphisms have been reported in the human gene[64–66], one of which spans a microsatellite repeat region in the 5′ untranscribed promoter region of the gene which can affect levels of NRAMP1 expression[67]. In a preliminary study conducted in 2000, Graham et al. detected a higher frequency of a novel allele 5 of the promoter region in PBC patients compared to normal controls and patients with other types of liver disease[68]. The effect of allele 5 on the levels of NRAMP1 expression is currently unknown.

Another purported susceptibility locus in PBC is the promoter region of the IL-10 gene. This immunomodulatory cytokine is known to play a critical role in the development of Th1-type responses of CD4$^+$ T cells, and thereby possibly controlling autoreactive cell-mediated response against the biliary epithelium. The promoter region of the IL-10 gene contains three known SNPs at positions -592, -819, and -1082. In a study conducted in England no associations were detected at position -592. Unfortunately, the SNPs at the other two locations were not yet discovered, and hence were not investigated. However, Matsushita et al. most recently evaluated the genetic polymorphisms at all three positions in two ethnic populations[69]. This study revealed that Italian PBC patients displayed a significantly higher frequency for the homozygous G/G genotype at position -1082 compared to that of ethnic-matched controls. On the contrary, Japanese PBC patients demonstrated no significant differences in the three SNPs analysed.

There have been several other candidate genes implicating susceptibility to PBC, including IL-10[70], CD40 ligand[71], CD14[72], endothelial nitric oxide synthase (eNOS)[73], early T-lymphocyte activation 1 (eta-1)/osteopontin[74]. However, no associations were detected in the polymorphisms of these candidate genes with the development of PBC.

CONCLUDING REMARKS

Epidemiological studies involving the familial prevalence of PBC have hinted at a genetic component of disease, yet the cumulative effort to dissect the genetic influence has been elusive. The majority of initial investigations seeking to identify genes associated with PBC have focused on those genes that encode the highly polymorphic MHC antigens. However, with the exception of HLA-DR8, no obvious associations of MHC genes have so far been discovered with the development of PBC. Clearly, the jury is still out concerning the correlation of HLA-DR8 molecule with disease onset. Thus, we favour the notion that PBC is a heterogeneous disease, where a multiple combination of genes within the genome are capable of causing similar or identical disease phenotype[9]. Furthermore, attempts at associating non-MHC genes with PBC have been essentially futile with the exception of several candidate genes showing modest associations. Some have proposed that negative results normally found with gene association studies are due to multiple factors involved in the inheritance of autoimmune disease susceptibility[75]. In other words, susceptibility arises from the combined impact of multiple contributing susceptibility genes, each potentially interacting with environmental factors. Thus, in such a complex system, small sample size rapidly diminishes the possibility of obtaining statistically significant associations. Ultimately, linkage analysis studies will be the preferred method in dissecting the genetic contributions in the development of PBC.

References

1. Carson DA. Genetic factors in the etiology and pathogenesis of autoimmunity. FASEB J. 1992;6:2800–5.
2. Miller FW. Genetics of autoimmune diseases. Exp Clin Immunogenet. 1995;12:182–90.
3. Kaplan MM. Primary biliary cirrhosis. N Engl J Med. 1996;335:1570–80.
4. Neuberger J. Primary biliary cirrhosis. Lancet. 1997;350:875–9.
5. Gershwin ME, Ansari AA, Mackay IR et al. Primary biliary cirrhosis: an orchestrated immune response against epithelial cells. Immunol Rev. 2000;174:210–25.
6. Leung PS, Coppel RL, Ansari A, Munoz S, Gershwin ME. Antimitochondrial antibodies in primary biliary cirrhosis. Semin Liver Dis. 1997;17:61–9.
7. Nakanuma Y, Yasoshima M, Tsuneyama K, Harada K. Histopathology of primary biliary cirrhosis with emphasis on expression of adhesion molecules. Semin Liver Dis. 1997;17:35–47.
8. Tsuji K, Watanabe Y, Van De Water J et al. Familial primary biliary cirrhosis in Hiroshima. J Autoimmun. 1999;13:171–8.
9. Tanaka A, Borchers AT, Ishibashi H, Ansari AA, Keen CL, Gershwin ME. Genetic and familial considerations of primary biliary cirrhosis. Am J Gastroenterol. 2001;96:8–15.
10. Bach N, Schaffner F. Familial primary biliary cirrhosis. J Hepatol. 1994;20:698–701.
11. Kim WR, Lindor KD, Locke GR 3rd et al. Epidemiology and natural history of primary biliary cirrhosis in a US community. Gastroenterology. 2000;119:1631–6.
12. Metcalf JV, Bhopal RS, Gray J, Howel D, James OF. Incidence and prevalence of primary biliary cirrhosis in the city of Newcastle upon Tyne, England. Int J Epidemiol. 1997;26:830–6.

13. Parikh-Patel A, Gold E, Mackay IR, Gershwin ME. The geoepidemiology of primary biliary cirrhosis: contrasts and comparisons with the spectrum of autoimmune diseases. Clin Immunol. 1999;91:206–18.
14. Hamlyn AN, Macklon AF, James O. Primary biliary cirrhosis: geographical clustering and symptomatic onset seasonality. Gut. 1983;24:940–5.
15. Myszor M, James OF. The epidemiology of primary biliary cirrhosis in northeast England: an increasingly common disease? Q J Med. 1990;75:377–85.
16. Brind AM, Bray GP, Portmann BC, Williams R. Prevalence and pattern of familial disease in primary biliary cirrhosis. Gut. 1995;36:615–17.
17. Jones DE, Watt FE, Metcalf JV, Bassendine MF, James OF. Familial primary biliary cirrhosis reassessed: a geographically-based population study. J Hepatol. 1999;30:402–7.
18. Danielsson A, Boqvist L, Uddenfeldt P. Epidemiology of primary biliary cirrhosis in a defined rural population in the northern part of Sweden. Hepatology. 1990;11:458–64.
19. Floreani A, Naccarato R, Chiaramonte M. Prevalence of familial disease in primary biliary cirrhosis in Italy. J Hepatol. 1997;26:737–8.
20. Gregersen PK. Discordance for autoimmunity in monozygotic twins. Are 'identical' twins really identical? Arthritis Rheum. 1993;36:1185–92.
21. Chohan MR. Primary biliary cirrhosis in twin sisters. Gut. 1973;14:213–14.
22. Kaplan MM, Rabson AR, Lee YM, Williams DL, Montaperto PA. Discordant occurrence of primary biliary cirrhosis in monozygotic twins. N Engl J Med. 1994;331:951.
23. Friedrich C. More on primary biliary cirrhosis in monozygotic twins. N Engl J Med. 1995; 332:336.
24. Ercilla G, Pares A, Arriaga F et al. Primary biliary cirrhosis associated with HLA-DRw3. Tissue Ant. 1979;14:449–52.
25. Miyamori H, Kato Y, Kobayashi K, Hattori N. HLA antigens in Japanese patients with primary biliary cirrhosis and autoimmune hepatitis. Digestion. 1983;26:213–17.
26. Onishi S, Sakamaki T, Maeda T. DNA typing of HLA class II genes; DRB1*0803 increases the susceptibility of Japanese to primary biliary cirrhosis. J Hepatol. 1994;21:1053–60.
27. Bassendine MF, Dewar PJ, James OF. HLA-DR antigens in primary biliary cirrhosis: lack of association. Gut. 1985;26:625–8.
28. Briggs DC, Donaldson PT, Hayes P, Welsh KI, Williams R, Neuberger JM. A major histocompatibility complex class III allotype (C4B 2) associated with primary biliary cirrhosis (PBC). Tissue Ant. 1987;29:141–5.
29. Johnston DE, Kaplan MM, Miller KB, Connors CM, Milford EL. Histocompatibility antigens in primary biliary cirrhosis. Am J Gastroenterol. 1987;82:1127–9.
30. Prochazka EJ, Terasaki PI, Park MS, Goldstein LI, Busuttil RW. Association of primary sclerosing cholangitis with HLA-DRw52a. N Engl J Med. 1990;322:1842–4.
31. Manns MP, Bremm A, Schneider PM et al. HLA DRw8 and complement C4 deficiency as risk factors in primary biliary cirrhosis. Gastroenterology. 1991;101:1367–73.
32. Morling N, Dalhoff K, Fugger L et al. DNA polymorphism of HLA class II genes in primary biliary cirrhosis. Immunogenetics. 1992;35:112–16.
33. Invernizzi P, Battezzati PM, Crosignani A et al. Peculiar HLA polymorphisms in Italian patients with primary biliary cirrhosis. J Hepatol. 2003;38:401–6.
34. Gores GJ, Moore SB, Fisher LD, Powell FC, Dickson ER. Primary biliary cirrhosis: associations with class II major histocompatibility complex antigens. Hepatology. 1987;7:889–92.
35. Underhill J, Donaldson P, Bray G, Doherty D, Portmann B, Williams R. Susceptibility to primary biliary cirrhosis is associated with the HLA-DR8-DQB1*0402 haplotype. Hepatology. 1992; 16:1404–8.
36. Gregory WL, Mehal W, Dunn AN et al. Primary biliary cirrhosis: contribution of HLA class II allele DR8. Q J Med. 1993;86:393–9.
37. Begovich AB, Klitz W, Moonsamy PV, Van de Water J, Peltz G, Gershwin ME. Genes within the HLA class II region confer both predisposition and resistance to primary biliary cirrhosis. Tissue Ant. 1994;43:71–7.
38. Wassmuth R, Depner F, Danielsson A et al. HLA class II markers and clinical heterogeneity in Swedish patients with primary biliary cirrhosis. Tissue Ant. 2002;59:381–7.
39. Begovich AB, McClure GR, Suraj VC et al. Polymorphism, recombination, and linkage disequilibrium within the HLA class II region. J Immunol. 1992;148:249–58.

40. Donaldson P, Agarwal K, Craggs A, Craig W, James O, Jones D. HLA and interleukin 1 gene polymorphisms in primary biliary cirrhosis: associations with disease progression and disease susceptibility. Gut. 2001;48:397–402.
41. Zhang L, Weetman AP, Bassendine M, Oliveira DB. Major histocompatibility complex class-II alleles in primary biliary cirrhosis. Scand J Immunol. 1994;39:104–6.
42. Bittencourt PL, Palacios SA, Farias AQ et al. Analysis of major histocompatibility complex and CTLA-4 alleles in Brazilian patients with primary biliary cirrhosis. J Gastroenterol Hepatol. 2003;18:1061–6.
43. Mella JG, Roschmann E, Maier KP, Volk BA. Association of primary biliary cirrhosis with the allele HLA-DPB1*0301 in a German population. Hepatology. 1995;21:398–402.
44. Underhill JA, Donaldson PT, Doherty DG, Manabe K, Williams R. HLA DPB polymorphism in primary sclerosing cholangitis and primary biliary cirrhosis. Hepatology. 1995;21:959–62.
45. Seki T, Kiyosawa K, Ota M et al. Association of primary biliary cirrhosis with human leukocyte antigen DPB1*0501 in Japanese patients. Hepatology. 1993;18:73–8.
46. Seldin MF, Amos CI, Ward R, Gregersen PK. The genetics revolution and the assault on rheumatoid arthritis. Arthritis Rheum. 1999;42:1071–9.
47. Aitman TJ, Todd JA. Molecular genetics of diabetes mellitus. Baillieres Clin Endocrinol Metab. 1995;9:631–56.
48. Gregory WL, Daly AK, Dunn AN et al. Analysis of HLA-class-II-encoded antigen-processing genes TAP1 and TAP2 in primary biliary cirrhosis. Q J Med. 1994;87:237–44.
49. Wilson AG, di Giovine FS, Blakemore AI, Duff GW. Single base polymorphism in the human tumour necrosis factor alpha (TNF alpha) gene detectable by NcoI restriction of PCR product. Hum Mol Genet. 1992;1:353.
50. Wilson AG, Symons JA, McDowell TL, McDevitt HO, Duff GW. Effects of a polymorphism in the human tumor necrosis factor alpha promoter on transcriptional activation. Proc Natl Acad Sci USA. 1997;94:3195–9.
51. Kroeger KM, Carville KS, Abraham LJ. The −308 tumor necrosis factor-alpha promoter polymorphism effects transcription. Mol Immunol. 1997;34:391–9.
52. Wu WS, McClain KL. DNA polymorphisms and mutations of the tumor necrosis factor-alpha (TNF-alpha) promoter in Langerhans cell histiocytosis (LCH). J Interferon Cytokine Res. 1997;17:631–5.
53. Gordon MA, Oppenheim E, Camp NJ, di Giovine FS, Duff GW, Gleeson D. Primary biliary cirrhosis shows association with genetic polymorphism of tumour necrosis factor alpha promoter region. J Hepatol. 1999;31:242–7.
54. Tanaka A, Quaranta S, Mattalia A, Coppel R, Rosina F, Manns M, Gershwin ME. The tumor necrosis factor-alpha promoter correlates with progression of primary biliary cirrhosis. J Hepatol. 1999;30:826–9.
55. Jones DE, Watt FE, Grove J et al. Tumour necrosis factor-alpha promoter polymorphisms in primary biliary cirrhosis. J Hepatol. 1999;30:232–6.
56. Agarwal K, Jones DE, Daly AK et al. CTLA-4 gene polymorphism confers susceptibility to primary biliary cirrhosis. J Hepatol. 2000;32:538–41.
57. Kershenobich D, Rojkind M, Quiroga A, Alcocer-Varela J. Effect of colchicine on lymphocyte and monocyte function and its relation to fibroblast proliferation in primary biliary cirrhosis. Hepatology. 1990;11:205–9.
58. Van de Water J, Turchany J, Leung PS et al. Molecular mimicry in primary biliary cirrhosis. Evidence for biliary epithelial expression of a molecule cross-reactive with pyruvate dehydrogenase complex-E2. J Clin Invest. 1993;91:2653–64.
59. Tanaka A, Nalbandian G, Leung PS et al. Mucosal immunity and primary biliary cirrhosis: presence of antimitochondrial antibodies in urine. Hepatology. 2000;32:910–15.
60. Reynoso-Paz S, Leung PS, Van De Water J et al. Evidence for a locally driven mucosal response and the presence of mitochondrial antigens in saliva in primary biliary cirrhosis. Hepatology. 2000;31:24–9.
61. Garred P, Brygge K, Sorensen CH, Madsen HO, Thiel S, Svejgaard A. Mannan-binding protein-levels in plasma and upper-airways secretions and frequency of genotypes in children with recurrence of otitis media. Clin Exp Immunol. 1993;94:99–104.
62. Kelly P, Jack DL, Naeem A et al. Mannose-binding lectin is a component of innate mucosal defense against *Cryptosporidium parvum* in AIDS. Gastroenterology. 2000;119:1236–42.

63. Matsushita M, Miyakawa H, Tanaka A et al. Single nucleotide polymorphisms of the mannose-binding lectin are associated with susceptibility to primary biliary cirrhosis. J Autoimmun. 2001;17:251–7.
64. Liu J, Fujiwara TM, Buu NT et al. Identification of polymorphisms and sequence variants in the human homologue of the mouse natural resistance-associated macrophage protein gene. Am J Hum Genet. 1995;56:845–53.
65. Blackwell JM, Barton CH, White JK et al. Genomic organization and sequence of the human NRAMP gene: identification and mapping of a promoter region polymorphism. Mol Med. 1995;1:194–205.
66. Buu NT, Cellier M, Gros P, Schurr E. Identification of a highly polymorphic length variant in the 3'UTR of NRAMP1. Immunogenetics. 1995;42:428–9.
67. Blackwell JM. Structure and function of the natural-resistance-associated macrophage protein (Nramp1), a candidate protein for infectious and autoimmune disease susceptibility. Mol Med Today. 1996;2:205–11.
68. Graham AM, Dollinger MM, Howie SE, Harrison DJ. Identification of novel alleles at a polymorphic microsatellite repeat region in the human NRAMP1 gene promoter: analysis of allele frequencies in primary biliary cirrhosis. J Med Genet. 2000;37:150–2.
69. Matsushita M, Tanaka A, Kikuchi K et al. Association of single nucleotide polymorphisms of the interleukin-10 promoter gene and susceptibility to primary biliary cirrhosis: immunogenetic differences in Italian and Japanese patients. Autoimmunity. 2002;35:531–6.
70. Zappala F, Grove J, Watt FE et al. No evidence for involvement of the interleukin-10 −592 promoter polymorphism in genetic susceptibility to primary biliary cirrhosis. J Hepatol. 1998;28:820–3.
71. Higuchi M, Horiuchi T, Kojima T et al. Analysis of CD40 ligand gene mutations in patients with primary biliary cirrhosis. Scand J Clin Lab Invest. 1998;58:429–32.
72. Corpechot C, Poupon R. Promoter polymorphism of the CD14 endotoxin receptor gene and primary biliary cirrhosis. Hepatology. 2002;35:242–3.
73. Selmi C, Zuin M, Biondi ML et al. Genetic variants of endothelial nitric oxide synthase in patients with primary biliary cirrhosis: association with disease severity. J Gastroenterol Hepatol. 2003;18:1150–5.
74. Kikuchi K, Tanaka A, Miyakawa H et al. Eta-1/osteopontin genetic polymorphism and primary biliary cirrhosis. Hepatol Res. 2003;26:87–90.
75. Wanstrat A, Wakeland E. The genetics of complex autoimmune diseases: non-MHC susceptibility genes. Nat Immunol. 2001;2:802–9.

3
Infectious aetiology of primary biliary cirrhosis

R. JOPLIN

INTRODUCTION: INFECTIOUS AETIOLOGY OF PRIMARY BILIARY CIRRHOSIS?

Considerable circumstantial evidence supports the hypothesis that primary biliary cirrhosis (PBC) is the result of an autoimmune reaction[1,2]. Associations between PBC and other organ-specific autoimmune disorders exist and circulating auto-antibodies to well-characterized, highly conserved autoantigens are present[3,4]; however, a number of observations have long suggested involvement of an infectious component in the aetiology of PBC[5].

1. Sequence homology exists between autoantigens recognized by PBC-specific autoantibodies and prokaryotic antigens, suggesting a possible role for molecular mimicry with an infectious agent[6].
2. Unlike most other autoimmune conditions, PBC responds poorly to corticosteroid therapy[7].
3. Geographical clustering of PBC is observed, with migrant populations assuming the incidence of the indigenous population[8].
4. Recurrent PBC has been demonstrated in the allograft following liver transplantation for PBC[9].
5. Aggressive immunosuppressive therapy following liver transplantation for PBC is associated with earlier recurrence of clinical manifestations of PBC[10].
6. Th1 cytokines (e.g. gamma interferon) predominate over Th2 in the PBC liver, suggesting response to infection[11].
7. Transmission of PBC between genetically and non-genetically linked individuals has been reported[12].

Although specific prokaryotic agents have been proposed as implicated in PBC (including *Mycobacterium gordonae*[13], *Escherichia coli*[14,15] and *Salmonella*) these reports remain unsubstantiated[16–18]. Infection (viral or bacterial) could act as a trigger for the onset of PBC through molecular mimicry between T-cell recognition of an infectious agent and B-cell epitopes of highly conserved antigens in the host[19].

ANTIGENS RECOGNIZED BY AUTOANTIBODIES IN PBC

The close association between PBC and autoantibodies with specificity for mitochondrial antigens (antimitochondrial antibodies – AMA) has been established for several decades. These antigens are components of three functionally related mitochondrial multienzyme complexes, the 2-oxo-acid dehydrogenase complexes (2-OADC)[20]. Each complex is composed of multiple copies of three enzymes termed E1, E2 and E3, and the major antigen pyruvate dehydrogenase complex (PDC) contains a fourth component, E3 binding protein (E3bp, known previously as component X). Antibodies to PDC-E2 and PDC-E3bp can be detected in the serum of more than 95% of patients with PBC[21], but individual patients may have autoreactivity to several components of the 2-OADC[22].

In addition to, or in place of AMA, patients with PBC frequently have antibodies to a range of nuclear antigens[23]. Although present in a smaller proportion of patients these antinuclear antibodies (ANA) appear to be equally specific for PBC. The 2-OADC antigens recognized by AMA are present in all aerobic cells where they are localized to the mitochondrial inner membrane[20]. Immunostaining of tissues with antibodies to the mitochondrial and nuclear antigens produces a characteristic staining pattern corresponding to the appropriate organelle. When AMA is used for immunostaining, a particulate staining pattern is observed, corresponding to the intracellular distribution of mitochondria. The intracellular location the PBC autoantigens isolates them from the immune system and it has therefore been difficult to predict a primary role for these antigens in PBC. Historically the autoantibodies have been regarded as secondary epiphenomena resulting from tissue damage and release of intracellular contents, or as a response to crossreaction with a prokaryotic agent.

While the autoantigens in PBC are ubiquitous and present in all nucleated cells, paradoxically tissue damage in PBC is limited to ductular epithelium, with biliary epithelium apparently the major target. However, it is now established that, in patients with PBC, epitopes of the mitochondrial antigens are not restricted to mitochondria but show aberrant distribution on a number of tissues.

1. Biliary epithelium of PBC patients shows diffuse high-intensity intracellular distribution of PDC-E2, PDC-E3bp and OGDC-E2 on BEC of intact ducts and regenerative ductules with localization of antigen to the plasma membrane[24–26]. In normal and other liver disease controls only intracellular mitochondrial staining was seen.
2. Salivary gland epithelium of PBC patients has also been described as having high intensity of PDC-E2 on ductular epithelium[27,28].
3. Perihepatic lymph nodes of PBC patients, but not controls, show high-intensity diffuse distribution of PDC-E2 in a subset of cells suggested to be sinus macrophages[29].

Thus, in addition to intrahepatic biliary ducts (known to be dominant targets in PBC), other tissues including salivary gland epithelium and lymphoid tissue also show aberrant distribution of the major autoantigen, PDC-E2. The aberrant distribution of PDC-E2 on BEC in PBC has been found to occur very early in the natural history of the disease[30] and is also observed on BEC in biopsies of liver allografts from patients who have undergone liver transplantation for PBC[31]. These findings are consistent with the concept of changes in distribution of PDC-E2 corresponding with early events both in the generation of primary PBC and recurrence of PBC in the allograft. Furthermore, the observation of aberrant distribution of autoantigen in the allograft might suggest the presence of an extrahepatic agent that, following transplantation, is capable of inducing PBC-specific changes in normal (donor) liver.

ROLE OF ANTIGENS RECOGNIZED BY AMA IN PBC

In-vivo studies suggest that AMA are not pathogenetic; immunization of a range of laboratory animals with PDC-E2 resulted in generation of AMA but not biliary tract disease[32]. However, under normal circumstances mitochondrial antigens recognized by AMA would be shielded by the plasma membrane from immune cells and molecules. Translocation of autoantigen from mitochondrion to plasma membrane, such as was observed in the biliary epithelium of patients with PBC, may be essential for immunopathology to occur. Alternatively, selective infection of cellular targets by a crossreactive prokaryote could explain the higher intensity of autoantigen observed in some cells.

A major handicap in studying the role of autoantigens in PBC has been the lack of an appropriate model with which to conduct investigations. Histological studies of biopsy material, explanted liver and post-mortem tissues have proven useful, but dynamic processes are difficult to determine using fixed material. *In-vivo* models, however, also have associated problems. No natural animal model of PBC is known, and while numerous *in-vivo* models have been proposed, none possesses the full complement of features that characterize PBC[33–36]. Lack of an acceptable *in-vivo* model has led to studies aimed at establishing *in-vitro* models of PBC utilizing human cells. Such studies were previously impossible, as obtaining adequate cell numbers from biopsy material was prohibitive. However, adequate yield of cell numbers for *in-vitro* studies can be obtained from the larger volumes of tissue available through liver transplantation programmes.

Human intrahepatic biliary epithelial cells (BEC) can now be isolated with high purity from the livers of patients with PBC and controls[37,38]. The isolated cells can subsequently be maintained in tissue culture and utilized for dynamic studies[39]. Studies of human BEC maintained *in vitro* have demonstrated these cells to be immunologically active, and they express and respond to immunologically important molecules[40–44]. Such *in-vitro* technology was also used in an in-depth study of the subcellular distribution of PDC-E2 in BEC purified from patients with PBC and controls. BEC specifically from patients with PBC, but not controls, showed intense staining for PDC-E2 associated with the plasma membrane of BEC. Use of purified BEC permitted realization of PDC-E2 as associated with the external aspect of the plasma membrane where it would be

A

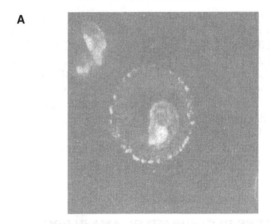

B

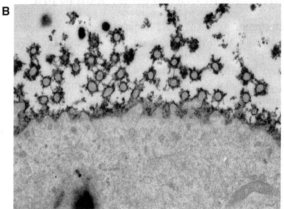

Figure 1 Biliary epithelial cells purified from the liver of patients with PBC and stained with antibodies to PDC-E2. Plasma membrane distribution of PDC-E2 visualized (**A**) by immunofluorecsence and (**B**) by electron microscopy

accessible to immune cells and molecules (Figure 1)[45]. However, studies to characterize the intracellular and plasma membrane antigens of BEC purified from PBC liver, and recognized by antibody to PDC-E2, failed to detect any non-human, crossreactive molecule[46].

ABERRANT DISTRIBUTION OF PDC-E2 IS INDUCED ON NORMAL BEC CULTURED WITH HOMOGENATES OF PERIHEPATIC LYMPH NODES FROM PATIENTS WITH PBC: AN *IN-VITRO* MODEL OF PBC?

To investigate whether aberrant distribution of PDC-E2 could be induced on normal BEC, BEC were purified from normal liver (obtained from donor organs) and non-PBC controls and incubated *in vitro* with homogenates of perihepatic

Table 1 Increase in PDC-E2 on normal BEC induced by lymph node and viral agents. Increase in PDC-E2 assessed by immunostaining of BEC proteins on Western blots using anti-PDC-E2 and expressed relative to BEC cultured without homogenate

Incubation medium	No. of experiments	Mean intensity (range)	p-Value
Homogenates			
PBC lymph node	17	**2.38** (1.2–6.4)	0.01
OLD lymph node	12	0.89 (0.31–1.44)	n.s.
Normal lymph node	10	0.78 (0.42–1.64)	n.s.
Conditioned media			
5-day supernatant:			
PBC-conditioned media	4	**2.19** (1.07–3.14)	0.04
5-day supernatant:			
control-conditioned media	4	1.06 (0.93–1.21)	n.s.
5-day supernatant:			
PBC-conditioned media	13	**3.0** (0.4–6.4)	0.028
Irradiated 5-day supernatant:			
PBC-conditioned media	4	0.96 (0.67–1.24)	n.s.
Viruses			
MMTV	7	**2.1** (1.4–2.8)	0.04
Control viruses	3	1.04	n.s.

OLD = other liver disorder.

lymph nodes from PBC patients. Increased intensity and plasma membrane distribution of PDC-E2 was observed on the treated cells (more than two-fold increase in BEC incubated with PBC homogenates relative to controls) (Table 1)[47]. Change in intensity and distribution of PDC-E2 was also observed when normal BEC were cultured in serially passaged conditioned media supernatants from BEC previously exposed to homogenates of lymph nodes from patients with PBC (Table 1)[48]. An exposure period of around 5 days was required prior to the development of aberrant PDC-E2 in normal BEC, suggesting that a dynamic rather than passive mechanism was involved in the transmissible process. Furthermore, induction of aberrant distribution and intensity of PDC-E2 on normal BEC was abrogated by gamma-irradiation (to 30 Gy) of the PBC tissue homogenate or serially cultured media (Table 1)[48].

The results of these studies suggested the presence of a transmissible factor in the perihepatic lymph nodes of patients with PBC. That this process was abrogated by gamma-irradiation could be regarded as evidence supportive of the hypothesis that the transmissible factor contained nucleic acids, and is consistent with involvement of an infectious agent in the PDC-E2 inductive process.

CHARACTERIZATION OF THE TRANSMISSIBLE AGENT IN PBC PERIHEPATIC LYMPH NODES

In early attempts to identify an infectious agent, BEC freshly purified from patients with PBC and controls were examined by electron microscopy. While prokaryotic particles were not observed, virus-like structures were. Spherical structures of

100–120 nm diameter with a definable envelope and electron-dense core (consistent with size and morphology of mature retroviruses) were observed associated with BEC purified from patients with PBC at a frequency of approximately 1 per 100 cells (a total of approximately 1000 cells were analysed). Only one such particle was observed in an equivalent number of BEC from patients with other liver diseases.

Further studies to characterize possible viral structures associated with PBC were undertaken using BEC purified from the livers of patients with PBC and controls, and lymph node homogenates and conditioned media from transmission experiments in which PBC homogenates induced aberrant PDC-E2 on normal BEC.

1. cDNA libraries were constructed from BEC extracted from the livers of PBC patients and normal (organ donor) controls[49].
2. Pellets centrifuged from media conditioned by PBC lymph node homogenates were negatively stained and examined by electron microscopy.
3. Media conditioned by PBC lymph node homogenates were examined for reverse transcriptase activity.

RETROVIRAL SEQUENCES CAN BE CLONED FROM BEC AND PERIHEPATIC LYMPH NODES OF PATIENTS WITH PBC

A 125 base-pair PCR product was obtained from the PBC library which was not represented in normal BEC cDNA. Eight clones derived from the PCR product were sequenced and were found to share 97% homology with each other and with HUMREVTRAC, which codes for human reverse transcriptase[49]. Further searches of sequence databases also revealed a 95–100% homology with murine mammary tumour virus (MMTV) genes. Additional sequences cloned from the DNA of a PBC patient's perihepatic lymph node were also shown to share identity with MMTV and with human proviral sequences isolated from breast cancer tissues[48].

MMTV PROTEIN IS PRESENT IN LYMPH NODE BUT NOT LIVER OF PATIENTS WITH PBC AND IN NORMAL BEC CULTURED WITH HOMOGENATES OF PBC LYMPH NODES

Immunostaining of lymph node and liver samples from patients with PBC and controls with an anti-MMTV monoclonal antibody ($p27^{CA}$, that recognizes MMTV capsid protein) revealed no reactivity in liver samples but 75% of PBC perihepatic lymph nodes contained positively stained cells (<10% in controls). Distribution of $p27^{CA}$ was similar to the aberrant PDC-E2 observed previously in lymph nodes and double immunofluorescence staining for $p27^{CA}$ and PDC-E2 revealed coincidence of viral protein and aberrant PDC-E2 in a subset of lymph node cells. Only those cells showing aberrant PDC-E2, also showed coincident positivity for $p27^{CA}$.

MEDIA CONDITIONED BY PBC LYMPH NODE HOMOGENATES HAVE REVERSE TRANSCRIPTASE ACTIVITY

All media conditioned by PBC lymph node homogenates had evidence of reverse transcriptase activity. The buoyant density of particles associated with reverse transcriptase activity was investigated by linear sucrose gradient studies. Reverse transcriptase activity was found to be associated with retrovirus RNA sequences at a buoyant density of 1.15–1.17 g/ml, where enveloped retroviruses usually co-sediment. None of the control samples had demonstrable human retrovirus RNA by RT-PCR, and in just one control supernatant a single fraction was found to be reverse transcriptase positive. Negative staining of pellets centrifuged from media conditioned by cells previously cultured with PBC lymph node homogenates revealed spherical, 110–120 nm diameter particles with an electron-dense nuclear core. By RT-PCR no evidence was found for retrovirus in BEC before co-culture with lymph node homogenates, but samples were positive in seven of 10 BEC from PBC lymph node homogenate-treated cultures as compared to two of 15 BEC incubated with control homogenates. Using immunofluorescence with FITC labelled anti-p27^{CA}, three of three BEC co-cultivated with PBC lymph node homogenates demonstrated a green punctate, cytoplasmic signal. BEC samples cultured with control homogenates showed no reactivity.

MMTV INDUCES ABERRANT PDC-E2 ON NORMAL BEC *IN VITRO*

The above studies suggested that the retroviral activity associated with perihepatic lymph nodes from patients with PBC and MMTV share features in common. The hypothesis that MMTV might be able to induce aberrant PDC-E2 on normal BEC was therefore tested. Supernatants from the MMTV-producing cell line, MM5MT, and from cell lines infected with control viruses were incubated with normal BEC. MM5MT supernatants induced a two-fold increase in PDC-E2 in normal BEC in a similar fashion to PBC lymph nodes and the PBC-conditioned supernatants (Table 1). No increase in PDC-E2 was observed when supernatants from control viruses were used. BEC co-cultured with MM5MT supernatants demonstrated a green punctate, cytoplasmic signal, suggesting uptake of MMTV by BEC. Untreated BEC showed no such reactivity.

The series of studies described suggest that the majority of patients with PBC have evidence of retroviral infection of perihepatic lymph nodes; however, immunohistochemistry failed to identify viral protein in liver. Although incubation of normal BEC with homogenates of PBC lymph nodes induced both aberrant distribution of PDC-E2 and evidence of retroviral infection, these studies do not directly demonstrate an inductive role for MMTV or related retrovirus in PBC. However, association between PBC and retroviral infection might provide solutions to a number of previously unexplained characteristic features of PBC.

1. Female preponderance of PBC: MMTV replication is partly regulated by a progesterone-responsive glucocorticoid regulatory element in the promoter region of the MMTV LTR[50].

2. Weak genetic associations: while most autoimmune conditions have strong genetic links those present in PBC are weak and may represent host susceptibility to retroviral infection; PBC may become manifest only in genetically predisposed individuals.
3. Poor efficacy of conventional immunosuppressive therapy in PBC.
4. Earlier recurrence of PBC following liver transplantation in the presence of aggressive immunosuppression.
5. Geographical and familial clustering of PBC.

SUMMARY AND CONCLUSIONS

Autoantibodies that recognize specific intracellular antigens including key metabolic mitochondrial enzymes are present in the serum of patients with PBC. The major mitochondrial antigen, PDC-E2, is aberrantly distributed on biliary epithelium and in perihepatic lymph nodes of patients with PBC. An *in-vitro* model of PBC was developed in which aberrant distribution of PDC-E2 was induced on normal biliary epithelium by incubating biliary epithelial cells (BEC) purified from normal liver with homogenates of lymph nodes from patients with PBC. Examination of the cells, homogenates and conditioned media from these studies revealed particulate structures having morphology and size consistent with retroviruses. Furthermore, reverse transcriptase activity co-sedimented with particles corresponding to 110–120 nm retroviruses. Subtraction of cDNA libraries constructed from normal and PBC BEC libraries generated sequences specific to PBC which shared sequence homology with murine mammary tumour virus (MMTV). Incubation of normal BEC with supernatants from MMTV-infected cells induced aberrant distribution of PDC-E2 in normal BEC. The data support a view, long held by some, that PBC may result from reaction to an infectious agent. While an inductive mechanism remains unproven the data suggest a close association between retroviral infection and the tissues of PBC patients that also show aberrant distribution of mitochondrial autoantigens. The availability of the *in-vitro* technologies described has permitted development of a model of PBC with which to test Koch's postulates *in vitro*.

Acknowledgements

The author is grateful for the support of Professor J. M. Neuberger and the PBC Foundation, UK.

References

1. Joplin RE, Neuberger JM. Immunopathology of primary biliary cirrhosis. Eur J Gastroenterol Hepatol. 1999;11:587–93.
2. Jones DEJ, Bassendine MF. Primary biliary cirrhosis. J Intern Med. 1997;241:345–8.
3. Fussey SPM, Guest JR, James OFW, Bassendine MF, Yeaman SJ. Identification and analysis of the major M2 auto-antigens in primary biliary cirrhosis. Proc Natl Acad Sci USA. 1988;85: 8654–8.

4. Coppel RL, Mcneilage LJ, Surh CD et al. Primary structure of the human M2 mitochondrial auto-antigen of primary biliary cirrhosis – dihydrolipoamide acetyltransferase. Proc Natl Acad Sci USA. 1988;85:7317–21.

5. Tanaka A, Prindiville TP, Gish R et al. Are infectious agents involved in primary biliary cirrhosis? A PCR approach. J Hepatol. 1999;31:664–71.

6. Fussey SPM, Lindsay JG, Fuller C et al. Autoantibodies in primary biliary cirrhosis – analysis of reactivity against eukaryotic and prokaryotic 2-oxo acid dehydrogenase complexes. Hepatology. 1991;13:467–74.

7. Leuschner U. Medical treatment of vanishing bile duct syndrome. In: Alvaro D, Benedetti A, Strazzabosco M, editors. Vanishing Bile Duct Syndrome: Pathophysiology and Treatment. Dordrecht: Kluwer, 1997:213–23.

8. Anand AC, Elias E, Neuberger JM. End-stage primary biliary cirrhosis in a first generation migrant South Asian population. Eur J Gastroenterol Hepatol. 1996;8:663–6.

9. Hubscher SG, Elias E, Buckels JAC, Mayer AD, McMaster P, Neuberger JM. Primary biliary cirrhosis – histological evidence of disease recurrence after liver transplantation. J Hepatol. 1993;18:173–84.

10. Dmitrewski J, Hubscher SG, Mayer AD, Neuberger JM. Recurrence of primary biliary cirrhosis in the liver allograft: the effect of immunosuppression. J Hepatol. 1996;24:253–7.

11. Harada K, Van de Water J, Leung PSC et al. *In situ* nucleic acid hybridization of cytokines in primary biliary cirrhosis: Predominance of the Th1 subset. Hepatology. 1997;25:791–6.

12. Jones DEJ, Watt FE, Metcalf JV, Bassendine MF, James OFW. Familial primary biliary cirrhosis reassessed: a geographically-based population study. J Hepatol. 1999;30:402–7.

13. Vilagut L, Pares A, Rodes J et al. Mycobacteria – related to the aetiopathogenesis of primary biliary cirrhosis? J Hepatol. 1996;24:125.

14. Hopf U, Stemerowicz R, Rodloff A et al. Relation between *Escherichia coli* R(rough) forms in gut, lipid-A in liver, and primary biliary cirrhosis. Lancet. 1989;2:1419–22.

15. Butler P, Valle F, Hamiltonmiller JMT, Brumfitt W, Baum H, Burroughs AK. M2 Mitochondrial antibodies and urinary rough mutant bacteria in patients with primary biliary cirrhosis and in patients with recurrent bacteriuria. J Hepatol. 1993;17:408–14.

16. Floreani A, Bassendine MF, Mitchison H, Freeman R, James OFW. No specific association between primary biliary cirrhosis and bacteriuria. J Hepatol. 1989;8:201–7.

17. O'Donohue J, Fidler H, Garcia-Barcelo M, Nouri-Aria K, Williams R, McFadden J. Mycobacterial DNA not detected in liver sections from patients with primary biliary cirrhosis. J Hepatol. 1998;28:433–8.

18. Burke D, Jackson D, Gould K, Freeman R, Bassendine MF, James OFW. Primary biliary cirrhosis (Pbc) – no evidence to support a role for enterobacteriaceae rough (R) mutants in its etiology. Hepatology. 1991;14:A62.

19. Coppel RL, Gershwin ME. Primary biliary cirrhosis – the molecule and the mimic. Immunol Rev. 1995;144:17–49.

20. Yeaman SJ, Fussey SPM, Mutimer DJ, James OFW, Bassendine MF. M2 auto-antigens in primary biliary cirrhosis. Lancet. 1989;1:103.

21. Leung PSC, Coppel RL, Ansari A, Munoz S, Gershwin ME. Antimitochondrial antibodies in primary biliary cirrhosis. Semin Liver Dis. 1997;17:61–9.

22. Leung PSC, Van de Water J, Coppel RL, Gershwin ME. Molecular characterization of the mitochondrial autoantigens in primary biliary cirrhosis. Immunol Res. 1991;10:518–27.

23. Luettig B, Boeker KHW, Schoessler W et al. The antinuclear autoantibodies Sp100 and gp210 persist after orthotopic liver transplantation in patients with primary biliary cirrhosis. J Hepatol. 1998;28:824–8.

24. Joplin R, Wallace LL, Johnson GD et al. Subcellular localization of pyruvate-dehydrogenase dihydrolipoamide acetyltransferase in human intrahepatic biliary epithelial cells. J Pathol. 1995;176:381–90.

25. VandeWater J, Ansari AA, Surh CD et al. Evidence for the targeting by 2-oxo-dehydrogenase enzymes in the T-cell response of primary biliary cirrhosis. J Immunol. 1991;146:89–94.

26. Joplin R, Gershwin ME. Ductular expression of autoantigens in primary biliary cirrhosis. Semin Liver Dis. 1997;17:97–103.

27. Reynoso-Paz S, Leung PSC, Van de Water J et al. Evidence for a locally driven mucosal response and the presence of mitochondrial antigens in saliva in primary biliary cirrhosis. Hepatology. 2000;31:24–9.

28. Tsuneyama K, Van de Water JV, Yamazaki K et al. Primary biliary cirrhosis an epithelitis: evidence of abnormal salivary gland immunohistochemistry. Autoimmunity. 1997;26:23–31.
29. Joplin R, Lindsay JG, Hubscher SG et al. Distribution of dihydrolipoamide acetyltransferase (E2) in the liver and portal lymph-nodes of patients with primary biliary cirrhosis – an immuno-histochemical study. Hepatology. 1991;14:442–7.
30. Tsuneyama K, Van de Water J, Leung PSC et al. Abnormal expression of the E2 component of the pyruvate-dehydrogenase complex on the luminal surface of biliary epithelium occurs before major histocompatibility complex class-Ii and Bb1/B7 expression. Hepatology. 1995;21:1031–7.
31. Van de Water J, Gerson LB, Ferrell LD et al. Immunohistochemical evidence of disease recurrence after liver transplantation for primary biliary cirrhosis. Hepatology. 1996;24:1079–84.
32. Krams SM, Surh CD, Coppel RL, Ansari A, Ruebner B, Gershwin ME. Immunization of experimental animals with dihydrolipoamide acetyltransferase, as a purified recombinant polypeptide, generates mitochondrial antibodies but not primary biliary cirrhosis. Hepatology. 1989;9:411–16.
33. Quaranta S, Shulman H, Paganin S et al. Is GVHD a model of PBC? Characterization of autoantibodies in GVHD. Hepatology. 1998;28:1516.
34. Tsuneyama K, Kono N, Hoso M et al. Aly/aly mice: a unique model of biliary disease. Hepatology. 1998;27:1499–507.
35. Jones DEJ, Palmer JM, Kirby JA et al. Experimental autoimmune cholangitis: a mouse model of immune-mediated cholangiopathy. Liver. 2000;20:351–6.
36. Sasaki M, Long SA, Van de Water J et al. The SJL/J mouse is not a model for PBC. Hepatology. 2002;35:1284–6.
37. Joplin R, Strain AJ, Neuberger JM. Immuno-isolation and culture of biliary epithelial cells from normal human liver. In Vitro Cell Devel Biol. 1989;25:1189–92.
38. Joplin R, Strain AJ, Neuberger JM. Biliary epithelial cells from the liver of patients with primary biliary cirrhosis – isolation, characterization, and short-term culture. J Pathol. 1990;162:255–60.
39. Ishida Y, Smith S, Wallace L et al. Ductular morphogenesis and functional polarization of normal human biliary epithelial cells in three-dimensional culture. J Hepatol. 2001;35:2–9.
40. Leon MP, Bassendine MF, Gibbs P, Thick M, Kirby JA. Immunogenicity of biliary epithelium: study of the adhesive interaction with lymphocytes. Gastroenterology. 1997;112:968–77.
41. Leon MP, Kirby JA, Gibbs P, Thick M, Bassendine MF. Cytotoxic immune lysis of human intrahepatic biliary epithelial cells: Modulation by ICAM-1 blockade. Hepatology. 1996;23:T41.
42. Leon MP, Kirby JA, Gibbs P, Burt AD, Bassendine MF. Immunogenicity of biliary epithelial cells – study of the expression of B7 molecules. J Hepatol. 1995;22:591–5.
43. Leon MP, Spickett G, Jones DEJ, Bassendine MF. Cd4+ T-cell subsets defined by isoforms of Cd45 in primary biliary cirrhosis. Clin Exp Immunol. 1995;99:233–9.
44. Morland CM, Fear J, Mcnab G, Joplin R, Adams DH. Promotion of leukocyte transendothelial cell migration by chemokines derived from human biliary epithelial cells in vitro. Proc Assoc Am Phys. 1997;109:372–82.
45. Joplin R, Lindsay JG, Johnson GD, Strain A, Neuberger J. Membrane dihydrolipoamide acetyltransferase (E2) on human biliary epithelial cells in primary biliary cirrhosis. Lancet. 1992;339:93–4.
46. Joplin RE, Wallace LL, Lindsay JG, Palmer JM, Yeaman SJ, Neuberger JM. The human biliary epithelial cell plasma membrane antigen in primary biliary cirrhosis: pyruvate dehydrogenase X? Gastroenterology. 1997;113:1727–33.
47. Sadamoto T, Joplin R, Keogh A, Mason A, Carman W, Neuberger J. Expression of pyruvate-dehydrogenase complex PDC-E-2 on biliary epithelial cells induced by lymph nodes from primary biliary cirrhosis. Lancet. 1998;352:1595–6.
48. Xu LZ, Shen ZW, Guo LS et al. Does a betaretrovirus infection trigger primary biliary cirrhosis? Proc Natl Acad Sci USA. 2003;100:8454–9.
49. Shih A, Misra R, Rush MG. Detection of multiple, novel reverse-transcriptase coding sequences in human nucleic acids – relation to primate retroviruses. J Virol. 1989;63:64–75.
50. Dickson C, Smith R, Peters G. In vitro synthesis of polypeptides encoded by the long terminal repeat region of mouse mammary tumor virus DNA. Nature. 1981;291:511–13.

4
Gender and primary biliary cirrhosis: is microchimerism an aetiological factor?

D. E. J. JONES

INTRODUCTION

From the earliest descriptions of the disease[1] to recent epidemiological studies it has been clear that primary biliary cirrhosis (PBC) is a condition which predominantly affects women[2,3]. In this review the impact of gender on our understanding of PBC will be discussed in terms of the clues with which the gender predominance might provide us regarding the pathogenesis of disease, touching on the practical issues faced in the clinical management of male and female patients.

PBC AS A FEMALE-PREDOMINANT DISEASE

In a recent comprehensive study of the epidemiology of PBC in the northeast of England (studying a total of 770 patients) the ratio of female to male prevalent cases rose from 9.1:1 at the study outset (1987) to 11.5:1 at the study finish (1994)[2]. The female to male ratio for incident cases through the course of the study was 9.4:1. This, one of the largest and most recent studies of the epidemiology of PBC, confirms the clinical impression that the disease is one which predominantly (but not exclusively) affects women. The majority of autoimmune diseases show increased incidence and prevalence in female patients (13 of the 20 commonest in one comparative study, with two showing equal gender prevalence and five a (typically weak) male predominance[4]). Of these 20 conditions only one, Sjögren's syndrome, showed a greater female predominance than PBC (Figure 1).

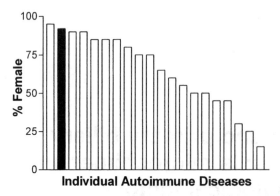

Figure 1 Percentages of the patient population who are female for the 20 commonest autoimmune diseases. Each bar denotes data for a single disease. PBC is denoted by the black bar. Data taken from Beeson[4]

THE ROLE PLAYED BY GENDER IN THE AETIOLOGY OF PBC

The marked female predominance of PBC raises interesting questions regarding the aetiology of the disease. Any model for disease aetiology must ultimately explain why the majority of (but critically not all) patients are female. At the theoretical level there are three potential explanations for the increased prevalence of PBC in females:

1. Increased risk of exposure to, or prevalence of, a disease-promoting factor in females.
2. Differences in the clinical phenotype of disease between males and females resulting in an increased likelihood of the disease being diagnosed in females.
3. Gender-specific differences in the nature or magnitude of the response to a risk or susceptibility factor common to males and females.

These potential mechanisms are, of course, not mutually exclusive.

POTENTIAL MECHANISMS FOR THE GENDER IMBALANCE IN PBC

Increased risk of exposure to, or prevalence of, a disease-promoting factor in females

One obvious potential explanation for the increased susceptibility of females to PBC would be that women are exposed at an increased level to a disease-promoting factor. Given the conventional view that PBC represents an example of a complex polygenic disorder (in which disease results from a complex interaction between environmental and genetic factors) the putative female susceptibility factor could be genetic or environmental in nature. The genetic basis of PBC susceptibility has been reviewed extensively elsewhere, and further discussion lies outside the scope of this chapter[5]. Suffice to say that none of the currently identified disease-associated loci in PBC is X or Y chromosome encoded.

With regard to female-predominant environmental disease triggers, attention has focused on the urogenital tract and, in particular, on the potential role played by pregnancy-associated factors in increasing disease susceptibility (accepting of course that there cannot be an obligate role for pregnancy-associated phenomena given that the disease can develop in men). One area of recent interest in the literature has been the concept that fetal microchimerism might contribute to disease susceptibility.

Fetal microchimerism

It is now becoming clear that even normal pregnancy results in a two-way traffic of cells from maternal to fetal circuits[6] and, importantly, vice-versa[7], the presence of small numbers of retained allogeneic cells of fetal origin in the maternal circulation being termed fetal microchimerism. Fetal cells entering the maternal circulation, which typically belong to the $CD34^+$ haematological precursor subset, appear to have the potential to persist for many years[8].

The similarities between graft-versus-host disease (GvHD) and the connective tissue disease scleroderma/systemic sclerosis led to the hypothesis that fetal microchimerism might, through a process analogous to GvHD, give rise to the tissue damage seen in scleroderma. The epidemiology of scleroderma, a condition with a marked female predominance[4] which typically develops in the post-childbearing years, appeared to be supportive of the hypothesis. The hypothesis was tested by looking for the presence of fetal-derived DNA in the peripheral blood of scleroderma patients and matched controls. The technical problem of distinguishing between DNA of maternal and fetal origin was solved by using molecular biology approaches (typically fluorescence *in-situ* hybridization (FISH) or nested (PCR)) to identify Y chromosome DNA in the tissues of female scleroderma patients who had had a previous male fetus pregnancy (and who were not part of a male/female twin pair or had had previous organ transplantation or blood transfusion; potential confounding routes for microchimerism development). Such studies suggested that, although microchimerism was seen in a proportion of normal female controls with a previous male pregnancy, the frequency in the population of fetal microchimerism, and, indeed, the levels of retention of fetal male cells seen in individual subjects, were significantly higher in scleroderma patients than in matched controls[9,10]. The conclusion of these studies was that fetal microchimerism is associated with scleroderma and may play an aetiological role.

Extension of the fetal microchimerism model to PBC was a logical step given the similar disease epidemiology, the clinical association between PBC and systemic sclerosis/scleroderma[11], and the fact that the histological features of PBC (in particular the vanishing bile ducts) are redolent, as was the case with systemic sclerosis/scleroderma, with those seen in GvHD. The association between fetal microchimerism and PBC has now been extensively studied[12–18]. The tissues studied have included both liver and peripheral blood mononuclear cells (PBMC), and the experimental designs adopted (nested PCR or FISH for Y chromosome DNA in female patients and controls with a previous male fetus pregnancy) have closely mimicked those adopted in the earlier systemic sclerosis/scleroderma studies. The individual studies are summarized in Tables 1 and 2.

Table 1 Summary of studies of the frequency of fetal microchimerism in peripheral blood in PBC patients and matched controls

First author (ref.)	PBC patient number	Control number	Technique used	PBC FMC + (%)	Control FMC + (%)
Invernizzi[13]	36	36	PCR	13 (36)	11 (31)
Corpechot[14]	20	20	PCR	9 (45)	5 (25)
Fanning[15]	18	18	PCR	0 (0)	1 (6)
Selva-O'Callaghan[18]	14	14	(PCR)	1 (7)	0 (0)

Table 2 Summary of studies of the frequency of fetal microchimerism in liver tissue in PBC patients and matched controls

First author (ref.)	PBC patient number	Control number	Technique used	PBC FMC + (%)	Control FMC + (%)
Tanaka[12]	37	39	PCR	26 (70)	28 (72)
Corpechot[14]	15	25	PCR	5 (33)	8 (32)
Fanning[15]	19	20	ISH	8 (42)	0 (0)*
Rubbia-Brandt[17]	10	3	FISH	0 (0)	0 (0)
Schoniger-Hekele[16]	21	13	FISH	3 (14)	1 (8)

*$p < 0.05$.

Tanaka and colleagues used a PCR-based approach incorporating highly sensitive WAVE-based detection technology on liver biopsy material from 37 PBC patients and 39 controls (all subjects having given birth to a male child). Y-chromosome-derived DNA sequences were identified in 26 PBC patients (70%) and 28 controls (72%)[12]. The high level of detection seen in this study is likely to reflect the sensitivity of the detection system used. Invernizzi and colleagues, using nested PCR on peripheral blood samples from 36 female patients and controls with male offspring matched for age, age of last son and number of children, found Y-chromosome-specific DNA in 13 (36%) PBC patients and 11 (31%) controls[13]. Corpechot et al. studied both PBMC and liver biopsy material. PBMC and liver Y chromosome sequence DNA was detected using nested PCR. Microchimerism was seen in similar proportions of PBMC and liver tissue from PBC patients and controls (PBMC 9/20 vs 5/20; liver 5/15 vs 8/25)[14]. Fanning and colleagues again studied both PBMC and liver biopsy material. PBMC Y chromosome sequence DNA was detected using nested PCR, whilst an *in-situ* hybridization approach was adopted for liver tissue. Microchimerism was seen in only one control PBMC specimen (and in none of the PBC patients). Microchimerism was seemingly present in the liver of PBC patients (8/19 (42%)) but not controls (0/20, $p < 0.05$)[15]. This study, which is notable for being the only one demonstrating a significant increase in the fetal microchimerism rate in PBC patients when compared with controls, was also notable for the low level of detectable microchimerism seen in the control population selected (it is unclear whether or

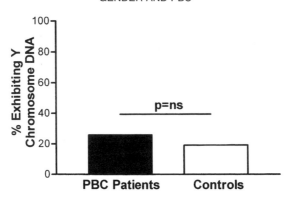

Figure 2 Cumulative data for the frequency of fetal microchimerism in blood from PBC patients and controls

not all the control subjects whose liver was studied had carried a male fetus pregnancy). Schoniger-Hekele et al. used nested PCR to demonstrate Y-chromosome genetic material in the liver tissue of 5/28 (18%) of PBC patients compared with 4/77 (5%) of chronic liver disease controls[16]. Other studies[17,18] failed to detect significant microchimerism in either patients or controls.

When the data from the individual studies are combined (Figures 2 and 3) no differences are seen in the population prevalences of fetal microchimerism between PBC patients and controls for either peripheral blood or liver tissue. Based on what is now a quite extensive literature we can conclude that fetal microchimerism does not occur at increased frequency in PBC patients, and that there are at present no data to support the theory that fetal microchimerism plays an aetiological role in PBC.

Other gender-specific risk factors

Early reports suggesting that PBC patients have an increased incidence of urinary tract infections (a clinical problem seen with an increased prevalence in females) have not been supported by follow-up studies[19,20]. More recently two groups in the USA and UK have adopted a case–control epidemiological approach to searching for disease risk factors[21,22]. These studies, although not designed to explore the role for gender-specific risk factors, can provide us with some important data. Neither study demonstrated any association between PBC and gender-specific surgery, gender-specific pathology or infectious disease or any aspect of reproductive and/or obstetric history.

A reasonable conclusion from these studies, taken together, is that no gender-specific risk factor for PBC has yet been identified which can account for the increased prevalence and incidence of PBC.

Different disease phenotype in females leading to diagnosis

A further theoretical explanation for the gender distribution of PBC would be a disparity in the clinical expression of the disease. There are two possibilities. The first is that PBC has a dramatically worse outcome in men, thereby reducing the prevalence of the disease and, accordingly, the proportion of men in any geographically based cohort. That this is not the case is emphatically demonstrated by the increased incidence of the disease (to go along with prevalence of the disease) seen in females in the key epidemiological studies[2,3]. It is worth noting that PBC does differ between male and female patients in one way which has an impact on individual prognosis. The incidence of hepatocellular carcinoma (HCC) appears to be significantly higher in male patients than in female patients (reflecting the experience in cirrhosis of all aetiologies)[23]. The incidence of HCC remains, however, even in male PBC patients, at a level that does not meaningfully influence the mortality rate of the whole PBC population.

The second phenotypic explanation for the gender distribution of PBC would be that the condition has a more clinically apparent phenotype resulting in a greater likelihood of clinical presentation and the diagnosis being made in female patients. Direct comparative studies of the clinical expression of PBC and male and female patients have been limited. The limited data available suggest, however, that there are no differences in the symptom spectrum, rate of progression and clinical expression of PBC between male and female patients (with the exception of the previously outlined HCC incidence difference)[24-26].

Increased or altered response to a common trigger in females

Recent improvements in our understanding of the normal mechanisms of regulation of the immune system suggest that sex-hormone-mediated effects on the immune response may play a significant role in the pathogenesis of autoimmunity. Both androgens and oestrogens are potent immune modulators, able to negatively regulate both the thymus and bone marrow[27,28]. Critically, however, androgens and oestrogens have contrasting effects on different immune cell populations (including regulatory cells). Data from murine models of autoimmune disease such as experimental autoimmune encephalomyelitis (EAE, a model with features redolent of multiple sclerosis) clearly demonstrate that disease susceptibility is increased in female animals compared to males, that removal of the testes increases susceptibility whilst removal of the ovaries confers protection, and that

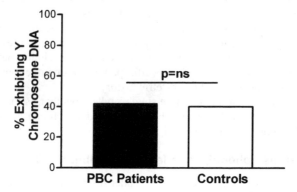

Figure 3 Cumulative data for the frequency of fetal microchimerism in liver tissue from PBC patients and controls

sex hormone replacement therapy in castrated animals confers a degree of susceptibility appropriate to the 'gender' of the sex hormone given[29]. The identities of the cell types demonstrating the key response to oestrogens for the modulation of autoimmunity (antigen-presenting cells or T cells themselves) at present remain unclear. Certainly, oestrogen receptor is expressed by all lymphocyte subsets[30]. Perhaps the most plausible hypothesis is that the key effect of oestrogen on potentially autoreactive immune responses is at the level of control of thymic deletion of autoreactive T cells. At present no data are available regarding differences in immune function between males and females in the direct context of PBC.

CONCLUSION

The incidence and prevalence of PBC are both significantly higher in females than in males. With the exception of an increased risk of HCC in male patients with stage IV disease (cirrhosis) disease phenotype appears to be similar in the two gender groups. There is, at present, no evidence to suggest that the gender imbalance results from increased exposure to a disease trigger in females. In particular, there is no evidence to support the hypothesis that fetal microchimerism may contribute to disease pathogenesis. Perhaps the most plausible model for the female predominance in PBC is that, following exposure to a disease trigger which itself shows no gender specificity (the potential identity of such a trigger is a source of much current debate), the nature of the response induced in males and females varies under the control of sex hormones. In this model an androgen-modulated immune system would normally retain the capacity to regulate or delete the potentially autoreactive immune cells triggered. An oestrogen-modulated immune system would be less able to regulate the response, resulting in a greater frequency of induced pathological autoimmunity.

References

1. Addison T, Gull W. On a certain affliction of the skin-vitiligoides – a planus tuberosa. Guys Hosp Rev. 1857;7:268–84.
2. James OFW, Bhopal R, Howel D, Gray J, Burt AD, Metcalf JV. Primary biliary cirrhosis once rare, now common in the UK? Hepatology. 1999;30:390–4.
3. Kim WR, Lindor KD, Locke GR et al. Epidemiology and natural history of primary biliary cirrhosis in a US community. Gastroenterology. 2000;119:1631–6.
4. Beeson PB. Age and sex associations of 40 autoimmune diseases. Am J Med. 1994;96:457–62.
5. Jones DEJ, Donaldson PT. Genetic factors in the pathogenesis of primary biliary cirrhosis. Clin Liver Dis. 2003;7:841–64.
6. Lo YMD, Lo ESF, Watson N, Nokes L, Sargent IL, Thilaganathan B, Wainscoat JS. Two-way traffic between mother and fetus: biologic and clinical implications. Blood. 1996;88:4390–5.
7. Bianchi D, Williams JM, Sullivan LM, Hanson FW, Klinger KW, Shuber AP. PCR quantitation of fetal cells in maternal blood in normal and aneuploid pregnancies. Am J Human Genet. 1996;61:822–9.
8. Bianchi D, Zickwolf G, Weil G, Sylvester S, Demaria M. Male fetal progenitor cells persist in maternal blood for as long as 27 years. Proc Natl Acad Sci USA. 1996;93:705–8.
9. Nelson JL, Furst DE, Maloney S et al. Microchimerism and HLA-compatible relationships of pregnancy in scleroderma. Lancet. 1998;351:540–1.
10. Evans P, Lambert N, Maloney S, Furst D, Moore J, Nelson J. Long-term fetal microchimerism in peripheral blood mononuclear cell subsets in healthy women and women with scleroderma. Blood. 1999;93:2033–7.

11. Watt FE, Bassendine MF, James OFW, Jones DEJ. A population based study of autoimmunity in primary biliary cirrhosis (PBC) patients and their families: evidence for a shared susceptibility. J Hepatol. 2001;34:211.

12. Tanaka A, Lindor K, Gish R et al. Fetal microchimerism alone does not contribute to the induction of primary biliary cirrhosis. Hepatology. 1999;30:833–8.

13. Invernizzi P, De Andreis C, Sirchia SM et al. Blood fetal microchimerism in primary biliary cirrhosis. Clin Exp Immunol. 2000;122:418–22.

14. Corpechot C, Barbu V, Chazouillieres O, Poupon R. Fetal microchimerism in primary biliary cirrhosis. J Hepatol. 2000;33:696–700.

15. Fanning PA, Jonsson JR, Clouston AD et al. Detection of male DNA in the liver of female patients with primary biliary cirrhosis. J Hepatol. 2000;33:690–5.

16. Schoniger-Hekele M, Muller C, Ackermann J et al. Lack of evidence for involvement of fetal microchimerism in pathogenesis of primary biliary cirrhosis. Dig Dis Sci. 2002;47:1909–14.

17. Rubbia-Brandt L, Philippeaux MM, Chavez S, Mentha G, Borisch B, Hadengue A. FISH for Y chromosome in women with primary biliary cirrhosis: lack of evidence for leucocyte microchimerism. Hepatology. 1999;30:821–2.

18. Selva-O'Callaghan A, Prades EB, Fuste LC, Blasco VV, Laque RS, Vilardell-Tarres M. Fetal microchimerism in patients with primary biliary cirrhosis. Med Clin. 2002;119:770–2.

19. Burroughs AK, Rosenstein IJ, Epstein O, Hamilton-Miller JM, Brumfitt W, Sherlock S. Bacteriuria and primary biliary cirrhosis. Gut. 1984;25:133–7.

20. Floreani A, Bassendine MF, Mitchison H, Freeman R, James OFW. No specific association between primary biliary cirrhosis and bacteriuria. J Hepatol. 1989;8:201–7.

21. Howel D, Fischbacher CM, Bhopal RS, Gray J, Metcalf JV, James OFW. An exploratory population-based case–control study of primary biliary cirrhosis. Hepatology. 2000;31:1055–60.

22. Parikh-Patel A, Gold EB, Wormann H, Krivy KE, Gershwin ME. Risk factors for primary biliary cirrhosis in a cohort of patients from the United States. Hepatology. 2001;33:16–21.

23. Jones DEJ, Metcalf JV, Collier JD, Bassendine MF, James OFW. Hepatocellular carcinoma in primary biliary cirrhosis and its impact on outcomes. Hepatology. 1997;26:1138–42.

24. Nalbandian G, Van de Water J, Gish R et al. Is there a serological difference between men and women with primary biliary cirrhosis? Am J Gastroenterol. 1999;94:2482–6.

25. Lucey MR, Neuberger JM, Williams R. Primary biliary cirrhosis in men. Gut. 1986;27:1373–6.

26. Rubel LR, Rabin L, Seeff LB, Licht H, Cuccherini BA. Does primary biliary cirrhosis in men differ from primary biliary cirrhosis in women? Hepatology. 1984;4:671–7.

27. Okuyama R, Abo T, Seki S et al. Estrogen administration activates extrathymic T cell differentiation in the liver. J Exp Med. 1992;175:661–9.

28. Olsen NJ, Olson G, Viselli SM, Gu X, Kovacs WJ. Androgen receptors in thymic epithelium modulate thymus size and thymocyte development. Endocrinology. 2001;142:1278–83.

29. Vorskuhl RR, Pitchekian-Halabi H, Mackenzie-Graham A, McFarland HF, Raine CS. Gender differences in autoimmune demyelination in the mouse: implications for multiple sclerosis. Ann Neurol. 1996;39:724–33.

30. Tornwall J, Carey AB, Fox RI, Fox HS. Estrogens in autoimmunity: expression of estrogen receptors in thymic and autoimmune T-cells. J Gend Spec Med. 1999;2:33–40.

Section II
Histology and immunology of primary biliary cirrhosis and autoimmune cholestatic disease

5
Histology of autoimmune cholestatic liver diseases

V. J. DESMET

INTRODUCTION

The category of autoimmune cholestatic liver diseases comprises the entities known as primary biliary cirrhosis (PBC), primary sclerosing cholangitis (PSC), and overlap syndromes between each of these with autoimmune hepatitis[1,2]. The latter (overlap) group is described in Chapter 14 of this volume.

PBC and PSC are 'vanishing bile duct' diseases, characterized by (apparently at least partially) autoimmune-based destruction and disappearance of intrahepatic bile ducts, resulting in chronic impairment of bile flow or cholestasis. It follows that the histological features in liver biopsies of patients with PBC or PSC comprise changes due to chronic cholestasis in general, besides portal alterations and bile duct lesions characteristic for the individual diseases. These are described below under the headings: liver changes of chronic cholestasis; portal and bile duct lesions in PBC; portal and bile duct lesions in PSC[3,4].

HISTOPATHOLOGY OF CHRONIC CHOLESTASIS

A group of changes represent elementary lesions of chronic cholestasis in general, including parenchymal, periportal and architectural changes. Where the chronic cholestatic condition is due to a disease characterized by disappearance of the intrahepatic bile ducts, progressive ductopenia is part of the picture. The nature and extent of the cholestatic changes, as well as the ductopenia, are not static, and progress over time.

Parenchymal lesions of chronic cholestasis

Diseases characterized by progressive ductopenia, such as PBC and PSC, represent conditions of incomplete cholestasis, during which retention of bilirubin (histological bilirubinostasis) and clinical jaundice are not part of the symptoms during (very) long periods of time (months or years). They appear only in the later decompensating phase of the disorder, or during complications (e.g. super-imposed drug-induced cholestasis). The parenchymal lesions of chronic cholestasis comprise cholestatic liver cell rosettes, clusters of xanthomatous cells in portal tracts or in the lobular parenchyma, feathery degeneration of hepatocytes, bile infarcts (in later stages), and progressive periportal cholate-stasis[4]. As mentioned, bilirubinostasis is a later and unfavourable lesion.

Periportal and architectural features of chronic cholestasis

A striking feature in most cases of chronic bile retention (with the unexplained exception of some patients with PSC), is so-called 'ductular reaction'. This lesion is recognized as an increased number of ductular profiles in the periphery of and around the portal tracts, gradually extending into the periportal parenchyma and accompanied by oedema, neutrophil polymorphonuclear leucocyte infiltration, and progressive periductular fibroplasia[5]. The wedge-shaped periportal extension of the ductular reaction, often in combination with periportal parenchymal features of cholate-stasis, creates an irregular portal–parenchymal interface, termed 'biliary piecemeal necrosis'[6]. Progressive periductular fibrosis eventually leads to fibrous linkage of adjacent portal tracts. Such a stage of 'biliary fibrosis' (portal–portal septal fibrosis) is a potentially reversible lesion, to be distinguished from biliary cirrhosis[7].

Biliary cirrhosis is the final stage in disturbance of the lobular architecture, additionally characterized by portal–central fibrous septa and more obvious parenchymal nodularity. The periportal and architectural changes form the base for staging in chronic cholestatic liver disease: portal (stage 1), periportal (stage 2), septal (stage 3) and cirrhotic stage (stage 4)[8]. Staging of PBC in needle biopsy specimens may be subject to considerable sampling error, due to the irregular distribution of the lesions throughout the liver[9]. Immunostaining for cytokeratin 7, revealing increasing positivity of the parenchyma with progression of cholestasis, may be a useful adjunct in staging of PBC[10].

Ductopenia

Bile-duct loss or ductopenia is recognized as the absence of an interlobular bile duct, most easily recognized as a hepatic artery branch without accompanying interlobular bile duct of similar size ('widowed artery')[11]. The degree of ductopenia is evaluated by calculating the percentage of portal tracts with missing ducts, or by calculating the bile duct-to-portal tract ratio. The normal ratio in healthy liver[12] varies between 0.9 and 1.8. Originally, ductopenia was defined[12] as absence of interlobular bile ducts in at least 50% of portal tracts or a bile duct/portal tract ratio below 0.5. Earlier stages can be diagnosed as ductopenia in adequate liver specimens (comprising at least 10 portal tracts).

PRIMARY BILIARY CIRRHOSIS

Besides features of chronic cholestasis, the liver biopsy of patients suffering from PBC also reveals lesions characteristic of this disease, mostly confined to the portal tracts and interlobular bile ducts. It should be mentioned from the out-set that these histopathological alterations are identical in so-called 'autoimmune cholangitis' or 'antimitochondrial antibody-negative PBC'[13].

It has been repeatedly emphasized that PBC, a term coined by Ahrens et al. in 1950[14], is a misnomer, since the disease corresponds to cirrhosis only in its final, terminal stage. Alternative names such as 'chronic non-suppurative destructive cholangitis'[15] granulomatous cholangitis[16] and 'autoimmune cholangitis'[17] have not attained popularity; a recent proposal has been 'primary cholangiohepatitis'[18].

The early portal lesion consists of mononuclear inflammatory cell infiltration with destructive injury of small intrahepatic bile ducts, preferably interlobular ducts measuring 40–80 μm in diameter. The lining cholangiocytes reveal cyto-plasmic swelling and vacuolization, irregularity of the apical border, or show eosinophilic cytoplasmic condensation and nuclear pycnosis. Apoptosis is a mechanism of death of cholangiocytes[19,20]. Besides degenerative features, the bile duct epithelium also shows proliferative changes[21].

Bile duct damage and portal inflammation are not homogeneously spread throughout the liver, so that a needle liver biopsy may fail to include the lesions[22].

The most characteristic lesion is the development of epithelioid granulomas, often in close association with the bile ducts ('granulomatous cholangitis')[6]. The epithelioid cells may be more loosely arranged than in a classical compact granuloma, and may be admixed with foamy macrophages[23].

Lymphocytes permeate between the bile duct lining cholangiocytes; finally the basement membrane ruptures. Disintegrating and ruptured bile ducts are sur-rounded by lymphocytes, plasma cells, epithelioid cells, variable numbers of eosinophils, and foamy macrophages. Hyaline deposits may appear in the portal areas, sometimes within lymphoid aggregates[24].

The bile duct damage appears to be related, amongst others things, to infiltrat-ing CD57[+] CD3[+] natural killer cells[25,26]. In the inflamed periductal areas the size and the number of lymphatics is increased[27], whereas the peribiliary capillary plexus becomes involved, resulting in sclerosis and reduction of the plexus[28–30].

Remnants of bile duct epithelium may be identifiable as single epithelial cells, better revealed by immunostaining for cytokeratin 7, or as small deposits of amorphous, PAS-positive material. Finally, the bile duct segment disappears completely, leaving only a focal scar-like condensation of portal mesenchyme or a cluster of lymphocytes at the site of the vanished duct.

With further progression of the disease[31], the number of interlobular (and small septal) ducts decreases. Progressive ductopenia induces chronic cholestasis of increasing severity with associated parenchymal and fibrotic changes. A note-worthy feature of the liver parenchyma in precirrhotic stages of PBC is the development of parenchymal nodularity, similar to nodular regenerative hyper-plasia[32–34]. This may play a role in the development of clinically notable portal hypertension before the cirrhotic stage[35]. The nodularity itself may be the result of portal phlebosclerosis secondary to portal and ductal inflammation[36].

A considerable number of studies have been devoted to immunohistochemical investigations of liver biopsies of patients with PBC in order to further elucidate immunological mechanisms in the pathogenesis of bile duct damage and destruction. These include immunohistochemical demonstration of lymphocyte subsets, antigen-presenting cells, possible target antigens, major histocompatibility antigens, cytokines, chemokines and apoptosis-related factors. These investigations were recently summarized in several reviews[26,37–39].

Histological differential diagnosis of PBC requires consideration and exclusion of several chronic liver diseases. These include predominantly chronic hepatitis and several other vanishing bile duct disorders. The most diagnostic feature is the combination of granulomatous cholangitis with features of chronic cholestasis. The later stages (biliary fibrosis and cirrhosis) are less characteristic and difficult to differentiate from other vanishing bile duct disorders, especially PSC.

A problem for the pathologist is the diagnosis of recurrent PBC after liver transplantation. Bile duct injury in the liver allograft may result from acute or cellular rejection, from viral infection (in particular *de-novo* or reactivation of hepatitis C and CMV infection), and from disease recurrence in patients who received their liver transplant for end-stage PBC. The diagnosis of recurrent PBC rests on the demonstration of the most suggestive feature: the florid duct lesion of granulomatous cholangitis[37], often with plasmocytosis in the earlier biopsy specimens[40].

PRIMARY SCLEROSING CHOLANGITIS (PSC)

As is the case for PBC, PSC has also to be recognized as a specific disease on the basis of portal and bile duct alterations in a background of more or less evident (or advanced) cholestatic features. PSC is a disease which may affect large and small bile ducts in combination (the classical type of PSC), or in a minority of cases only small bile ducts (so-called small duct PSC)[41]. The term 'large ducts' refers here to cholangiographically demonstrable (extrahepatic and intrahepatic) larger ducts, whereas the term 'small ducts' refers to smaller intrahepatic bile ducts not demonstrable by the usual imaging techniques; the latter are the diagnostic territory of the histopathologist: small septal and interlobular ducts visualized by light microscopy.

Cholangiography or other imaging techniques and liver biopsy examination are complementary in the diagnosis of PSC. Imaging results inform about the involvement of larger ducts, whereas liver biopsy allows evaluation of smaller bile duct lesions, ductopenia, and grade and stage of chronic cholestatic liver disease[42–44].

The lesions of larger intrahepatic ducts and of the extrahepatic biliary tree reflect the changes seen on imaging: annular scars or fibrous cords which alternate with tubular or saccular cholangiectases; ulcerations with or without cholangitic abscesses, intrahepatic stones and large perihilar scars[37]. Histopathological study of surgical or endoscopic specimens of the extrahepatic bile ducts is not very helpful in establishing the diagnosis of PSC[45,46].

The distinctive bile duct lesion in PSC is a fibro-obliterative cholangitis, characterized by a concentric periductal ('onion-skin type') fibrosis, possibly with degeneration and atrophy of the cholangiocytic lining, and eventual replacement of the bile duct by a fibrous cord. This lesion, accompanied by ductopenia and signs of chronic cholestasis, is virtually diagnostic of PSC. However, this lesion may be found only in less than 40% of liver needle biopsies.

The early intrahepatic histopathological lesions (portal stage or stage 1) are confined within the portal tracts, and consist of a mixed inflammatory infiltrate (lymphocytes, plasma cells, neutrophils) which tends to predominate around the interlobular bile ducts. Small interlobular ducts may show degenerative changes of cholangiocytes. These early portal lesions are not specific; but in a patient with inflammatory bowel disease even minimal changes such as portal oedema and some ductular reaction should raise a strong suspicion of early PSC[46].

Some portal oedema and incipient periductal fibrosis may be present. Epithelioid granulomas are not considered part of the lesions and, if present, are thought to reflect associated pathology (sarcoidosis, drug-induced liver injury, etc.)[47,48]. An increase in the number of mast cells is observed in the bile duct wall in long-standing sclerosing cholangitis[49].

Portal tracts enlarge, with disruption of the limiting plates (stage 2 or periportal stage). In many instances focal ductular reaction with associated neutrophilic infiltrate (active cholangiolitis) predominates. In apparently more florid cases the portal inflammation is quite dense and is associated with interface hepatitis simulating chronic hepatitis. However, in this stage there are often already signs of periportal cholate stasis, with cytokeratin 7 expression and rhodanin- and orcein-positive granules in periportal hepatocytes, indicating chronic cholestatic disease.

In many cases the inflammation is milder and appears to have subsided; the portal connective tissue becomes more collagenized and irradiates with thin extensions and short septa into the surrounding parenchyma, giving the portal tracts a stellate appearance.

Concentric periduct fibrosis and focal ductopenia may be present, and PAS-diastase staining often reveals thickening of the basement membrane around remaining, sometimes atrophic-appearing, ducts[50].

Further progression of the disease is reflected in increasing periportal fibrosis with development of portal–portal septa (biliary fibrosis or stage 3) and finally true cirrhosis (stage 4).

Stages 3 and 4 are usually associated with marked features of chronic cholestasis, reflected in ductular reaction, periseptal interface hepatitis, periportal cholate stasis (cytokeratin 7 expression, accumulation of copper and copper-binding protein, Mallory body formation), and a progressive reduction in the number of interlobular ducts[51].

The interlobular ducts may disappear without leaving a trace; often their former site is indicated either by small clusters of lymphocytes and macrophages, or – as mentioned above – by rounded scars. These fibrous, cord-like scars are more prominent in PSC than in PBC and than in secondary sclerosing cholangitis[37]. Some unusual cases of PSC are characterized by prominent, hypertrophic scars left over from disappeared bile ducts[52,53], suggesting a peculiar reactivity of the portal connective tissue in such cases ('keloid cholangitis')[54].

Immunohistochemical studies have focused on cholestatic lesions and features related to immunological mechanisms[37,55,56].

Patients with PSC are at an increased risk for developing cholangiocarcinoma in up to 20% of patients[57]. The concomitant or sequential demonstration of bile duct cell dysplasia, carcinoma *in situ* and foci of microinvasive carcinoma in various segments of the biliary system suggest a multicentric origin[58]. The presence of biliary dysplasia can be used as a marker for current or developing biliary malignancy; the criteria for biliary dysplasia can be agreed upon and the entity is recognizable in liver biopsies[59]. The diagnostic histopathologist should be alerted to search for and to report this lesion in biopsies from patients with PSC, as it raises a high degree of suspicion for development of cholangiocarcinoma. Immunohistochemical staining for carcinoembryonic antigen (CEA) may be helpful: dysplastic biliary epithelium shows both cytoplasmic and luminal staining for CEA, whereas normal bile duct cells display only apical positivity[60].

The differential diagnosis of PSC requires careful consideration from several other chronic liver diseases. The more characteristic portal and bile duct alterations in any vanishing bile duct disease are found in the early stages and tend to diminish or even disappear as the disease progresses. It hence follows that later stages resemble each other with common features of biliary fibrosis or cirrhosis, ductopenia and lesions of chronic cholestasis[48].

The inflammatory infiltrate tends to be mild in PSC and is usually more severe in PBC[46], but this is not really helpful in individual cases. In a series of 318 patients with either PBC or PSC, studied several years ago, distinction was reliable in only 28% of cases[61]. Cholestasis is an early and more frequent finding in PSC than in PBC[62]. In the cirrhotic stage of PSC the biopsies usually reveal unequivocal biliary features, with garland-shaped regenerative nodules and signs of chronic cholestasis[46]. Periductal concentric fibrosis and duct replacement by fibrous cords favour PSC; in contrast, epithelioid granulomas are mostly found in PBC. Further histological mimics of PSC are idiopathic adulthood ductopenia, lymphoma-associated ductopenia, drug-induced and toxic ductopenia and iatrogenic sclerosing cholangitis[63].

The staging of PSC is based on the liver biopsy findings, and not on large duct abnormalities as they appear on cholangiograms. This is justified by the observation that the progression of the disease towards liver transplantation or death is determined primarily by the changes in the hepatic parenchyma, not by large-duct changes[46]. The staging criteria for PSC are identical to those for PBC.

Two special variants of PSC deserve mention: childhood PSC and small-duct PSC.

Several series of paediatric patients with PSC have been reported in recent years[64-67]. Autoimmune features appear to be more common in children, with an autoimmune hepatitis/sclerosing cholangitis overlap syndrome[67]. Histologically, the combination of cholangitic changes and interface hepatitis is more frequent, though not exclusive, to those patients with bile duct damage on ERCP.

Three recent studies have addressed the problem of small-duct PSC[68-70]. A thoughtful summary of these investigations appeared in an editorial by Chapman[71], with the following conclusions. In contrast to the initial report by Wee and Ludwig[72], which suggested that patients with small duct PSC would progress to large duct PSC and cholangiocarcinoma, the long-term follow-up of such patients turns out differently. The results from all three studies are remarkably similar. The clinical course of the disease is much more benign in the small duct group. No patients in the series presented have developed cholangiocarcinoma, and only a small minority progressed to large duct PSC. The results suggest that small duct PSC is indeed a rare condition, might represent a distinct clinical entity, and in the majority of cases does not represent an early form of classical PSC[71].

References

1. Woodward J, Neuberger J. Autoimmune overlap syndromes. Hepatology. 2001;33:994–1002.
2. Chazouillères O. The variant forms of cholestatic diseases involving small bile ducts in adults. J Hepatol. 2000;32(Suppl. 2):16–18.
3. Desmet VJ. Chronic cholestasis. In: Hoofnagle JH, Goodman Z, editors. Liver Biopsy. Interpretation for the 1990s, Thorofare: Slack, 1991:25–38.
4. Desmet VJ. Histopathology of cholestasis. Verh Dtsh Ges Pathol. 1995;79:233–40.
5. Desmet V, Roskams T, Van Eyken P. Ductular reaction in the liver. Pathol Res Pract. 1995;191:513–24.
6. Ludwig J. New concepts in biliary cirrhosis. Semin Liver Dis. 1987;7:293–301.
7. Desmet VJ. Cirrhosis: aetiology and pathogenesis: cholestasis. In: Boyer JL, Bianchi L, editors. Liver Cirrhosis. Falk Symposium 44. Lancaster: MTP, 1987:101–18.
8. Ludwig J, La Russo NF, Wiesner RH. The syndrome of primary sclerosing cholangitis. In: Popper H, Schaffner F, editors. Progress in Liver Diseases, Vol. IX. Philadelphia: WB Saunders, 1990:555–66.
9. Garrido MC, Hubscher SG. Accuracy of staging in primary biliary cirrhosis. J Clin Pathol. 1996;49:556–9.
10. Yabushita K, Yamamoto K, Ibuki N et al. Aberrant expression of cytokeratin 7 as a histological marker of progression in primary biliary cirrhosis. Liver. 2001;21:50–5.
11. Crawford AR, Lin XZ, Crawford JM. The normal adult human liver biopsy: a quantitative reference standard. Hepatology. 1998;28:323–31.
12. Alagille D, Odièvre M, Gautier M, Dommergues JP. Hepatic ductular hypoplasia associated with characteristic facies, vertebral malformations, retarded physical, mental and sexual development and cardiac murmur. J Pediatr. 1975;86:63–71.
13. Goodman ZD, McNally P, Davis DR, Ishak KG. Autoimmune cholangitis: a variant of primary biliary cirrhosis. Clinicopathologic and serologic correlations in 200 cases. Dig Dis Sci. 1995;40:1232–42.
14. Ahrens T, Payne MA, Kunkel HG, Eisenmenger WJ, Blondheim SH. Primary biliary cirrhosis. Medicine. 1950;29:299–364.
15. Rubin E, Schaffner F, Popper H. Primary biliary cirrhosis: chronic non-suppurative destructive cholangitis. Am J Pathol. 1965;46:387–407.
16. Ludwig J, Czaja AJ, Dickson R, La Russo NF, Wiesner RH. Manifestations of nonsuppurative cholangitis in chronic hepatobiliary diseases: morphologic spectrum, clinical correlations and terminology. Liver. 1984;4:105–16.
17. Heathcote J. Autoimmune cholangitis. Gut. 1997;40:440–2.
18. Nakanuma Y, Harada K. Primary cholangiohepatitis as an alternative name for primary biliary cirrhosis. Pathol Int. 2003;53:412–14.
19. Harada K, Ozaki S, Gershwin ME, Nakanuma Y. Enhanced apoptosis relates to bile duct loss in primary biliary cirrhosis. Hepatology. 1997;26:1399–405.
20. Tinmouth J, Lee M, Wanless IR, Tsui FWL, Inman R, Heathcote EJ. Apoptosis of biliary epithelial cells in primary biliary cirrhosis and primary sclerosing cholangitis. Liver. 2002;22:228–34.
21. Nakanuma Y, Harada K. Florid duct lesion in primary biliary cirrhosis shows highly proliferative activities. J Hepatol. 1993;19:216–21.
22. Scheuer PJ. Ludwig symposium on biliary disorders – part II. Pathologic features and evolution of primary biliary cirrhosis and primary sclerosing cholangitis. Mayo Clin Proc. 1998;73:179–83.
23. Nakanuma Y, Ohta G. Quantitation of hepatic granulomas and epithelioid cells in primary biliary cirrhosis. Hepatology. 1983;3:423–7.
24. Portmann B, Popper H, Neuberger J, Williams R. Sequential and diagnostic features in primary biliary cirrhosis based on serial histologic study in 209 patients. Gastroenterology. 1985;88:1777–90.
25. Harada K, Isse K, Tsuneyama K, Ohta H, Nakanuma Y. Accumulating CD57+ CD3+ natural killer T cells are related to intrahepatic bile duct lesions in primary biliary cirrhosis. Liver Int. 2003;23:94–100.

26. Nakanuma Y, Tsuneyama K, Sasaki M, Harada K. Destruction of bile ducts in primary biliary cirrhosis. Baillieres Best Pract Res Clin Gastroenterol. 2000;14:549–70.
27. Yamauchi Y, Ikeda R, Michitaka K, Hiasa Y, Horiike N, Onji M. Morphometric analysis of lymphatic vessels in primary biliary cirrhosis. Hepatol Res. 2002;24:107–13.
28. Washington K, Clavien PA, Killenberg P. Peribiliary vascular plexus in primary sclerosing cholangitis and primary biliary cirrhosis. Hum Pathol. 1997;28:791–975.
29. Kobayashi S, Nakanuma Y, Matsui O. Intrahepatic peribiliary vascular plexus in various hepato-biliary diseases. A histological survey. Hum Pathol. 1994;25:940–6.
30. Matsunaga Y, Terada T. Peribiliary capillary plexus around interlobular bile ducts in various chronic liver diseases: an immunohistochemical and morphometric study. Pathol Int. 1999;49: 869–73.
31. Locke III GR, Therneau TM, Ludwig J, Dickson ER, Lindor KD. Time course of histological progression in primary biliary cirrhosis. Hepatology. 1996;23:52–6.
32. Nakanuma Y, Ohta G. Nodular hyperplasia of the liver in primary biliary cirrhosis of early histological stages. Am J Gastroenterol. 1987;82:8–10.
33. Colina F, Pinedo F, Solis JA, Moreno D, Nevado M. Nodular regenerative hyperplasia of the liver in early histological stages of primary biliary cirrhosis. Gastroenterology. 1992;102: 1319–24.
34. Chazouillères O, Andreani T, Legendre C, Poupon R, Darnis F. Hyperplasie nodulaire régénérative du foie et cirrhose biliaire primitive. Une association fortuite? Gastroenterol Clin Biol. 1986; 10:764–6.
35. Navasa M, Parés A, Bruguera M, Caballeria J, Bosch J, Rodés J. Portal hypertension in primary biliary cirrhosis. Relationship with histological features. J Hepatol. 1987;5:292–8.
36. Wanless IR. Understanding non-cirrhotic portal hypertension: ménage à foie (editorial). Hepatology. 1988;8:192–3.
37. Portmann BC, Nakanuma Y. Diseases of the bile ducts. In: MacSween RNM, Burt AD, Portmann BC, Ishak KG, Scheuer PJ, Anthony PP, editors. Pathology of the Liver, 4th edn. London: Churchill Livingstone, 2002:435–506.
38. Desmet VJ, Roskams T. Immunological reaction patterns in the liver. In: Moreno-Otero R, Abillos A, Garcia-Monzon C, editors. Immunology and the Liver: Cytokines, Madrid: Accion Medica, 2002:45–64.
39. Reynoso-Paz S, Coppel RL, Mackay IR, Bass NM, Ansari AA, Gershwin ME. The immunobiology of bile and biliary epithelium. Hepatology. 1999;30:351–7.
40. Khettry U, Anand N, Paul PN et al. Liver transplantation for primary biliary cirrhosis: a long-term-pathologic study. Liver Transplant. 2003;9:87–96.
41. Ludwig J. Small-duct primary sclerosing cholangitis. Semin Liver Dis. 1991;11:11–17.
42. Sapey T, Turlin B, Canva-Delcambre V et al. Value of liver biopsy and endoscopic retrograde cholangiography in patients with chronic anicteric cholestasis: a retrospective study of 79 patients. Gastroenterol Clin Biol. 1999;23:178–85.
43. Angula P, Lindor KD. Primary sclerosing cholangitis. Hepatology. 1999;30:325–32.
44. Harnois D, Lindor KD. Primary sclerosing cholangitis: evolving concepts in diagnosis and treatment. Dig Dis. 1997;15:23–41.
45. Ludwig J, La Russo NF, Wiesner RH. Primary sclerosing cholangitis. In: Peters RL, Craig JR, editors. Liver Pathology. Contemporary Issues in Surgical Pathology, Vol. 8. New York: Churchill Livingstone, 1986:193–213.
46. Ludwig J. Histopathology of primary sclerosing cholangitis. In: Manns MP, Stiehl A, Chapman RW, Wiesner RH, editors. Primary Sclerosing Cholangitis. Dordrecht: Kluwer, 1998:14–21.
47. Ludwig J, Colina F, Poterucha JJ. Granulomas in primary sclerosing cholangitis. Liver. 1995; 15:307–12.
48. Desmet VJ. Histopathology of chronic cholestasis and adult ductopenic syndrome. In: Lindor KD, Dickson ER, editors. Clinics in Liver Disease, Vol. 2, No. 2. Primary Biliary Cirrhosis, Primary Sclerosing Cholangitis and Adult Cholangiopathies, Philadelphia: WB Saunders, 1998:249–64.
49. Tsuneyama K, Kono N, Yamashiro M et al. Aberrant expression of stem cell factor on biliary epithelial cells and peribiliary infiltration of c-kit-expressing mast cells in hepatolithiasis and primary sclerosing cholangitis: a possible contribution to bile duct fibrosis. J Pathol. 1999;189:609–14.
50. Fleming KA. Interlobular bile duct basement membrane thickening – a specific marker for primary sclerosing cholangitis (PSC)? J Pathol. 1993;169(Suppl.).

51. Casali AM, Carbone G, Cavalli G. Intrahepatic bile duct loss in primary sclerosing cholangitis: a quantitative study. Histopathology. 1998;32:449–53.
52. MacSween RNM, Burt AD, Haboubi NY. Unusual variant of primary sclerosing cholangitis. J Clin Pathol. 1987;40:541–5.
53. Bhathal PS, Powell LW. Primary intrahepatic obliterating cholangitis: a possible variant of sclerosing cholangitis. Gut. 1969;10:886–93.
54. Desmet VJ. Intrahepatic bile ducts under the lens. J Hepatol. 1985;1:545–59.
55. Van Eyken P, Desmet V. Immunohistology of primary sclerosing cholangitis. In: Meyer zum Büschenfelde KH, Hoofnagle J, Manns M, editors. Immunology and Liver. Lancaster: Kluwer, 1993:307–17.
56. Dienes HP, Lohse AW, Gerken G et al. Bile duct epithelia as target cells in primary biliary cirrhosis and primary sclerosing cholangitis. Virchows Archiv. 1997;431:119–24.
57. Broomé U, Olsson R, Lööf L et al. Natural history and prognostic factors in 305 Swedish patients with primary sclerosing cholangitis. Gut. 1996;38:610–15.
58. Wee A, Ludwig J, Coffey RJ, La Russo N, Wiesner R. Hepatobiliary carcinoma associated with primary sclerosing cholangitis and chronic ulcerative colitis. Human Pathol. 1985;16:719–26.
59. Fleming KA, Boberg KM, Glaumann H, Bergquist A, Smith D, Clausen OPF. Biliary dysplasia as a marker of cholangiocarcinoma in primary sclerosing cholangitis. J Hepatol. 2001;34:360–5.
60. Miros M, Kerlin P, Walker N, Harper J, Lynch S, Strong R. Predicting cholangiocarcinoma in patients with primary sclerosing cholangitis before transplantation. Gut. 1991;32:1369–73.
61. Wiesner RH, La Russo NF, Ludwig J, Dickson ER. Comparison of the clinicopathologic features of primary sclerosing cholangitis and primary biliary cirrhosis. Gastroenterology. 1985;88:108–14.
62. Farrant JM, Hayllar KM, Wilkinson ML et al. Natural history and prognostic variables in primary sclerosing cholangitis. Gastroenterology. 1991;100:1710–17.
63. Kim WR, Ludwig J, Lindor KD. Variant forms of cholestatic diseases involving small bile ducts in adults. Am J Gastroenterol. 2000;95:1130–8.
64. Roberts EA. Primary sclerosing cholangitis in children. J Gastroenterol Hepatol. 1999;14: 588–93.
65. Floreani A, Zancan L, Melis A, Baragiotta A, Chiaramonte M. Primary sclerosing cholangitis (PSC): clinical, laboratory and survival analysis in children and adults. Liver. 1999;19:228–33.
66. Feldstein AE, Perrault J, El-Youssif M, Lindor KD, Kreese DK, Angulo P. Primary sclerosing cholangitis in children: a long-term follow-up study. Hepatology. 2003;38:210–17.
67. Gregorio GV, Portmann B, Karani J et al. Autoimmune hepatitis/sclerosing cholangitis overlap syndrome in childhood: a 16-year prospective study. Hepatology. 2001;33:544–53.
68. Angulo P, Maor-Kendler Y, Donling JG, Lindor K. Small duct primary sclerosing cholangitis prevalence and natural history. Gastroenterology. 2000;120:A33.
69. Bjornsson E, Cullen S, Fleming K et al. Patients with small duct primary sclerosing cholangitis have a favourable long term prognosis. Hepatology. 2001;34:A733.
70. Broomé U, Glaumann H, Lindström E et al. Natural history and outcome in 32 Swedish patients with small duct primary sclerosing cholangitis (PSC). J Hepatol. 2002;36:586–9.
71. Chapman RW. Editorial. Small duct primary sclerosing cholangitis. J Hepatol. 2002;36:692–4.
72. Wee A, Ludwig J. Pericholangitis in chronic ulcerative colitis: primary sclerosing cholangitis of the small bile ducts? Ann Intern Med. 1985;102:581–7.

6
Mechanisms of biliary epithelial cell apoptosis in primary biliary cirrhosis

D. H. ADAMS and S. C. AFFORD

INTRODUCTION

Canaliculi between pairs of hepatocytes form the terminal branches of the biliary tree into which hepatocytes secrete bile. The canaliculi drain into intrahepatic bile ducts, true ductular structures formed by a distinct epithelial cell, the cholangiocyte. These intrahepatic bile ducts drain into larger segmental ducts and eventually form an interconnecting branching system which transports bile from the liver into the gut. The intrahepatic bile ducts are found in portal tracts between the liver lobules. Together with branches of the hepatic artery and the portal veins the intrahepatic bile ducts form the portal triad. The biliary system is continuous with the gastrointestinal tract and thus exposed to microbial agents in the gut lumen. It is thus critical that mechanisms are present to prevent ascending infection via the biliary system.

Protection is afforded by several mechanisms. The continuous bile flow discourages ascending infection by luminal bacteria[5] but, if microbial agents do gain access to the biliary epithelium, several mechanisms have evolved to limit the infection. The portal tracts contain elements required to generate both innate and cognate immune responses against invading pathogens including resident cytotoxic lymphocytes[6]. These bile duct-associated T cells display cytolytic activity, and can lyse intestinal epithelial cell lines, suggesting that they share characteristics with intestinal intraepithelial lymphocytes and are able to act as a first line of defence to antigens entering via the biliary tract. In addition cholangiocytes respond to inflammatory damage or exposure to microbial products by secreting cytokines and chemokines that stimulate an inflammatory response[7–9] including the recruitment of monocytes and lymphocytes[10,11]. Thus the epithelium itself plays a role in promoting the chronic inflammatory response that characterizes primary biliary cirrhosis (PBC).

The biliary epithelium can be infected by several pathogens, and although microbes rarely cause direct bile duct damage they may be contributing factors to bile duct loss[12–14]. If bile ducts are infected the immune system needs to be able to selectively kill infected cholangiocytes. The mechanisms involved in these processes are poorly understood, although there is evidence that, when they are deficient, as is the case in HIV infection or X-linked hyperIgM syndrome, cholangiocyte apoptosis is dysregulated and susceptibility to biliary infections increases[14–16]. In primary biliary cirrhosis the cholangiocytes are the targets for immune attack and significant cholangiocyte destruction compromises the integrity of the biliary system, leading to progressive cholestasis and a vicious irreversible cycle of inflammation and bile duct loss[17–21]. The progressive loss of bile ducts is associated with lymphocyte infiltration of the portal tracts and apoptosis of cholangiocytes (Figure 1)[22–27]. The liver responds to injury by undergoing a proliferative response leading to restoration of normal liver architecture and function, and antiproliferative mechanisms have evolved to limit this response and to prevent the development of a malignancy[28]. As a consequence both cholangiocytes and hepatocytes are highly sensitive to apoptotic death[29], including that mediated by effector leucocytes. This response is beneficial when it allows the immune system to rapidly clear infected epithelial cells, but when it is triggered inappropriately, or allowed to continue after clearance of the offending pathogen, it can result in irreversible inflammatory bile duct damage and loss[30].

TUMOUR NECROSIS FACTOR RECEPTOR (TNFr) SUPERFAMILY MEMBERS IN CHOLANGIOCYTE APOPTOSIS

Hepatocytes are intrinsically sensitive to apoptotic death mediated via activation of members of the TNFr superfamily particularly Fas (CD95)[31–34]. Fas is widely expressed on hepatocytes and up-regulated during inflammation[35] when direct activation of Fas leads to massive hepatocyte damage and fulminant liver failure[36]. More recent evidence suggests that cholangiocytes also up-regulate Fas in response to chronic inflammation and are also highly susceptible to Fas-mediated death[30]. The ability of Fas engagement to kill cells by apoptosis has led to the development of regulatory mechanisms by which Fas activation is controlled by other molecules, acting in a paracrine or autocrine fashion. Fas-mediated apoptosis can be amplified by activation of other TNFr family members, thereby providing a mechanism for controlling Fas-mediated responses[37]. One of the first examples of this mechanism was described in hepatocytes and involves the activation of another closely related member of the TNFr family, CD40[35]. We have now demonstrated a similar role for CD40 in cholangiocyte apoptosis in PBC[30] (Figures 2 and 3).

Activation of CD40 on the cell surface of cholangiocytes triggers autocrine Fas ligand (CD95L) up-regulation leading to autocrine and paracrine activation of Fas. The requirement for Fas in this model is demonstrated by the ability to block the effects of CD40 activation by neutralizing either Fas or FasL (Figure 4). Under basal conditions cholangiocytes express little CD40 in vivo, but expression is up-regulated in response to inflammation, and in-vitro CD40

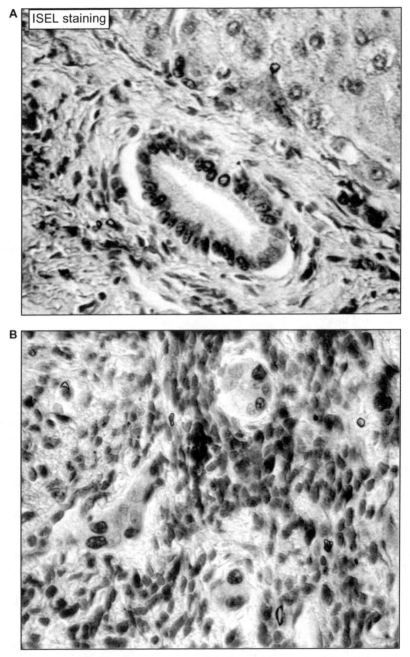

Figure 1 In normal non-inflamed liver the bile ducts show little evidence of cholangiocyte apoptosis; however, in PBC, bile ducts surrounded by an inflammatory infiltrate of CD3-positive T cells frequently contain cholangiocytes undergoing apoptosis revealed by *in situ* DNA end-labelling and nuclear morphology (panels **A** and **B**). Reproduced in part from reference 30 with permission

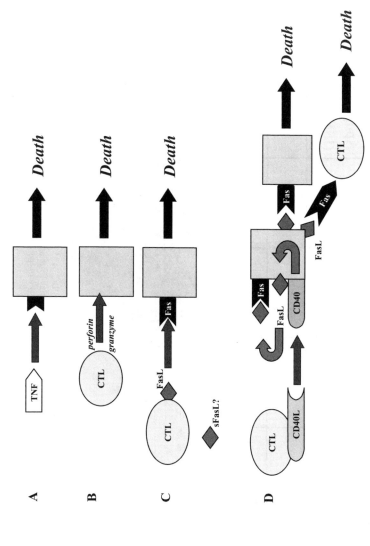

Figure 2 Cytotoxic T lymphocytes (CTL) can kill cholangiocytes via several pathways. **A**: Soluble factors including TNF-α may directly induce apoptosis. **B**: CTL can use granzymes and perforin pathways to directly trigger apoptosis in target cells. **C**: CTL express cell surface FasL which allows them to directly activate the death-inducing receptor Fas expressed on inflamed cholangiocytes; in addition soluble FasL may also be secreted and may also activate this pathway. **D**: CD40 on cholangiocytes can be activated by CD40L on CTL leading to autocrine expression of FasL and amplification of Fas-dependent apoptosis by autocrine and paracrine pathways. The expression of Fas on CTL may also allow FasL-expressing cholangiocytes to induce apoptosis in the effector T cells

A

	Bile ducts FAS	Bile ducts FasL	CTL Fas L	Bile ducts Apoptosis (ISEL)	CTL Apoptosis (ISEL)
Normal	+/−	−	−	−	−
PBC	+++	+	++	++	+/−

B

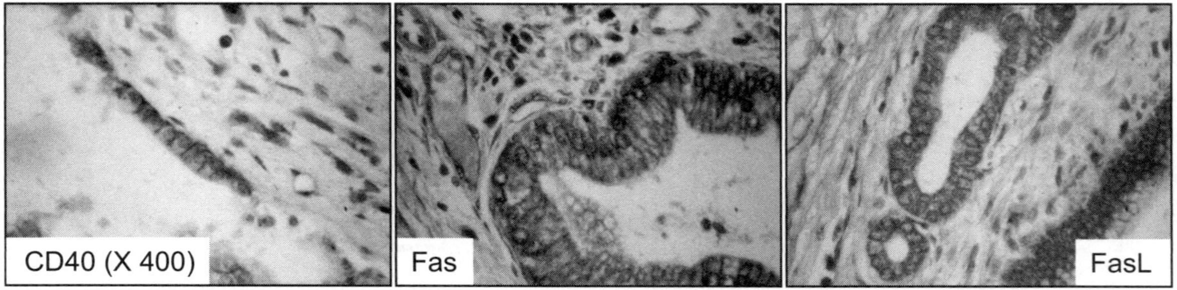

Figure 3 CD40, Fas and Fasl all increase on intrahepatic bile ducts in PBC. **A:** Semi-quantitative immunohistochemistry staining for Fas, FasL ligand and apoptosis (ISEL) on bile ducts and infiltrating effector lymphocytes in normal liver and PBC. **B:** Staining for CD40, Fas and FasL, confirming that the same ducts express all three molecules in PBC. Reproduced in part from reference 30 with permission

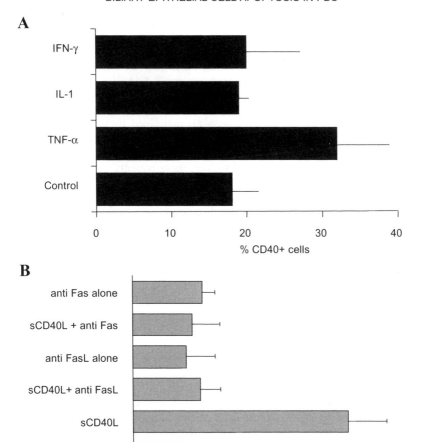

Figure 4 **A**: TNF-α increases CD40 expression on biliary epithelial cells in culture. **B**: Activation of CD40 on cholangiocytes with soluble CD40 ligand leads to a marked increase in apoptosis, which can be prevented by pretreatment with blocking antibodies against either Fas or FasL. Reproduced in part from reference 30 with permission

expression increases in response to cytokines including TNF-α[30] (Figures 3 and 4). *In vitro*, soluble CD40 ligand (CD40L, CD154, gp39) or crosslinking antibodies can both activate CD40-mediated Fas-dependent killing. In inflammatory liver diseases, including PBC, CD40L expression is increased at sites of active bile duct inflammation where it is restricted to macrophages and infiltrating effector lymphocytes. Thus activation of this amplification mechanism will occur only in the presence of a chronic inflammatory infiltrate. Since the reports of cooperative interactions between CD40 and Fas, studies in other models have shown that activation of other TNFr family members[37], including TNFR2, CD30 and CD40, can lead to apoptosis mediated via autocrine or paracrine activation of TNFR1. Our data suggest these mechanisms also apply to cholangiocytes.

There is compelling support for the importance of CD40-mediated Fas-dependent cell death in the liver. Genetic perturbations of the CD40/CD40L system have a number of liver-specific consequences. CD40L-deficient mice are unable to clear certain biliary infections, resulting in persistent cholangitis[16], and humans with the X-linked hyperIgM syndrome are also deficient in functional CD40L and display a similar phenotype characterized by a failure to clear cryptosporidial infections of the biliary tract. This ultimately leads to persistent chronic infection and a cholangiopathy with features similar to sclerosing cholangitis and cholangiocyte dysplasia predisposing these patients to the development of cholangiocarcinoma[14].

The consequences of CD40 activation in the inflammatory environment are likely to be more far-reaching than the destruction of cholangiocytes via Fas-mediated apoptosis. The CD40/CD40L system plays a pivotal role in modulating many facets of the inflammatory response, and overexpression of CD40 ligand leads to a massive inflammatory response[38–40]. Signals mediated via CD40 modulate a wide range of biological functions including stimulating adhesion molecule expression, chemokine secretion and extracellular matrix deposition, as well as the provision of costimulatory signals which promote T-cell/B-cell interactions and proliferation.

MECHANISMS OF CHOLANGIOCYTE APOPTOSIS

There are a number of ways in which cholangiocytes can be eliminated via apoptotic mechanisms, in addition to direct activation of cell surface Fas. TNF-α, which is produced by mononuclear cells and endothelial cells in the inflamed liver, can kill cholangiocytes directly[31], as well as by activating Fas and cytolytic T lymphocytes express perforin and potent apoptosis-inducing proteolytic enzymes called granzymes, which they inject into target cells, resulting in caspase activation and apoptosis. There is circumstantial evidence that this pathway is also involved in cholangiocyte apoptosis in PBC[41,42]. Although ursodeoxycholic acid (UDCA) is cytoprotective[43] other bile acids, particularly tauroursodeoxycholate (TDC) and glycochenodeoxycholate (GCDC), can induce apoptosis directly via several mechanisms[44]. Thus in PBC several mechanisms may contribute and amplify bile duct loss[45] (Figure 2).

WHAT DRIVES PERSISTENT INFLAMMATION AND BILE DUCT DAMAGE IN PBC?

The persistent expression of CD40L on infiltrating lymphocytes in PBC contrasts with *in-vitro* studies of T lymphocytes in which CD40L expression in response to activation is usually transient. Little is known concerning the regulation of CD40 ligand expression and the factors which may maintain its expression *in vivo*. It is likely that chronic inflammation alters the microenvironment in favour of persistent CD40L expression[70], and this process may involve the

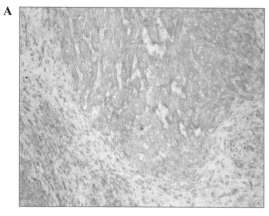

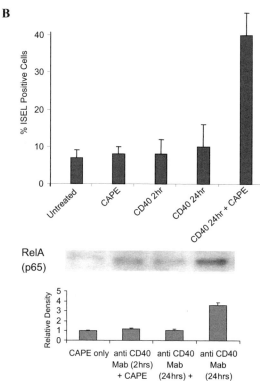

Figure 5 **A**: CD40 is also increased on sinusoidal endothelium in PBC; however, activation of CD40 on isolated human sinusoidal endothelial cells leads to endothelial cell proliferation and no increase in apoptosis unless NFκB is inhibited. **B**: Levels of apoptosis (ISEL) in the upper panel after treatment with CD40 ligand or the NFκB inhibitor caffeic acid (CAPE). In the absence of CAPE no increase in endothelial cells apoptosis is seen with CD40 activation, whereas levels of apoptosis similar to those seen in cholangiocytes are observed in NFκB activation and are prevented by pretreatment with CAPE. Reproduced in part from reference 78, used with permission

activation of specific signal transduction pathways and transcription factors including nuclear factor kappa B (NFκB)-dependent mechanisms and the novel AT hook transcription factor AKNA 1[71]. Persistent CD40L expression may be a critical factor in driving and sustaining chronic inflammation in PBC and providing the signal for effector cell amplification of target cell apoptosis[72]. In addition CD40 is up-regulated on endothelium in the inflamed liver but, in contrast to cholangiocytes, activation of CD40 on endothelium leads to increased adhesion molecule and chemokine expression and endothelial cell proliferation rather than apoptosis (Figure 5). We have recently reported that the different outcome of CD40 ligation on these cell types is a consequence of the relative activation of transcription factors, particularly NFκB and AP-1[78]. Thus in cholangiocytes CD40 ligation leads to transient NFκB activation followed by sustained AP-1 activation, whereas in endothelial cells NFκB activation is sustained in the face of minimal AP-1 activation (Figure 6). Furthermore, CD40/CD40L interactions are also likely to have direct effects on the infiltrating CD40L-bearing effector cells. Intracellular signalling via CD40L in T lymphocytes leads to JNK, p38 and lck activation, which are likely to have profound effects on cell survival and activation, although the downstream functional consequences of such pathways in the context of tissue leucocytes are not known[73].

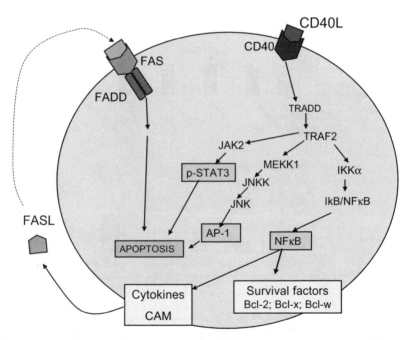

Figure 6 Intracellular signalling in response to CD40 activation will determine cellular fate. Activation of NFκB leads initially to an increase in FasL, but if sustained it leads to the expression of protective anti-apoptotic genes. Sustained NFκB activation is a feature of CD40 activation on endothelial cells, whereas activation of STAT-3 and AP-1 promotes apoptosis and this pathway dominates in cholangiocytes activated by CD40 engagement

CONCLUSIONS

Cholangiocytes are the target of immune-mediated attack in PBC and other biliary diseases. They contribute actively to local inflammation by secreting cytokines and chemokines capable of recruiting and localizing effector cells within portal tracts. In chronic inflammatory diseases of the bile ducts this results in the establishment of tertiary lymphoid structures and continuing leucocyte recruitment and retention within the liver. Bile duct loss in PBC involves Fas-dependent apoptosis, and this may be amplified by complex autocrine and paracrine interactions involving other members of the TNF receptor superfamily, particularly CD40 and its ligand. A better understanding of these processes may lead to novel therapeutic approaches aimed at switching off the chronic inflammatory response and protecting bile ducts from apoptosis.

Acknowledgements

The authors acknowledge support from clinical members of the Liver Unit at the Queen Elizabeth Hospital. Financial support for research cited in this chapter was received from the BBSRC, the Wellcome Trust, the MRC, the Sir Jules Thorn Trust and the Genetics Institute, Boston, USA.

References

1. Knolle PA, Gerken G. Local control of the immune response in the liver. Immunol Rev. 2000;174:21–34.
2. Seki S, Habu Y, Kawamura T et al. The liver as a crucial organ in the first line of host defense: the roles of Kupffer cells, natural killer (NK) cells and NK1.1 Ag+ T cells in T helper 1 immune responses. Immunol Rev. 2000;174:35–46.
3. Friedman SL. Molecular regulation of hepatic fibrosis, an integrated cellular response to tissue injury. J Biol Chem. 2000;275:2247.
4. Lalor PF, Adams DH. The liver: a model of organ-specific lymphocyte recruitment. Expert Rev Mol Med. 2002;2002:1–15.
5. Bjornsson ES, Kilander AF, Olsson RG. Bile duct bacterial isolates in primary sclerosing cholangitis and certain other forms of cholestasis – a study of bile cultures from ERCP. Hepatogastroenterology. 2000;47:1504.
6. Probert CS, Christ AD, Saubermann LJ et al. Analysis of human common bile duct-associated T cells: evidence for oligoclonality, T cell clonal persistence, and epithelial cell recognition. J Immunol. 1997;158:1941–8.
7. Morland CM, Fear J, McNab G, Joplin R, Adams DH. Promotion of leukocyte transendothelial cell migration by chemokines derived from human biliary epithelial cells *in vitro*. Proc Assoc Am Phys. 1997;109:372.
8. Goddard S, Williams A, Morland C et al. Differential expression of chemokines and chemokine receptors shapes the inflammatory response in rejecting human liver transplants. Transplantation. 2001;72:1957.
9. Shields PL, Morland CM, Salmon M, Qin S, Hubscher SG, Adams DH. Chemokine and chemokine receptor interactions provide a mechanism for selective T cell recruitment to specific liver compartments within hepatitis C-infected liver. J Immunol. 1999;163:6236.
10. Colletti LM, Green ME, Burdick MD, Strieter RM. The ratio of ELR+ to ELR− CXC chemokines affects the lung and liver injury following hepatic ischemia/reperfusion in the rat. Hepatology. 2000;31:435.
11. Wang H, Gao X, Fukumoto S, Tademoto S, Sato K, Hirai K. Differential expression and regulation of chemokines JE, KC, and IP-10 gene in primary cultured murine hepatocytes. J Cell Physiol. 1999;181:361.

12. Bach N, Thung SN, Schaffner F. The histological features of chronic hepatitis C and autoimmune chronic hepatitis: a comparative analysis. Hepatology. 1992;15:572.

13. Scheuer PJ, Ashrafzadeh P, Sherlock S, Brown D, Dusheiko GM. The pathology of hepatitis C. Hepatology. 1992;15:567.

14. Hayward AR, Levy J, Facchetti F et al. Cholangiopathy and tumors of the pancreas, liver and biliary tree in boys with X-linked immunodeficiency and hyper-IgM. J Immunol. 1997;158:977.

15. Lefkowitch JH. The liver in AIDS. Semin Liver Dis. 1997;17:335.

16. Stephens J, Cosyns M, Jones M, Hayward A. Liver and bile duct pathology following *Cryptosporidium parvum* infection of immunodeficient mice [In process citation]. Hepatology. 1999;30:27.

17. Harada K, Ozaki S, Gershwin ME, Nakanuma Y. Enhanced apoptosis relates to bile duct loss in primary biliary cirrhosis. Hepatology. 1997;27:1399.

18. Kaneko H, Oda M, Yokomori H et al. Immunohistochemical microscopic analysis of bile-duct destruction in primary biliary-cirrhosis – involvement of intercellular-adhesion molecules. Int Hepatol Commun. 1994;2:271.

19. Kim WR, Ludwig J, Lindor KD. Variant forms of cholestatic diseases involving small bile ducts in adults. Am J Gastroenterol. 2000;95:1130.

20. Tjandra K, Sharkey KA, Swain MG. Progressive development of a Th1-type hepatic cytokine profile in rats with experimental cholangitis. Hepatology. 2000;31:280.

21. Sherlock S. The syndrome of disappearing intrahepatic bile ducts. Lancet. 1987;2:493.

22. Sherlock S. Primary biliary cirrhosis, primary sclerosing cholangitis, and autoimmune cholangitis. Clin Liver Dis. 2000;4:97.

23. Scheuer PJ. Ludwig Symposium on biliary disorders – part II. Pathologic features and evolution of primary biliary cirrhosis and primary sclerosing cholangitis. Mayo Clin Proc. 1998;73:179.

24. Dienes HP, Lohse AW, Gerken G et al. Bile duct epithelia as target cells in primary biliary cirrhosis and primary sclerosing cholangitis. Virchows Arch. 1997;431:119.

25. Joplin R, Gershwin ME. Ductular expression of autoantigens in primary biliary cirrhosis. Semin Liver Dis. 1997;17:97.

26. Kita H, Mackay IR, Van de Water J, Gershwin ME. The lymphoid liver: considerations on pathways to autoimmune injury. Gastroenterology. 2001;120:1485.

27. Leon MP, Bassendine MF, Wilson JL, Ali S, Thick M, Kirby JA. Immunogenicity of biliary epithelium: investigation of antigen presentation to CD4+ T cells. Hepatology. 1996;24:561.

28. Fausto N. Liver regeneration. J Hepatol. 2000;32:19.

29. Patel T, Steer CJ, Gores GJ. Apoptosis and the liver: a mechanism of disease, growth regulation, and carcinogenesis. Hepatology. 1999;30:811.

30. Afford SC, Ahmed-Choudhury J, Randhawa S et al. CD40 activation-induced, Fas-dependent apoptosis and NF-kappaB/AP-1 signaling in human intrahepatic biliary epithelial cells. FASEB J. 2001;15:2345–54.

31. Bradham CA, Plumpe J, Manns MP, Brenner DA, Trautwein C. Mechanisms of hepatic toxicity. I. TNF-induced liver injury. Am J Physiol. 1998;275:G387.

32. Galle PR, Hofmann WJ, Walczak H et al. Involvement of the CD95 (APO-1/Fas) receptor and ligand in liver damage. J Exp Med. 1995;182:1223.

33. Leist M, Gantner F, Kunstle G et al. The 55-kD tumor necrosis factor receptor and CD95 independently signal murine hepatocyte apoptosis and subsequent liver failure. Mol Med. 1996; 2:109–24.

34. Strand S, Hofmann WJ, Grambihler A et al. Hepatic failure and liver cell damage in acute Wilson's disease involve CD95 (APO-1/Fas) mediated apoptosis. Nat Med. 1998;4:588.

35. Afford SC, Rhandawa S, Eliopoulos AG, Hubscher SG, Young LS, Adams DH. CD40 activation induces apoptosis in cultured human hepatocytes via induction of cell surface FasL expression and amplifies Fas mediated hepatocyte death during allograft rejection. J Exp Med. 1999; 189:441–6.

36. Ogasawara J, Watanabe-Fukunaga R, Adachi M et al. Lethal effect of the anti-Fas antibody in mice [published erratum appears in Nature. 1993;365:568]. Nature. 1993;364:806.

37. Grell M, Zimmermann G, Gottfried E et al. Induction of cell death by tumour necrosis factor (TNF) receptor 2, CD40 and CD30: a role for TNF-R1 activation by endogenous membrane-anchored TNF. EMBO J. 1999;18:3034.

38. Mehling A, Loser K, Varga G et al. Overexpression of CD40 ligand in murine epidermis results in chronic skin inflammation and systemic autoimmunity. J Exp Med. 2001;194:615–28.
39. Van Kooten C. Immune regulation by CD40-CD40-l interactions – 2; Y2K update. Front Biosci. 2000;5:D880–693.
40. Henn V, Slupsky JR, Grafe M et al. CD40 ligand on activated platelets triggers an inflammatory reaction of endothelial cells. Nature. 1998;391:591.
41. Harada K, Ozaki S, Gershwin ME, Nakanuma Y. Enhanced apoptosis relates to bile duct loss in primary biliary cirrhosis. Hepatology. 1997;26:1399.
42. Balkow S, Kersten A, Tran TT et al. Concerted action of the FasL/Fas and perforin/granzyme A and B pathways is mandatory for the development of early viral hepatitis but not for recovery from viral infection. J Virol. 2001;75:8781–91.
43. Colell A, Coll O, Garcia-Ruiz C et al. Tauroursodeoxycholic acid protects hepatocytes from ethanol-fed rats against tumor necrosis factor-induced cell death by replenishing mitochondrial glutathione. Hepatology. 2001;34:964–71.
44. Higuchi H, Bronk SF, Takikawa Y et al. The bile acid glycochenodeoxycholate induces trail-receptor 2/DR5 expression and apoptosis. J Biol Chem. 2001;276:38610.
45. Jaeschke H, Gores GJ, Cederbaum AI, Hinson JA, Pessayre D, Lemasters JJ. Mechanisms of hepatotoxicity. Toxicol Sci. 2002;65:166–76.
46. Adams DH, Hubscher SG, Shaw J et al. Increased expression of ICAM-1 on bile ducts in primary biliary cirrhosis and primary sclerosing cholangitis. Hepatology. 1991;14:426.
47. Ayres R, Neuberger JM, Shaw J, Adams DH. Intercellular adhesion molecule-1 and MHC antigens on human intrahepatic bile duct cells: effect of pro-inflammatory cytokines. Gut. 1993;34:1245.
48. Leon MP, Bassendine MF, Gibbs P, Thick M, Kirby JA. Immunogenicity of biliary epithelium: study of the adhesive interaction with lymphocytes. Gastroenterology. 1997;112:968.
49. Frasca L, Marelli-Berg F, Imami N et al. Interferon-gamma-treated renal tubular epithelial cells induce allospecific tolerance. Kidney Int. 1998;53:679.
50. Marelli-Berg FM, Weetman A, Frasca L et al. Antigen presentation by epithelial cells induces anergic immunoregulatory CD45RO+ T cells and deletion of CD45RA+ T cells. J Immunol. 1997;159:5853.
51. Desmet VJ, Gerber M, Hoofnagle JH, Manns M, Scheuer PJ. Classification of chronic hepatitis: diagnosis, grading and staging. Hepatology. 1994;19:1513.
52. Hjelmstrom P, Fjell J, Nakagawa T, Sacca R, Cuff CA, Ruddle NH. Lymphoid tissue homing chemokines are expressed in chronic inflammation. Am J Pathol. 2000;156:1133–8.
53. Kratz A, Campos-Neto A, Hanson MS, Ruddle NH. Chronic inflammation caused by lympho-toxin is lymphoid neogenesis. J Exp Med. 1996;183:1461.
54. Ruddle NH. Lymphoid neo-organogenesis: lymphotoxin's role in inflammation and development. Immunol Res. 1999;19:119.
55. Grant AJ, Goddard S, Ahmed-Choudhury J et al. Hepatic expression of secondary lymphoid chemokine (CCL21) promotes the development of portal-associated lymphoid tissue in chronic inflammatory liver disease. Am J Pathol. 2002;33:288–91.
56. Grant AJ, Lalor P, Hubscher SG, Briskin M, Adams DH. MAdCAM-1 expression is increased in primary sclerosing cholangitis and supports lymphocyte adhesion to hepatic endothelium: a mechanism to explain the recruitment of mucosal lymphocytes to the liver in inflammatory liver disease. Hepatology. 2001;33:1065–72.
57. Murakami J, Shimizu Y, Kashii Y et al. Functional B-cell response in intrahepatic lymphoid follicles in chronic hepatitis C. Hepatology. 1999;30:143.
58. Freemont AJ. Functional and biosynthetic changes in endothelial cells of vessels in chronically inflamed tissues: evidence for endothelial control of lymphocyte entry into diseased tissues. J Pathol. 1988;155:225.
59. Buckley CD, Amft N, Bradfield PF et al. Persistent induction of the chemokine receptor CXCR4 by TGF-beta 1 on synovial T cells contributes to their accumulation within the rheumatoid synovium. J Immunol. 2000;165:3423.
60. Hjelmstrom P. Lymphoid neogenesis: de novo formation of lymphoid tissue in chronic inflammation through expression of homing chemokines. J Leukoc Biol. 2001;69:331.
61. Rappaport AM, MacPhee PJ, Fisher MM, Phillips MJ. The scarring of the liver acini (cirrhosis). Tridimensional and microcirculatory considerations. Virchows Arch A Pathol Anat Histopathol. 1983;402:107.

62. Gunn MD, Tangemann K, Tam C, Cyster JG, Rosen SD, Williams LT. A chemokine expressed in lymphoid high endothelial venules promotes the adhesion and chemotaxis of naive T lymphocytes. Proc Natl Acad Sci U S A. 1998;95:258.

63. Cyster JG. Chemokines and the homing of dendritic cells to the T cell areas of lymphoid organs [comment]. J Exp Med. 1999;189:447.

64. Sallusto F, Lenig D, Forster R, Lipp M, Lanzavecchia A. Two subsets of memory T lymphocytes with distinct homing potentials and effector functions [see comments]. Nature. 1999;401:708.

65. Fan L, Reilly CR, Luo Y, Dorf ME, Lo D. Cutting edge: ectopic expression of the chemokine TCA4/SLC is sufficient to trigger lymphoid neogenesis. J Immunol. 2000;164:3955–9.

66. Vassileva G, Soto H, Zlotnik A et al. The reduced expression of 6Ckine in the plt mouse results from the deletion of one of two 6Ckine genes. J Exp Med. 1999;190:1183.

67. Briskin M, Winsor-Hines D, Shyjan A et al. Human mucosal addressin cell adhesion molecule-1 is preferentially expressed in intestinal tract and associated lymphoid tissue. Am J Pathol. 1997;151:97.

68. Farstad IN, Halstensen TS, Kvale D, Fausa O, Brandtzaeg P. Topographic distribution of homing receptors on B and T cells in human gut-associated lymphoid tissue: relation of L-selectin and integrin alpha 4 beta 7 to naive and memory phenotypes. Am J Pathol. 1997;150:187.

69. Hillan KJ, Hagler KE, MacSween RN et al. Expression of the mucosal vascular addressin, MAdCAM-1, in inflammatory liver disease. Liver. 1999;19:509.

70. Murakami K, Ma W, Fuleihan R, Pober JS. Human endothelial cells augment early CD40 ligand expression in activated CD4+ T cells through LFA-3-mediated stabilization of mRNA. J Immunol. 1999;163:2667.

71. Siddiqa A, Sims-Mourtada JC, Guzman-Rojas L et al. Regulation of CD40 and CD40 ligand by the AT-hook transcription factor AKNA. Nature. 2001;410:383–7.

72. Buckley CD, Pilling D, Lord JM, Akbar AN, Scheel-Toellner D, Salmon M. Fibroblasts regulate the switch from acute resolving to chronic persistent inflammation. Trends Immunol. 2001; 22:199.

73. Brenner B, Koppenhoefer U, Grassme H, Kun J, Lang F, Gulbins E. Evidence for a novel function of the CD40 ligand as a signalling molecule in T-lymphocytes. FEBS Lett. 1997;417:301.

74. Taylor PC, Williams RO, Maini RN. Immunotherapy for rheumatoid arthritis. Curr Opin Immunol. 2001;13:611.

75. Feldmann M, Maini RN. Anti-TNF alpha therapy of rheumatoid arthritis: what have we learned? Annu Rev Immunol. 2001;19:163.

76. Graca L, Honey K, Adams E, Cobbold SP, Waldmann H. Cutting edge: anti-CD154 therapeutic antibodies induce infectious transplantation tolerance [In process citation]. J Immunol. 2000; 165:4783.

77. Harlan DM, Kirk AD. The future of organ and tissue transplantation: can T-cell costimulatory pathway modifiers revolutionize the prevention of graft rejection? J Am Med Assoc. 1999; 282:1076.

78. Ahmed-Choudhury J, Russell CL, Randhawa S, Young LS, Adams DH, Afford SC. Differential induction of NF-κB and AP-1 activity following CD40 ligation is associated with primary human hepatocyte apoptosis or intrahepatic endothelial cell proliferation. Mol Biol Cell. 2003;14:1334–45.

7
Role of autoantibodies and autoantigens in primary biliary cirrhosis

C. P. STRASSBURG

INTRODUCTION

Primary biliary cirrhosis (PBC) is a chronic inflammatory, cholestatic disease of the liver with an unknown cause. The clinical observation of a broad array of immune-mediated symptoms and phenomena suggests the disease to be of autoimmune aetiology, in the course of which small interlobular and septal bile ducts are progressively and irreversibly destroyed[1]. As in other autoimmune diseases, PBC affects women in over 90% of cases, and is associated with varying extrahepatic autoimmune syndromes occurring in up to 84%. These extrahepatic manifestations of immune-mediated disease include the dry gland syndrome (sicca syndrome with xerophthalmia and xerostomia) but also collagen diseases, autoimmune thyroid disease, glomerulonephritis and ulcerative colitis.

The detection of circulating antimitochondrial antibodies (AMA) is the single most important serological test for the diagnosis of PBC, in particular when clinical serological and histological signs of cholestatic disease and evidence of bile duct destruction are not yet present[2]. Specific AMA are detectable in over 95% of patients with PBC, and are yet another indicator of autoimmune mechanisms underlying this condition[3,4]. In 20–50% of patients suffering from PBC, antinuclear antibodies (ANA) are also detectable, and contribute to the definition of this disease[2,5–7]. Although none of these autoantibodies is tissue-, organ- or species-specific, AMA are highly disease-specific. Frequently, in particular in early disease, a clinical suspicion or the establishment of the diagnosis of PBC is based upon the detection of specific AMA as a single finding. Intense effort has been aimed at characterizing the molecular targets of PBC-associated AMA in order to improve and develop disease-specific serological test strategies[8].

AMA IN PBC

PBC-specific autoantibodies are directed against the ketoacid dehydrogenase complex (OADC). The OADC consists of three major antigens: pyruvate dehydrogenase (PDH), branched-chain ketoacid dehydrogenase (BCKD), and ketoglutarate dehydrogenase (OGD)[3,8,9]. Every enzyme in itself consists of three subunits with individual enzymatic activities: E1 (decarboxylase), E2 (dihydro lipoamide acyltransferase), and E3 (lipoamide dehydrogenase).

In 95% of all North American and European sera, and 65% of all Japanese PBC sera, AMA are directed against the E2 subunit of PDH (PDH-E2). PDH-E2 represents the 74 kDa autoantigen identified first as part of the M2 antigen fraction. AMA mainly belong to the IgM class of immunoglobulins, but IgA, IgG1 and IgG3 class autoantibodies are also regularly detected. The further analysis of PBC sera has demonstrated that 53–55% are reactive with the E2 subunit of BCKD (BCKD-E2), which corresponds to the earlier-identified 52 kDa antigen of M2. In addition, 39–88% of PBC sera display autoantibodies directed against the E2 unit of OGD (OGD-E2), corresponding to the 48 kDa component of M2. Reactivity of these three major subspecies of PBC-specific AMA has a number of common features: immunoreactivity favours epitopes on the E2 subunit in all three cases, the recognized epitopes are of considerable sizes and are conformation-dependent, and they are localized within the lipoyl domain of the molecules. Epitopes have been characterized for PDH-E2 (93 amino acids)[3,10], BCKD-E2 (227 amino acids)[11], and OGD-E2 (81 amino acids)[12]. Autoantibodies against PDH-E2 occur together with anti-BCKD-E2 in 60% of cases. In about 10–20% of PBC patients anti-BCKD-E2 autoantibodies are detected alone, the significance of which is not clear. It remains undisputed that autoantibodies against PDH-E2 are among the most interesting immunological features of PBC characterizing the B-cell response in this disease.

CHARACTERIZATION OF AUTOREACTIVE B-CELL RESPONSES

Numerous studies have been undertaken to elucidate the epitope reactivity of AMA against the major PBC-associated autoantigens[13]. These studies have revealed that all of the identified major epitopes reside in the lipoyl domains of the proteins and involve large amino acid portions, indicating conformation-dependent epitopes. These studies have involved PDH-E2, E3-binding protein, BCKD-E2 and OGD-E2. Knowledge of the dominant B-cell epitopes is designed to identify candidate regions which may also be of significance for T-cell immunoreactivity and may provide insight into the crossreactivity, and thus the aetiology, of the immune response observed in PBC. We have recently focused on the BCKD-E2 protein because a number of PBC sera display exclusive reactivity with this protein[14]. Truncation experiments of *in-vitro*-translated protein have been designed to avoid the problems of Western blot analysis, which leads to the linearization of target proteins and therefore limits the analysis of conformation-dependent epitope reactivity. Full-length protein was capable of binding all BCKD-E2-positive PBC sera, which dropped to 0% when only the first 63 amino acids (aa) of the protein were analysed. As expected, 85% reactivity was reached when aa 1–142 were employed, which span the entire lipoyl domain. However, a non-lipoyl domain fragment located between aa 143 and 421 was capable of binding to 59% of BCKD-E2 sera, indicating that a major non-lipoyl domain-dependent epitope is recognized in PBC patients[14]. Applied to patient sera there were no differences between lipoyl and non-lipoyl domain reactive sera with respect to requirement of liver transplantation. However, a subgroup of seven patients with an overlap syndrome with autoimmune hepatitis showed a preferential inhibition of the N-terminal aa 1–144 peptide (6/7) while only one of six reacted with the non-lipoyl domain aa 143–421 peptide. Interestingly 11% of the tested sera exclusively reacted with the full-length mature protein, indicating that additional larger epitopes are likely to exist.

B-CELL EPITOPES AND T-CELL REACTIVITY IN PBC

When PBC biopsies are assessed it is obvious that an intense cellular reaction is present in the portal tracts and is focused on the bile ducts. To establish a relationship with humoral autoimmunity peptide specificities of the PDH-E2 antigen were studied, leading to the identification of autoreactive CD4$^+$ clones proliferating in response to an aa motif located between 163 and 176, as well as aa 36–49[15,16]. With respect to the OGDH-E2 molecule a CD4$^+$ cell motif was identified between aa 100 and 113. When these motifs are aligned a common aa sequence of ExETDK is found. The analysis of T-cell precursor frequencies showed a 100-fold higher incidence in the liver and regional lymph nodes of PBC patients as compared to peripheral blood. They were also lower in more advanced stages of PBC and absent in primary sclerosing cholangitis (PSC). Interestingly, the B-cell epitopes on PDH-E2 map to a similar region between aa 164–183 and aa 38–57, demonstrating an overlap of B- and CD4$^+$ T-cell epitopes.

Similarly CD8$^+$ cells are a prominent feature of the cellular infiltrate observed in the liver biopsies of PBC patients. A recent analysis identified a CD8$^+$ cell epitope between aa 159 and 167 (KLSEGDLLA)[17]. These cell clones responded to stimulation with full-length PDH-E2, and PDH-E2 complexed with purified AMA from PBC patients as well as with monoclonal antibody[18]. As seen for CD4$^+$ cells, aa 159–167 peptide-stimulated precursor frequencies were 10-fold higher in PBC livers and in early stages of PBC. Combined these data show that autoantibody epitopes align with both CD4$^+$ and CD8$^+$ cell epitopes and share a common peptide motif ExETDK, which is also shared to some extent with PDH-E2 of *Escherichia coli* (ExDK). This points to a favoured hypothesis of mimicry in the pathogenesis of PBC.

Taken together epitope analyses show a defined B-cell response and a PDH-E2 driven cellular response in the liver involving presentation by antigen-presenting cells and dendritic cells aimed at the biliary epithelium (Figure 1). The antigen recognition shows a remarkable overlap in this process.

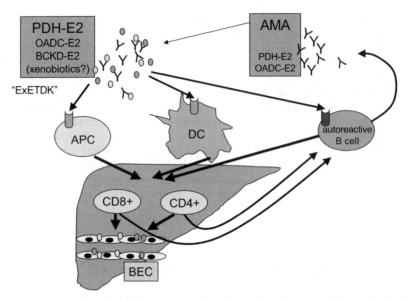

Figure 1 Graphic representation of a model of the immune attack on the biliary epithelium in primary biliary cirrhosis based on B-cell and T-cell data discussed in the text. In this model B- and T-cells act synergistically to produce biliary damage. A role of the diagnostic AMA found in PBC patients to be specifically directed against PDH-E2 or crossreactive antigens is suggested also for the pathogenesis of the disease. APC, antigen presenting cells; DC, dendritic cells; BEC, biliary epithelial cells

PDH-E2 ANTIGEN AND THE BILIARY EPITHELIAL CELL

Expression of PDH-E2 or crossreactive antigens on biliary epithelial cells (BEC) is therefore the logical next question in the understanding of the autoimmune process underlying PBC. Expression of PDH-E2 has been documented in BEC in several studies, and also in livers of patients after liver transplantation with recurrent disease[19–21]. In addition AMA, as well as PDH-E2, BCKD-E2 and OADC-E2, have been detected in the bile as well as in urine[22,23], which may indicate a mucosa-driven expression and secretion of these antigens, or their internalization as immune complexes. Studies with monoclonal antibodies have been able to stain BEC of PBC patients but not of normal controls[24,25]. In addition, since these mAb recognize different epitopes as natural AMA, but still stain a protein present in BEC, this may in fact be full-length PDH-E2, or a highly crossreactive molecule. The potential reasons for PDH-E2 expression in BEC may be the result of an increased protein synthesis or decreased degradation, differential subcellular targeting in PBC, novel molecules such as xenobiotics or adducts of these, or they may represent internalized immune complexes of AMA and PDH-E2 (or crosseactive) antigen.

A number of data point to an important role of immune complexes. When cytotoxic T-cell clones are stimulated this is achieved more efficiently with PDH-E2 immune complexes at 10-fold lower antigen concentrations[17]. From the point of view of interplay of B- and T-cell immunology this is an important observation because it establishes a role for autoantibodies to participate in the immune attack on the BEC. In this process internalization of complexes may ensue. It also raises the question of whether autoreactive B cells may function as antigen-presenting cells, which has been shown in other models of autoimmunity. These data close the link between B-cell autoreactivity and T-cell reactivity, aberrant expression of the target antigen and the histologically evident pathology in PBC livers. Stimulation of autoreactivity may thus enfold via three avenues involving immune complexes which activate antigen-presenting cells, dendritic cells and B cells functioning as antigen-presenting cells. AMA may therefore not only represent epiphenomena useful for the serological diagnosis of PBC, but may represent decisive players in the immune attack on the bile duct.

ANA AND PBC

In PBC sera the detection of ANA is a common finding, present in up to 50% of patients. Although ANA are found in a wide variety of diseases, including autoimmune hepatitis and rheumatological conditions, their specificity for certain autoantigens is striking in PBC. Antigens of the nuclear pore complex have emerged as secondary antigens in the serological diagnosis PBC[26,27]. Well characterized are autoantibodies against a 210 kDa glycoprotein of the nuclear membrane (gp210)[7,28] which are highly PBC-specific and occur in 10–47% of patients[29]. Nucleoporin p62 is targeted in 32% of PBC sera and also appears to be disease-specific[30]. In about 20% autoantibodies are detected against Sp100, a nucleoprotein of 100 kDa molecular weight[31,32]. Sp100 appears to exhibit a high specificity for PBC and has also been found to persist after orthotopic liver transplantation for PBC[33]. One study identified cyclin A as human autoantigen in hepatic and extrahepatic diseases[34]. Anti-cyclin A autoantibodies were detected in 7% of patients with PBC and more frequently in autoimmune hepatitis type 1. Other ANA with specificity for PBC include the lamin B receptor[35] and promyelocytic leukaemia-associated protein PML[36]. For most of these autoantigens the epitopes have been characterized and reported[37].

Although they occur in PBC, ANA show no crossreactivity with AMA. For gp210 the B-cell epitope is located between aa 1869 and 1883, and the CD4$^+$ cell epitope resides between aa 188 and 201. In a recent study the possibility of cellular mimicry between ANA and AMA was tested by generating CD4$^+$ cell clones selected by aa 163–176 peptide from PDH-E2[38]. Pulsing with LBR, p62 and centromere protein 62 led to no activation; however, Sp100 and gp210 peptides elicited the proliferation of PDH-E2-selected CD4$^+$ clones. This suggests mimicry initiation which goes beyond the identification of similar epitope motifs. Interestingly, in the same study, CD4$^+$ cell clones were identified which were stimulated with OGDC-E2, E3 binding protein as well as with BCKD-E2, despite initial selection with PDH-E2. One such clone proliferated in response to a peptide located within the non-lipoyl domain of BCKD-E2 which was recently identified by B-cell epitope mapping[14] (see above). These data suggest that crossreactivity of T-cell responses, as well as B-cell responses, may go beyond the similarities present at the amino acid sequence level, and may not be easily testable by classical peptide stimulation experiments.

CONCLUSION

AMA are a hallmark of PBC and are disease-specific when reactive with PDH-E2, OADC-E2 and BCKD-E2. They do not correlate with disease severity, course of disease, progression, or recurrence after liver transplantation. Beyond their diagnostic role in the establishment of the diagnosis of PBC they appear to have a pathophysiological role in the immune attack on the BEC. B- and T-cell epitopes on the PDH-E2 molecule map to similar regions. Via immune complexes and a potential role of B cells as antigen-presenting cells B and T cells appear to operate synergistically in the autoimmune process underlying PBC. In addition, crossreactivity of T cells is demonstrable between nuclear and mitochondrial antigens, for which there is no overlap of autoantibody epitope binding or sequence similarity. The future will show whether mimicry[20], or novel molecules such as xenobiotics[39,40], or infection[40] is the missing link which represents the driving force of the elucidated cell reactivities.

References

1. Strassburg CP, Manns MP. Autoimmune tests in primary biliary cirrhosis. Baillieres Best Pract Res Clin Gastroenterol. 2000;14:585–99.
2. Strassburg CP, Jaeckel E, Manns MP. Anti-mitochondrial antibodies and other immunological tests in primary biliary cirrhosis. Eur J Gastroenterol Hepatol. 1999;11:595–601.
3. Gershwin ME, Mackay IR. Primary biliary cirrhosis: paradigm or paradox for autoimmunity. Gastroenterology. 1991;100:822–33.
4. Gershwin ME, Coppel RL, Mackay IR. Primary biliary cirrhosis and mitochondrial autoantigens – insights from molecular biology. Hepatology. 1988;8:147–51.
5. Zuchner D, Sternsdorf T, Szostecki C, Heathcote EJ, Cauch-Dudek K, Will H. Prevalence, kinetics, and therapeutic modulation of autoantibodies against Sp100 and promyelocytic leukemia protein in a large cohort of patients with primary biliary cirrhosis. Hepatology. 1997;26: 1123–30.
6. Kurki P, Gripenberg M, Teppo AM, Salaspuro M. Profiles of antinuclear antibodies in chronic active hepatitis, primary biliary cirrhosis and alcoholic liver disease. Liver. 1984;4:134–8.
7. Lassoued K, Brenard R, Degos F et al. Antinuclear antibodies directed to a 200-kilodalton polypeptide of the nuclear envelope in primary biliary cirrhosis. A clinical and immunological study of a series of 150 patients with primary biliary cirrhosis. Gastroenterology. 1990;99: 181–6.
8. Van de Water J, Surh CD, Leung PS et al. Molecular definitions, autoepitopes, and enzymatic activities of the mitochondrial autoantigens of primary biliary cirrhosis. Semin Liver Dis. 1989; 9:132–7.
9. Gershwin ME, Rowley M, Davis PA, Leung P, Coppel R, Mackay IR. Molecular biology of the 2-oxo-acid dehydrogenase complexes and anti-mitochondrial antibodies. Prog Liver Dis. 1992; 10:47–61.
10. Van de Water J, Gershwin ME, Leung P, Ansari A, Coppel RL. The autoepitope of the 74-kD mitochondrial autoantigen of primary biliary cirrhosis corresponds to the functional site of dihydrolipoamide acetyltransferase. J Exp Med. 1988;167:1791–9.
11. Leung PS, Chuang DT, Wynn RM et al. Autoantibodies to BCOADC-E2 in patients with primary biliary cirrhosis recognize a conformational epitope. Hepatology. 1995;22:505–13.
12. Moteki S, Leung PS, Dickson ER et al. Epitope mapping and reactivity of autoantibodies to the E2 component of 2-oxoglutarate dehydrogenase complex in primary biliary cirrhosis using recombinant 2-oxoglutarate dehydrogenase complex. Hepatology. 1996;23:436–44.
13. Nishio A, Keeffe EB, Gershwin ME. Immunopathogenesis of primary biliary cirrhosis. Semin Liver Dis. 2002;22:291–302.
14. Csepregi A, Obermayer-Straub P, Kneip S et al. Characterization of a lipoyl domain-independent B-cell autoepitope on the human branched-chain acyltransferase in primary biliary cirrhosis and overlap syndrome with autoimmune hepatitis. Clin Dev Immunol. 2003;10:173–81.

15. Shimoda S, Van de Water J, Ansari A et al. Identification and precursor frequency analysis of a common T cell epitope motif in mitochondrial autoantigens in primary biliary cirrhosis. J Clin Invest. 1998;102:1831–40.
16. Shimoda S, Nakamura M, Shigematsu H et al. Mimicry peptides of human PDC-E2 163–176 peptide, the immunodominant T-cell epitope of primary biliary cirrhosis. Hepatology. 2000; 31:1212–16.
17. Kita H, Lian ZX, Van de Water J et al. Identification of HLA-A2-restricted CD8(+) cytotoxic T cell responses in primary biliary cirrhosis: T cell activation is augmented by immune complexes cross-presented by dendritic cells. J Exp Med. 2002;195:113–23.
18. Kita H, Matsumura S, He XS et al. Quantitative and functional analysis of PDC-E2-specific autoreactive cytotoxic T lymphocytes in primary biliary cirrhosis. J Clin Invest. 2002;109: 1231–40.
19. Joplin R, Gershwin ME. Ductular expression of autoantigens in primary biliary cirrhosis. Semin Liver Dis. 1997;17:97–103.
20. Van de Water J, Ishibashi H, Coppel RL, Gershwin ME. Molecular mimicry and primary biliary cirrhosis: premises not promises. Hepatology. 2001;33:771–5.
21. Joplin R, Wallace LL, Johnson GD et al. Subcellular localization of pyruvate dehydrogenase dihydrolipoamide acetyltransferase in human intrahepatic biliary epithelial cells. J Pathol. 1995; 176:381–90.
22. Nishio A, Van de Water J, Leung PS et al. Comparative studies of antimitochondrial autoantibodies in sera and bile in primary biliary cirrhosis. Hepatology. 1997;25:1085–9.
23. Tanaka A, Nalbandian G, Leung PS et al. Mucosal immunity and primary biliary cirrhosis: presence of antimitochondrial antibodies in urine. Hepatology. 2000;32:910–15.
24. Fukushima N, Nalbandian G, Van De Water J et al. Characterization of recombinant monoclonal IgA anti-PDC-E2 autoantibodies derived from patients with PBC. Hepatology. 2002;36:1383–92.
25. Migliaccio C, Nishio A, Van de Water J et al. Monoclonal antibodies to mitochondrial E2 components define autoepitopes in primary biliary cirrhosis. J Immunol. 1998;161:5157–63.
26. Bloch DB, Chiche JD, Orth D, de la Monte SM, Rosenzweig A, Bloch KD. Structural and functional heterogeneity of nuclear bodies. Mol Cell Biol. 1999;19:4423–30.
27. Worman HJ. Primary biliary cirrhosis and the molecular cell biology of the nuclear envelope. Mt Sinai J Med. 1994;61:461–75.
28. Nickowitz RE, Wozniak RW, Schaffner F, Worman HJ. Autoantibodies against integral membrane proteins of the nuclear envelope in patients with primary biliary cirrhosis. Gastroenterology. 1994;106:193–9.
29. Bandin O, Courvalin JC, Poupon R, Dubel L, Homberg JC, Johanet C. Specificity and sensitivity of gp210 autoantibodies detected using an enzyme-linked immunosorbent assay and a synthetic polypeptide in the diagnosis of primary biliary cirrhosis. Hepatology. 1996;23:1020–4.
30. Wesierska-Gadek J, Hohenuer H, Hitchman E, Penner E. Autoantibodies against nucleoporin p62 constitute a novel marker of primary biliary cirrhosis. Gastroenterology. 1996;110:840–7.
31. Szostecki C, Krippner H, Penner E, Bautz FA. Autoimmune sera recognize a 100 kD nuclear protein antigen (sp-100). Clin Exp Immunol. 1987;68:108–16.
32. Szostecki C, Will H, Netter HJ, Guldner HH. Autoantibodies to the nuclear Sp100 protein in primary biliary cirrhosis and associated diseases: epitope specificity and immunoglobulin class distribution. Scand J Immunol. 1992;36:555–64.
33. Luettig B, Boeker KH, Schoessler W et al. The antinuclear autoantibodies Sp100 and gp210 persist after orthotopic liver transplantation in patients with primary biliary cirrhosis. J Hepatol. 1998;28:824–8.
34. Strassburg CP, Alex B, Zindy F et al. Identification of cyclin A as a molecular target of antinuclear antibodies (ANA) in hepatic and non-hepatic autoimmune diseases. J Hepatol. 1996;25:859–66.
35. Lin F, Noyer CM, Ye Q, Courvalin JC, Worman HJ. Autoantibodies from patients with primary biliary cirrhosis recognize a region within the nucleoplasmic domain of inner nuclear membrane protein LBR. Hepatology. 1996;23:57–61.
36. Sternsdorf T, Guldner HH, Szostecki C, Grotzinger T, Will H. Two nuclear dot-associated proteins, PML and Sp100, are often co-autoimmunogenic in patients with primary biliary cirrhosis. Scand J Immunol. 1995;42:257–68.
37. Bluthner M, Schafer C, Schneider C, Bautz FA. Identification of major linear epitopes on the sp100 nuclear PBC autoantigen by the gene-fragment phage-display technology. Autoimmunity. 1999;29:33–42.

38. Shimoda S, Nakamura M, Ishibashi H et al. Molecular mimicry of mitochondrial and nuclear autoantigens in primary biliary cirrhosis. Gastroenterology. 2003;124:1915–25.
39. Long SA, Van de Water J, Gershwin ME. Antimitochondrial antibodies in primary biliary cirrhosis: the role of xenobiotics. Autoimmun Rev. 2002;1:37–42.
40. Selmi C, Balkwill DL, Invernizzi P et al. Patients with primary biliary cirrhosis react against a ubiquitous xenobiotic-metabolizing bacterium. Hepatology. 2003;38:1250–7.

Section III
Clinics of primary biliary cirrhosis

8
Clinical aspects and prognosis of primary biliary cirrhosis

J. KURTOVIC and S. M. RIORDAN

INTRODUCTION

Appreciation of the spectrum of clinical features of primary biliary cirrhosis (PBC) has evolved considerably over the past few decades, as a result of both the more widespread availability of biochemical and screening tests for this disorder and the recognition of a growing number of clinical associations. Although the substantial female predominance documented in early series remains true today, it has become clear that other so-called 'classical' clinical, biochemical and even immunological features of the disorder need not necessarily be present. Recognition of the extended clinical spectrum of PBC has resulted in a substantial increase in its reported prevalence. Far from the historical view of PBC as an uncommon condition, recent studies from the United Kingdom and United States indicate that PBC may affect up to 1 in 4000 women, including up to 1 in 1000 women over 40 years of age[1-5]. Only a small minority of patients nowadays present with liver failure, and most are even identified while asymptomatic[5,6]. Consequently, overall survival is now recognized to be substantially better than originally perceived[7].

This chapter reviews clinical and laboratory aspects of PBC at diagnosis in a variety of settings, including in patients with and without PBC-related symptoms, in females compared to males and in those with and without positive antimitochondrial antibody (AMA) titres. Familial PBC will be discussed and factors influencing prognosis will be considered. The prevalence of complicating hepatocellular carcinoma and its possible impact on overall survival, along with cardiovascular risk in the setting of the marked hypercholesterolaemia that may accompany chronic cholestasis, will also be addressed.

CLINICAL AND LABORATORY DATA AT DIAGNOSIS

Patients with PBC may experience a wide range of symptoms and, consequently, several patterns of presentation are recognized. As already alluded to, an increasing

Table 1 Prevalence of symptoms at diagnosis (%)

	Sherlock and Scheuer 1973[8]	Christensen et al. 1980[9]	Crowe et al. 1985[10]	Nyberg and Loof 1989[11]	Kim et al. 2000[5]	Prince et al. 2002[6]
Jaundice	33	12	11	4		3
Pruritus	57	47	35	26		19
Fatigue	0	8	5	11		21
Gastrointestinal bleeding/ascites	4	8	13	0		4
Abdominal pain	0	7	5	8		8
No PBC-related symptoms	4	16	32	49	80	61

number of patients are identified in the absence of any disease-related symptoms[5,6,8–11] (Table 1).

'Classical' mode of presentation

The 'classical' presentation of PBC with the combination of jaundice, pruritus, steatorrhoea and generalized xanthomas in middle-aged women, as described in the original report[7], is usually the consequence of advanced-stage disease. In this setting clinical jaundice, due to the progressive destruction of interlobular bile ducts, usually precedes other features of hepatic functional decompensation[12]. However, jaundice is not necessarily indicative of decompensated cirrhosis in patients with PBC. Complicating choledocholithiasis, as discussed later, has long been recognized as an alternative cause of jaundice in this group. A premature ductopenic variant of PBC, in which jaundice occurs in the setting of marked interlobular bile duct loss in the absence of advanced fibrosis or cirrhosis, has recently been reported in four Dutch patients, three of whom required liver transplantation within 7 years of diagnosis for progressive cholestasis and symptoms such as refractory pruritus. Cirrhosis had developed by the time of transplantation in one case, while the others still had non-cirrhotic disease[13]. Coombes-positive haemolytic anaemia, which may respond to treatment with ursodeoxycholic acid[14], is another uncommon cause of rapidly progressive jaundice in patients with PBC.

In addition to jaundice, severe bile duct damage in PBC results in impaired biliary excretion of conjugated bile salts, and this is the usual mechanism by which steatorrhoea occurs in patients with this disorder. Steatorrhoea may be marked, with faecal fat excretion of up to 68 g/day[15–17]. Deficiencies in fat-soluble vitamins are not uncommon, with the serum vitamin A and 25-hydroxyvitamin D levels reduced and the prothrombin time prolonged in 32.6%, 19.2% and 13.5% of patients, respectively, in one series[18]. The prolonged prothrombin time improved with vitamin K supplementation in the majority of cases, indicating that coagulopathy was predominantly due to vitamin K deficiency rather than hepatocellular dysfunction. Vitamin E deficiency was present in only 7.7% of patients. Variables most predictive of fat-soluble vitamin deficiency were an advanced histological stage of PBC, jaundice and hypoalbuminaemia[18]. Use of bile acid-binding resins such as cholestyramine for treatment of pruritus may exacerbate luminal bile salt deficiency and steatorrhoea in this setting. Conversely, as with jaundice, steatorrhoea may occasionally occur in the absence of advanced-stage PBC, as a result of associated exocrine pancreatic insufficiency or as a consequence of small intestinal bacterial overgrowth, which may complicate associated scleroderma, as discussed later.

Recent studies from the Mayo Clinic suggest that pruritus is similarly more likely to occur in patients with advanced disease, with the alkaline phosphatase level and Mayo risk score, as discussed later, identified as independent predictive factors[19]. Histological factors including extent of bile duct damage and portal granulomas were found to correlate with severity of pruritus in a French study in which clinical data were recorded on the day of the liver biopsy[20], although concerns remain over the reliability of available methods for comparing severity of this subjective symptom from patient to patient[21]. Little is known concerning the natural history of pruritus in patients with PBC. The probability of spontaneous improvement or resolution of pruritus at 1 year, as assessed by subjective methodology, is in the order of 23%, with the probability of developing pruritus over this time 27%[19]. The unpredictability of this phenomenon is shown by the fact that no significant correlation between pruritus status and trends in biochemical parameters of cholestasis has been identified[19]. Our experience is that pruritus often resolves, or at least improves, during the later stages of the disease. Diurnal and seasonal variations in the severity of pruritus are also common, with exacerbations at night and during winter, possibly due to increased dryness of the skin. Pruritus may first become evident or worsen during the third trimester of pregnancy, failing to resolve in the early post-partum period as would be expected with pregnancy-related cholestasis. The use of exogenous oestrogens can also trigger pruritus in PBC. As a consequence of chronic scratching, hyperpigmentation of the skin, most evident on the trunk and arms and due to an increased deposition of melanin, becomes increasingly marked[22].

Trends in modes of presentation

Jaundice and pruritus were by far the most common presenting symptoms in a series from the Royal Free Hospital, London, reported in 1973, together accounting for 90% of presentations[8]. The prevalence of each at diagnosis has fallen dramatically over the past 30 years, with jaundice and pruritus present in only 3% and 19% of patients, respectively, in a recent series[6]. Conversely, the prevalence of fatigue as a presenting symptom and the proportion of patients being diagnosed while asymptomatic have risen markedly[5,6,8–11] (Table 1).

Fatigue is unrelated to any objective marker of disease activity. Similarly, the occurrence of fatigue is not fully explained by the increased prevalences of sleep disturbance and depression that have been documented in this group[23]. The degree of fatigue experienced by PBC patients, as assessed by a validated fatigue impact score, is significantly greater than that experienced by age- and sex-matched community controls, and even by patients with another chronic liver disorder, namely autoimmune hepatitis[23]. The degree to which fatigue may interfere with normal daily activities has been estimated to be comparable to that reported by patients with end-stage renal failure[24,25]. Nonetheless, the prevalence and severity of fatigue may be overestimated in series involving patients attending specialist liver clinics, with a substantial proportion of community-based patients, in the order of 20%, reporting no impact of fatigue on their daily lives[23].

Up to 80% of patients in recently reported series have no PBC-related symptoms at the time of diagnosis[5,6], compared to only 4% some 30 years ago[8]. The diagnosis of PBC in this group is usually established after the chance finding of an abnormal physical sign, such as hepatomegaly, or, more often, an elevated serum alkaline phosphatase level during the course of an unrelated illness. Alternatively, patients may be diagnosed after biochemical and immunological screening is carried out, either as part of a routine health check or following the documentation of one of the many extrahepatic, predominantly autoimmune, disorders known to be associated with PBC. The most common of these associated conditions is Sjögren's syndrome, clinical features or immunological markers of which are present in around 75% of patients. Other common associations are with renal tubular acidosis (50%), gallstones (30%), a predominantly non-erosive arthritis (20%), thyroid dysfunction (15%), scleroderma (15%) and Raynaud's phenomenon (10%)[26]. Recent studies from Italy confirm previous reports of an association with coeliac disease[27,28], although no such association was evident in patients from Crete[29]. An association with psoriasis has recently been described[30]. Lichen planus is similarly increasingly recognized. Arthritis is the variable most responsible for the significantly reduced functional status of patients with PBC[31]. Recent data indicate that osteoporosis is not a specific complication of PBC, being no more prevalent than would be expected in a normal population of comparable age and sex[32].

Comparison of clinical and laboratory data at diagnosis in symptomatic and asymptomatic patients

Mahl et al.[33] at Yale compared clinical and laboratory features at diagnosis in 36 asymptomatic PBC patients to those in 243 counterparts with PBC-related symptoms. The prevalences of abnormal physical signs including jaundice (59%), hyperpigmentation (42%), hepatomegaly (74%) and splenomegaly (47%) were each significantly higher in the symptomatic group than in patients without PBC-related symptoms (6%, 13%, 50% and 12%, respectively). Laboratory indices of cholestasis, including the serum bilirubin and cholesterol levels, were significantly higher in symptomatic patients, while the serum albumin concentration was significantly lower in this group, implying more advanced disease in those presenting with PBC-related symptoms. These findings are in keeping with the results of histological studies from Sweden, the United Kingdom and the United States indicating that a significantly higher proportion of symptomatic patients at diagnosis have stage III or IV disease than their asymptomatic counterparts[11,33,34]. Nonetheless, a substantial proportion of asymptomatic patients still demonstrated abnormal physical signs and/or laboratory indices at diagnosis. For example, hepatomegaly was detectable at diagnosis in 50% of cases, while the median cholesterol value was in the hypercholesterolaemic range (6.5 mmol/L)[33]. Furthermore, stage III or IV disease was present at the time of diagnosis in 34–57% of the asymptomatic group[11,33,34].

Comparison of clinical and laboratory data at diagnosis in men and women

Whether men with PBC demonstrate the same clinical and laboratory features as women has been the subject of several studies. Rubel et al.[35] compared clinical and histological features in 30 men with 30 age-matched women, and found no significant differences between the two groups. Subsequently, Lucey et al.[36] compared clinical parameters at the time of diagnosis in 39 men and 191 women presenting to King's College Hospital, London over a 15-year period. The mean age and alkaline phosphatase levels at diagnosis were similar in each group. The distributions of early and advanced disease, as shown by both the serum bilirubin level and histological staging, were also comparable. Comparison of symptoms and signs at diagnosis showed that pruritus was present in significantly fewer men than women (45% versus 68%, respectively). Hyperpigmentation was also recorded significantly less often in males (35% versus 55%, respectively), probably related to the lower prevalence of pruritus and, hence, chronic scratching in this group. There were no gender-related differences in the frequencies of gastrointestinal haemorrhage, ascites, hepatomegaly, splenomegaly or xanthomas. Similar proportions of men and women had no liver-related symptoms at the time of diagnosis. Symptoms of associated Sjögren's syndrome were significantly less common in men than in women (15% versus 33%, respectively), in keeping with the known association of autoimmunity with female sex. More recently, Talwalkar et al.[19] reported that gender did not significantly influence the likelihood of pruritus in a series of 335 patients from the Mayo Clinic. Nonetheless, female patients were not stratified according to menopausal status in this study. This may be relevant, as the earlier study from King's College Hospital[36] found that differences in prevalence of pruritus in men and women were more marked in the premenopausal group, raising the possibility that the higher prevalence of pruritus in women was related to differences in levels of sex hormones.

Comparison of clinical and laboratory data at diagnosis according to AMA status

It has long been recognized that 5–10% of patients with clinical, histological and biochemical features typical of PBC are AMA-negative when tested by standard indirect immunofluorescence techniques[37,38]. Several studies have been performed to compare clinical, biochemical, serological and histological characteristics in these AMA-negative and -positive cases. A North American study of 17 AMA-negative patients and an equal number of AMA-positive patients matched for serum bilirubin concentration found that serum IgM concentrations were significantly less elevated in AMA-negative compared to -positive patients. Each of the AMA-negative group had serum positive for antinuclear antibody (ANA), usually in high titre (> 1 : 160), whereas only 3/17 (17.6%) AMA-positive patients were ANA-positive. Similarly, more of the AMA-negative group were positive for smooth muscle antibody (SMA) than were AMA-positive patients (7/17, 41.2% versus 1/17, 5.9%). Aside from these serological parameters, the AMA-positive and -negative patients were indistinguishable, with comparable symptoms, liver histology and prevalences of other autoimmune disorders[39]. Similar findings have been reported from the Mayo Clinic[40].

The concept of AMA-negative PBC as a distinct clinical entity depends fundamentally on the sensitivity of the methods used for AMA detection. Despite widespread clinical use, increasing experience suggests that immunofluorescence is rather insensitive. A number of studies have suggested that approximately 15–30% of patients who test AMA-negative by immunofluorescence become AMA-positive when their serum is re-tested by enzyme-linked immunoassay (ELISA) or immunoblot assays using purified bovine or porcine mitochondria as targets[39,41–43]. Other studies using cloned mitochondrial antigens, including hybrid-recombinant molecules, as targets in ELISA and immunoblot assays suggest that the true proportion of AMA-negative patients is even lower, with a positive AMA result found in 67–90% of patients who are AMA-negative by immunofluorescence[44,45].

In a study in which AMA status was determined by both immunofluorescence and immunoblotting, using bovine heart mitochondria as the target, Invernizzi et al.[41] compared clinical, biochemical, serological and histological features at diagnosis in 273 AMA-positive and 24 AMA-negative patients from an Italian centre. No significant differences were noted with respect to sex, age or prevalences of symptomatic disease, advanced histological stage or complications of cirrhosis, while the associations between AMA-negativity and both less elevated serum IgM levels (mean 409 mg/dl versus mean 591 mg/dl in AMA-positive patients) and increased prevalences of positive ANA (71% versus 31%, respectively) and SMA titres (37% versus 9%, respectively) were confirmed. Nonetheless, Muratori et al.[42] recently found that reactivity to gp210, a particular PBC-specific ANA directed against a transmembrane glycoprotein of the nuclear pore complex that may be associated with more severe PBC[46], was not significantly more prevalent in AMA-negative than -positive patients (15% versus 16%, respectively), despite overall ANA positivity being significantly more prevalent in the AMA-negative group (85% versus 48%, respectively).

FAMILIAL PBC

Instances of multiple cases of PBC occurring within single families clearly demonstrate that there is an inherited component to PBC[47]. Prevalence of the disorder among first-degree relatives has been found to range from 1.1% to 2.4% in the United Kingdom[30,34,48], while a 5.5% familial prevalence was reported in New York[49]. Notably, PBC is diagnosed in the daughters before their mothers in a substantial proportion of cases[48], probably as a consequence of increased awareness of the disease along with the more widespread availability of screening tests nowadays. Presumably for the same reasons, a greater proportion of daughters than their mothers are diagnosed while asymptomatic, at a younger age and with earlier stage disease[48]. Using population-based epidemiological methods, a positive family history was found in 6.4% of cases in the northeast of England, with a 2.3% prevalence in female offspring of patients with PBC. The relative risk for PBC among daughters of affected mothers was estimated to be 15[50].

PROGNOSIS

The natural history of PBC is extraordinarily variable. Nonetheless, a substantial proportion of patients develop liver failure, require liver transplantation or die prematurely of liver disease. As discussed later, mortality from non-liver-related causes is also increased[6]. PBC remains the third most common indication for liver transplantation in the United States, United Kingdom and Australia, either for complications of liver failure or, less commonly, for symptomatic reasons, such as intractable pruritus or profound fatigue. Post-liver transplant survival in patients transplanted for PBC is comparable to that in those transplanted for other aetiologies of cirrhosis, although recurrence of PBC has been documented in a minority of cases.

Prognostic models

Prognostic factors have been identified by workers at Yale[51], by a European consortium[52], at the Mayo Clinic[53] and, more recently, in Newcastle, United Kingdom[6] (Table 2). Patient age and the serum bilirubin level are common components of each of these models, with the serum albumin concentration identified as an important prognostic variable in three of these. Other prognostic factors variously include the presence of hepatomegaly or oedema, the prothrombin time, the alkaline phosphatase level, treatment with azathioprine and histological features such as central cholestasis, bridging fibrosis and cirrhosis. The most widely used prognostic model is that derived at the Mayo Clinic[53], which has been validated in both the tertiary referral setting[54] and in two recent studies of community-based and geographically defined patients[5,6].

Other laboratory indices of possible prognostic significance

Reactivity to gp210, as discussed earlier, was recently found in an Italian and Spanish series to be associated with more advanced PBC, as reflected by significantly higher bilirubin, alkaline phosphatase and γ-glutamyl transpeptidase levels and lower albumin concentrations. The Mayo risk score was also significantly higher in anti-gp210-positive patients[42] (Table 3). Such observations are consistent with data from Japan, where death from liver failure was more frequently observed in anti-gp210-positive PBC patients[46], and from Italy, where the presence of autoantibodies to the nuclear pore complex, including anti-gp210, was associated with more advanced PBC[55].

Table 2 Prognostic factors in PBC

Yale[51] (n = 280)	European[52] (n = 216)	Mayo Clinic[53] (n = 418)	Newcastle[6] (n = 770)
Age	Age	Age	Age
Bilirubin	Bilirubin	Bilirubin	Bilirubin
Hepatomegaly	Albumin	Albumin	Albumin
Bridging fibrosis/ cirrhosis	Azathioprine	Prothrombin time	Alkaline phosphatase
	Central cholestasis	Oedema	
	Cirrhosis		

Table 3 Laboratory markers of severity of PBC in relation to reactivity to gp210 (from ref. 42)

	Anti-gp210-positive (n = 15)	Anti-gp210-negative (n = 81)	p-Value
Mean bilirubin (mg/dl)	4.9	0.9	0.0001
Mean ALP (U/L)	4.3	1.9	0.0002
Mean GGT (U/L)	6.8	4.3	0.02
Mean albumin (g/L)	32	37	0.002
Mean Mayo risk score	6	4.5	0.0001

Recent data raise the possibility that particular human leucocyte antigen (HLA) and interleukin 1 (IL-1) gene polymorphisms may also be of prognostic significance in patients with PBC. In particular, the HLA DRB1*0801-DQA1* 0401-DQB1*0402 haplotype was associated with an increased risk of advanced and progressive disease. This haplotype was found in 24% of patients with late-stage histological disease compared to only 5% with early-stage disease and 3% of patients who showed no sign of clinical progression over a 10-year period. Conversely, the IL-1B* 1,1 genotype was associated with less severe and non-progressive disease, with this genotype identified in 77% of patients with early-stage disease and 71% of those with no sign of clinical progression over 10 years compared to 53% of patients with advanced-stage disease[56].

Conversely, available data indicate that survival is not significantly influenced by AMA status[39]. Neither was the particular profile of AMA positivity found to be of prognostic value in a recent North American series[57]. This contrasts with earlier findings from Europe suggesting that patients with both anti-M2 AMA (directed against the 2-oxoacid dehydrogenase complex located at the inner mitochondrial membrane) and anti-M4 AMA (directed against an antigen co-purifying with sulphite oxidase in the mitochondrial intermembrane space) ± anti-M8 AMA (the substrate of which remains unspecified) followed a more aggressive clinical course[58,59].

Natural history of asymptomatic patients at diagnosis

It is well established that symptomatic PBC is a progressive disorder in the majority of patients. An area of considerable clinical importance is the natural history of patients without PBC-related symptoms at diagnosis, given the increasing proportion of patients in this category. Here, we consider various aspects of the clinical course of such patients, including the proportion of those with normal liver-related biochemistry who will develop biochemical evidence of cholestasis, the proportion who will develop PBC-related symptoms and survival in relation to the development of such symptoms.

Development of cholestasis

The majority of asymptomatic patients with normal liver biochemistry at diagnosis will nonetheless have liver histology diagnostic of or compatible with PBC, and most will develop biochemical evidence of cholestasis over time. Metcalf et al.[60] in the United Kingdom followed 29 such patients for a median 17 years

Table 4 Proportion of asymptomatic patients at diagnosis who develop PBC-related symptoms

Authors/refs.	Location	n	Percentage developing symptoms	Mean/median follow-up (years)
Long et al. 1977[61]	Royal Free, UK	20	50	4.5
Mitchison et al. 1980[62]	Newcastle/King's, UK	95	36	5.8
Nyberg and Loof 1989[11]	Sweden	56	37	9.5
Balasubramanian et al. 1990[63]	Mayo Clinic, USA	37	89	7.6
Mahl et al. 1994[33]	Yale, USA	36	66	12.1
Metcalf et al. 1996[60]	Newcastle, UK	29	76	17.8
Springer et al. 1999[64]	Toronto, Canada	91	36	5.1

and found that 83% (24/29) developed cholestasis a median 5.6 years after the first detection of a positive AMA titre.

Development of symptoms

The proportion of asymptomatic patients who will subsequently develop PBC-related symptoms has been investigated in series from the United Kingdom, Sweden and the United States[11,33,60–64]. These studies demonstrate evidence of progressive disease in a substantial proportion of patients, with between 36% and 89% becoming symptomatic during mean/median follow-up periods ranging from 4.5 to 17.8 years (Table 4). The onset of symptoms may pre-date the development of cholestasis, as reflected in serum, with 45% of cases in a series from the United Kingdom conforming to this trend[60]. In keeping with the concept that initially asymptomatic PBC is a progressive disorder in the majority of cases, Prince et al.[6] recently found, using Kaplan–Meier methods in a large United Kingdom series of 770 patients followed for up to 28 years, that the proportion of asymptomatic patients fell from 61% at diagnosis to an estimated 17% at 10 years and as little as 5% at 20 years. The median time from diagnosis to the development of symptoms was found to be 2 years in a United Kingdom study in which median follow-up was 17.8 years[60] and 4.2 years in a North American series in which the median follow-up was 5.1 years[64].

Survival in relation to presence or absence of symptoms at diagnosis

Several studies have investigated survival in relation to the presence or absence of symptoms at diagnosis (Table 5). In studies of relatively small numbers of symptomatic patients reported in the 1950s and 1960s, Foulk et al.[65] and Sherlock[66] reported median survival of 6 and 5 years, respectively. In 1983 Roll et al.[51] at Yale reported that the estimated 10-year survival in a cohort of 243 symptomatic patients was 50%, while that in asymptomatic patients was over 90%. Some 16 years later Springer et al.[64] reported an estimated 10-year survival of 70% in a cohort of 91 initially asymptomatic patients in Toronto. Two other contemporary series report a 10-year survival of 57% and median survival of 9 years, respectively, in patient cohorts of whom 61–81% were asymptomatic at the time of diagnosis[5,6]. Forty-two per cent of deaths in one of these latter studies were directly attributable to liver disease, while 5.1% of patients (9% of those younger than 65 years at the time of diagnosis) underwent liver transplantation during follow-up of up to 28 years. Liver failure developed within 10 years of diagnosis in 26% of patients. Survival was substantially poorer in this cohort of PBC patients, most of whom had no PBC-related symptoms at diagnosis, than in age- and sex-matched controls, with a standardized mortality ratio of 2.87. Even when liver-related deaths were excluded, the standardized mortality ratio remained more than 50% greater than predicted[6].

Mahl et al.[33] have reported on an extended follow-up of the Yale cohort originally described by Roll et al.[51] and discussed above. Initially symptomatic and asymptomatic patients were followed for a median time from diagnosis of 6.4 years (range 0.04–24.2 years) and 12.1 years (range 1.1–19.2 years), respectively. Despite similar ages at diagnosis, median survival in the asymptomatic group was more than twice as long as in symptomatic patients (Figure 1). However, survival of patients asymptomatic at diagnosis is not normal, falling significantly below that of gender- and age-matched control groups after 6–12 years of follow-up[11,33,63,64]. This is probabaly due at least in part to the fact that a substantial proportion of patients asymptomatic at diagnosis ultimately become symptomatic, as already discussed, since, once this occurs, the survival rate of such patients becomes indistinguishable from that of patients who had been symptomatic

Table 5 Survival according to the presence or absence of PBC-related symptoms at diagnosis

Authors/refs.	Patients	Survival
Sherlock 1959[66]	n = 23, symptomatic	Mean survival 5 years
Foulk et al. 1964[65]	n = 49, symptomatic	Mean survival 6 years
Roll et al. 1983[51]	n = 243, symptomatic	50% 10-year survival
	n = 37, asymptomatic	>90% 10-year survival
Springer et al. 1999[64]	n = 91, asymptomatic	70% 10-year survival
Kim et al. 2000[5]	n = 46, 80% asymptomatic	57% 10-year survival
Prince et al. 2002[6]	n = 770, 61% asymptomatic	Median survival 9 years

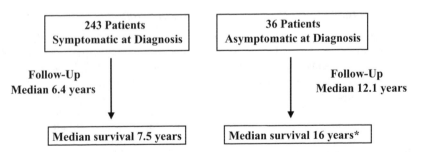

Figure 1 Survival according to the presence or absence of PBC-related symptoms at diagnosis (from ref. 33). *Initially asymptomatic patients who become symptomatic develop survival rate comparable to that of patients who are symptomatic at diagnosis

from the outset[33,62,64]. Median survival in the subgroup that remains persistently asymptomatic is significantly longer that in patients who develop symptoms[33,64], being comparable to that in healthy gender- and age-matched controls[64].

Impact of older age

Each of the prognostic models from Yale, the Mayo Clinic, Europe and the United Kingdom discussed earlier include older age as an independent adverse prognostic indicator. Nonetheless, there is increasing evidence that elderly patients who remain persistently asymptomatic may follow a particularly indolent clinical course.

Impact of gender

Available data indicate that overall survival does not differ significantly in men and women with PBC. Christensen et al.[9] reported no significant gender-related differences in the course of PBC in 25 men and 236 women, predominantly symptomatic at enrolment and followed for a median 18 months. Lucey et al.[36] similarly found no significant difference in survival in 39 men and 191 women, the majority with stage III or IV disease at the outset and with similar proportions of symptomatic to asymptomatic patients in each group, who were followed for a median 37 and 42 months, respectively.

Impact of hepatocellular carcinoma (HCC)

Differences in proportions of patients with early- and late-stage PBC and of men and women may have contributed to previous discrepant reports as to the prevalence of HCC in this disorder[67–70], since the presence of cirrhosis and male gender are, in general, important factors associated with HCC development.

An increased prevalence of HCC was documented in men (10.3% versus 1.6%), all with stage IV disease, in a series from the United Kingdom[36], while Jones et al.[68] similarly found an increased prevalence of HCC complicating advanced PBC in men in another United Kingdom study. An association between risk of HCC and advanced histological stage of PBC has been confirmed in two recent series[71,72]. The cumulative rate of development of HCC in patients with stage III or IV PBC at study enrolment (12.3% at 10 years) was significantly higher than that for patients with early-stage disease (7.3% at 10 years) in a Japanese series of 396 patients followed for 6–271 months[71]. All patients with HCC had progressed to stage III or IV disease by the time that HCC developed. A Spanish study of 140 patients with PBC followed for a mean period of 5.6 years found an incidence of HCC in the 45 with stage III or IV disease of 11.1%, similar to that in age- and sex-matched patients with hepatitis C virus-associated cirrhosis (15%). Conversely, none of the 95 patients with stage I or II PBC developed HCC during the study period[72]. As in earlier series, the incidence of HCC was higher in men than women in each of these latter studies[71,72].

Despite its increased prevalence, HCC does not affect overall survival in patients with PBC[71,72]. Presumably this is so because HCC develops only during the later stages of the clinical course, when other factors including liver failure and variceal bleeding, along with non-liver related co-morbidities, also influence outcome. These considerations probably also explain the fact that overall survival is not significantly different in men and women[36], as discussed above, despite the substantially higher prevalence of complicating HCC in men, even though an increased proportion of male deaths are attributable to this cause[68].

Risk of cardiovascular disease

As in other liver disorders in which cholestasis is a feature, reduced biliary excretion can lead to markedly raised serum cholesterol levels in patients with PBC, although disease progression is typically associated with falls towards normal of elevated cholesterol values, due to reduced hepatic synthesis of cholesterol at this stage. Despite hypercholesterolaemia, patients with PBC are not at increased risk of fatal or non-fatal cardiovascular events compared to age- and sex-matched controls[73-75]. Responsible mechanisms remain to be determined, although predominant increases in high-density lipoprotein and lipoprotein A1 levels, along with a modified low-density lipoprotein composition, may be contributory[73,76]. These findings have led some authors to surmise that patients with PBC may even be protected against cardiovascular disease[74,75,77]. This is certainly not our experience, however, as coronary artery disease is evident at angiography in a substantial proportion of our older PBC patients with advanced disease coming to liver transplantation assessment.

References

1. James OF, Bhopal R, Howel D, Gray J, Burt AD, Metcalf JV. Primary biliary cirrhosis once rare, now common in the United Kingdom? Hepatology. 1999;30:390–4.
2. Ray-Chadhuri D, Rigney E, McCormack K et al. Epidemiology of PBC in Sheffield updated: demographics and relation to water supply. Annual Meeting of the British Association for the Study of the Liver, London, England, 2001.
3. Kingham JG, Parker DR. The association between primary biliary cirrhosis and celiac disease: a study of relative prevalences. Gut. 1998;42:120–2.
4. Steinke D, Weston T, Morris A, Macdonald T, Dillon J. Incidence, prevalence and resource use of primary biliary cirrhosis in Tayside, Scotland. J Hepatol. 2001;31:532A.
5. Kim WR, Lindor KD, Locke GR et al. Epidemiology and natural history of primary biliary cirrhosis in a US community. Gastroenterology. 2000;119:1631–6.
6. Prince M, Chetwynd A, Newman W, Metcalf JV, James OFW. Survival and symptom progression in a geographically based cohort of patients with primary biliary cirrhosis: Follow-up for up to 28 years. Gastroenterology. 2002;123:1044–51.
7. Addison T, Gull W. On a certain affection of the skin, vitiligoidea-α plana, β tuberosa. Guy's Hosp Rep. 1851;7:265–76.
8. Sherlock S, Scheuer PJ. The presentation and diagnosis of 100 patients with primary biliary cirrhosis. N Engl J Med. 1973;289:674–8.
9. Christensen E, Crowe, Doniach D et al. Clinical pattern and course of disease in primary biliary cirrhosis based on an analysis of 236 patients. Gastroenterology. 1980;78:236–46.
10. Crowe J, Christensen E, Doniach D, Popper H, Tygstrup N, Williams R. Early features of primary biliary cirrhosis: an analysis of 85 patients. Am J Gastroenterol. 1985;80:466–8.
11. Nyberg A, Loof L. Primary biliary cirrhosis: clinical features and outcome with special reference to asymptomatic disease. Scand J Gastroenterol. 1989;24:57–64.
12. Heathcote J. The clinical expression of primary biliary cirrhosis. Semin Liver Dis. 1996;17:23–33.
13. Vleggar FP, van Buuren HR, Zondervan PE, ten Kate FJW, Hop WCJ, the Dutch Multicentre PBC study group. Jaundice in non-cirrhotic primary biliary cirrhosis: the premature ductopoenic variant. Gut. 2001;49:276–81.

14. Fuller SJ, Kumar P, Weltman M, Wiley JS. Autoimmune hemolysis associated with primary biliary cirrhosis responding to ursodeoxycholic acid as sole treatment. Am J Haematol. 2003; 72:31–3.
15. Herlong HF, Recker RR, Maddrey WC. Bone disease in primary biliary cirrhosis: histologic features and response to 25-hydroxyvitamin D. Gastroenterology. 1982;83:103–8.
16. Matloff DS, Kaplan MM, Neer RM, Goldberg MJ, Bitman W, Wolfe HJ. Osteoporosis in primary biliary cirrhosis: effects of 25-hydroxyvitamin D_3 treatment. Gastroenterology. 1982; 83:97–102.
17. Hodgson SF, Dickson ER, Wahner HW, Johnson KA, Mann KG, Riggs BL. Bone loss and reduced osteoblast function in primary biliary cirrhosis. Ann Intern Med. 1985;103:855–60.
18. Kaplan MM, Elta GH, Furie B, Sadowski JA, Russell RM. Fat-soluble vitamin nutriture in primary biliary cirrhosis. Gastroenterology. 1988;95:787–92.
19. Talwalkar JA, Souto E, Jorgensen RA, Lindor KD. Natural history of primary biliary cirrhosis. Clin Gastroenterol Hepatol. 2003;1:297–302.
20. Poupon R, Chazouilleres O, Balkau B, Poupon RE. Clinical and biochemical expression of the histopathological lesions of primary biliary cirrhosis: UDCA-PBC Group. J Hepatol. 1999;30: 408–12.
21. Bergasa NV. Studying pruritus in the 21st century. Clin Gastroenterol Hepatol. 2003;1:249–51.
22. Reynolds TB. The butterfly sign in patients with chronic jaundice and pruritus. Ann Intern Med. 1973;78:545–6.
23. Goldblatt J, Taylor PJS, Lipman T et al. The true impact of fatigue in primary biliary cirrhosis: a population study. Gastroenterology. 2002;122:1235–41.
24. Cauch-Dudek K, Abbey S, Stewart DE, Heathcote EJ. Fatigue and quality of life in primary biliary cirrhosis. Hepatology. 1995;22:108A.
25. Huet PM, Deslauriers J. Impact of fatigue on quality of life in patients with primary biliary cirrhosis. Gastroenterology. 1996;110:A1215.
26. Talwalkar JA, Lindor KD. Primary biliary cirrhosis. Lancet. 2003;362:53–61.
27. Volta U, Rodrigo L, Granito A et al. Celiac disease in autoimmune cholestatic liver disorders. Am J Gastroenterol. 2002;97:2609–13.
28. Floreani A, Betterle C, Baragiotta A et al. Prevalence of celiac disease in primary biliary cirrhosis and of antimitochondrial antibodies in adult celiac disease patients in Italy. Dig Liver Dis. 2002;34:258–61.
29. Chatzicostas C, Roussomoustakaki M, Drygiannakis D et al. Primary biliary cirrhosis and autoimmune cholangitis are not associated with celiac disease in Crete. BMC Gastroenterol. 2002;2:5.
30. Howel D, Fischbacher CM, Bhopal RS, Gray J, Metcalf JV, James OFW. An exploratory population-based case-control study of primary biliary cirrhosis. Hepatology. 2000;31:1055–60.
31. Parikh-Patel A, Gold EB, Utts J, Worman H, Krivy KE, Gershwin ME. Functional status of patients with primary biliary cirrhosis. Am J Gastroenterol. 2002;97:2871–9.
32. Newton J, Francis R, Prince M et al. Osteoporosis in primary biliary cirrhosis revisited. Gut. 2001;49:282–7.
33. Mahl TC, Shockcor W, Boyer JL. Primary biliary cirrhosis: survival of a large cohort of symptomatic and asymptomatic patients followed for 24 years. J Hepatol. 1994;20:707–13.
34. Myszor M, James OFW. The epidemiology of primary biliary cirrhosis in north-east England: an increasingly common disease? Q J Med. 1990;276:377–85.
35. Rubel LR, Rabin L, Seeff LF, Licht H, Cuccherini BA. Does primary biliary cirrhosis in men differ from primary biliary cirrhosis in women? Hepatology. 1984;4:671–7.
36. Lucey MR, Neuberger JM, Williams R. Primary biliary cirrhosis in men. Gut. 1986;27:1373–6.
37. Kaplan MM. Primary biliary cirrhosis. N Engl J Med. 1987;316:521–8.
38. Gershwin ME, Mackay IR. Primary biliary cirrhosis: paradigm or paradox for autoimmunity. Gastroenterology. 1991;100:822–33.
39. Michieletti P, Wanless IR, Katz A et al. Antimitochondrial antibody-negative primary biliary cirrhosis: a distinct syndrome of autoimmune cholangitis. Gut. 1994;35:260–5.
40. Lacerda MA, Ludwig J, Dickson ER et al. Antimitochondrial antibody-negative primary biliary cirrhosis. Am J Gastroenterol. 1995;90:247–9.
41. Invernizzi P, Crosignani A, Battezzatti PM et al. Comparison of the clinical features and clinical course of antimitochondrial antibody-positive and -negative primary biliary cirrhosis. Hepatology. 1997;25:1090–5.

42. Muratori P, Muratori L, Ferrari R et al. Characterization and clinical impact of antinuclear antibodies in primary biliary cirrhosis. Am J Gastroenterol. 2003;98:431–7.
43. Vergani D, Bogdanos D-P. Positive markers in AMA-negative PBC. Am J Gastroenterol. 2003; 98:241–2.
44. Moteki S, Leung PS, Coppel RL et al. Use of a designer triple expression hybrid clone for three different lipoyl domains for the detection of antimotochondrial autoantibodies. Hepatology. 1996;24:97–103.
45. Miyakawa H, Tanaka A, Kikuchi K et al. Detection of antimitochondrial autoantibodies in immunofluorescent AMA-negative patients with primary biliary cirrhosis using recombinant autoantigens. Hepatology. 2001;34:243–8.
46. Itoh S, Ichida T, Yoshida T et al. Autoantibodies against a 210 kDa glycoprotein of the nuclear pore complex as a prognostic marker in patients with primary biliary cirrhosis. J Gastroenterol Hepatol. 1998;13:257–65.
47. Mehal WZ, Gregory WL, Lo D et al. Defining the immunogenetic susceptibility to primary biliary cirrhosis. Hepatology. 1994;20:1213–19.
48. Brind AM, Bray GP, Portmann BC, Williams R. Prevalence and pattern of familial disease in primary biliary cirrhosis. Gut. 1995;36:615–17.
49. Bach N, Schaffner F. Prevalence of primary biliary cirrhosis in family members of affected patients. Gastroenterology. 1991;102:A776.
50. Jones DE, Watt FE, Metcalf JV, Bassendine MF, James OF. Familial primary biliary cirrhosis reassessed: a geographically-based population study. J Hepatol. 1999;30:402–7.
51. Roll J, Boyer JL, Barry D et al. The prognostic importance of clinical and histological features in asymptomatic and symptomatic primary biliary cirrhosis. N Engl J Med. 1983;308:1–7.
52. Christensen E, Altman DG, Neuberger J, De Stavola BL, Tygstrup N, Williams R. Updating prognosis in primary biliary cirrhosis using a time-dependent Cox regression model. Gastroenterology. 1993;105:1865–76.
53. Dickson ER, Grambsch PM, Fleming TR, Fisher LD, Langworthy A. Prognosis in primary biliary cirrhosis: model for decision making. Hepatology. 1989;10:1–7.
54. Grambsch PM, Dickson ER, Kaplan M, LeSage G, Fleming TR, Langworthy AL. Extramural cross-validation of the Mayo primary biliary cirrhosis survival model establishes its generalizability. Hepatology. 1989;10:846–50.
55. Invernizzi P, Podda M, Battezzati PM et al. Autoantibodies against nuclear pore complexes are associated with more active and severe liver disease in primary biliary cirrhosis. J Hepatol. 2001;34:366–72.
56. Donaldson P, Agarwal K, Craggs A, Craig W, James O, Jones D. HLA and interleukin 1 gene polymorphisms in primary biliary cirrhosis: associations with disease progression and disease susceptibility. Gut. 2001;48:397–402.
57. Joshi S, Cauch-Dudek K, Heathcote EJ, Lindor K, Jorgensen R, Klein R. Antimitochondrial antibody profiles: are they valid prognostic indicators in primary biliary cirrhosis? Am J Gastroenterol. 2002;97:999–1002.
58. Klein R, Kloppel G, Garbe W et al. Antimitochondrial antibody profiles determined at early stages of primary biliary cirrhosis differentiate between a benign and a progressive course of the disease: a retrospective analysis of 76 patients over 6–18 years. J Hepatol. 1991;12:21–7.
59. Klein R, Pointer H, Zilly W et al. Antimitochondrial antibody profiles in primary biliary cirrhosis distinguish at early stages between a benign and a progressive course: a prospective study in 200 patients followed for 10 years. Liver. 1997;17:119–28.
60. Metcalf JV, Mitchison HC, Palmer JM, Jones DE, Bassendine MF, James OFW. Natural history of early primary biliary cirrhosis. Lancet. 1996;348:1399–402.
61. Long RG, Scheuer PJ, Sherlock S. Presentation and course of asymptomatic primary biliary cirrhosis. Gastroenterology. 1977;72:1204–7.
62. Mitchison HC, Lucey MR, Kelly PJ, Neuberger JM, Williams R, James OFW. Symptom development and prognosis in primary biliary cirrhosis: a study in two centres. Gastroenterology. 1990;99:778–84.
63. Balasubramaniam K, Grambsch PM, Wiesner RH, Lindor KD, Dickson ER. Diminished survival in primary biliary cirrhosis. Gastroenterology. 1990;98:1567–71.
64. Springer J, Cauch-Dudek K, O'Rourke K, Wanless IR, Heathcote EJ. Asymptomatic primary biliary cirrhosis: a study of its natural history and prognosis. Am J Gstroenterol. 1999;94:47–53.

65. Foulk WT, Baggenstoss AH, Butt HR. Primary biliary cirrhosis: reevaluation by clinical and histologic study of 49 cases. Gastroenterology. 1964;47:354–74.
66. Sherlock S. Primary biliary cirrhosis (chronic intrahepatic obstructive jaundice). Gastroenterology. 1959;37:574–86.
67. Loof L, Adami HO, Sparen P et al. Cancer risk in primary biliary cirrhosis: a population-based study from Sweden. Hepatology. 1994;20:101–4.
68. Jones DE, Metcalf JV, Collier JD et al. Hepatocellular carcinoma in primary biliary cirrhosis and its impact on outcomes. Hepatology. 1997;26:1138–42.
69. Melia WM, Johnson PJ, Neuberger J et al. Hepatocellular carcinoma in primary biliary cirrhosis: detection by alfa-fetoprotein estimation. Gastroenterology. 1984;87:660–3.
70. Farinati F, Floreani A, De Maria N et al. Hepatocellular carcinoma in primary biliary cirrhosis. J Hepatol. 1994;21:315–16.
71. Shibuya A, Tanaka K, Mikyakawa H et al. for the PBC Forum 21. Hepatocellular carcinoma and survival in patients with primary biliary cirrhosis. Hepatology. 2002;35:1172–8.
72. Caballeria L, Pares A, Castells A, Gines A, Bru C, Rodes J. Hepatocellular carcinoma in primary biliary cirrhosis: similar incidence to that in hepatitis C virus-related cirrhosis. Am J Gastroenterol. 2001;96:1160–3.
73. Longo M, Crosignani, Battezzati PM et al. Hyperlipidaemic state and cardiovascular risk in primary biliary cirrhosis. Gut. 2002;51:265–9.
74. Crippin JS, Lindor KD, Jorgensen R et al. Hypercholesterolemia and atherosclerosis in primary biliary cirrhosis: what is the risk? Hepatology. 1992;15:858–62.
75. Van Dam GM, Gips CH. Primary biliary cirrhosis in the Netherlands. An analysis of associated diseases, cardiovascular risk and malignancies on the basis of mortality figures. Scand J Gastroenterol. 1997;32:77–83.
76. O'Kane MJ, Lynch PL, Callender ME, Trimble ER. Abnormalities of serum apo A1 containing lipoprotein particles in patients with primary biliary cirrhosis. Atherosclerosis. 1997;131:203–10.
77. Propst A, Propst T, Lechleitner M et al. Hypercholesterolemia in primary biliary cirrhosis is no risk factor for atherosclerosis. Dig Dis Sci. 1993;38:379–80.

9
Pathogenesis of pruritus and fatigue in cholestatic liver disease

M. G. SWAIN

OVERVIEW

Patients with cholestatic liver diseases commonly complain of fatigue and pruritus[1,2]; however, because these complaints are subjective in nature, and difficult to quantify, research into the pathogenesis of fatigue and pruritus in cholestasis has been significantly hampered. Moreover, the study of these symptoms has been made even more difficult by the problems associated with studying subjective human complaints in animal models of cholestasis. However, both pruritus and fatigue involve perception and as such by definition are related to neural activity.

In studying pruritus and fatigue one question clearly stands out: how does the cholestatic syndrome, with its complex combination of liver damage and retention of substances in the blood which are normally eliminated in bile, lead to changes in peripheral nerves as well as changes within the central nervous system (CNS)? In addition, how do these neural changes ultimately give rise to abnormal perceptions such as fatigue and pruritus (Figure 1)?

Therefore, any discussion of the pathogenesis of fatigue and pruritus in cholestasis needs to address this link between peripheral changes occurring in cholestasis with changes which must be occurring at the level of the neuron within the CNS. Moreover, the specific pathways of communication between the 'periphery' and the CNS need to be considered and defined.

PRURITUS IN CHOLESTATIC LIVER DISEASE

Clinical setting

Pruritus is commonly encountered in patients with cholestatic liver diseases such as primary biliary cirrhosis (PBC) and primary sclerosing cholangitis (PSC),

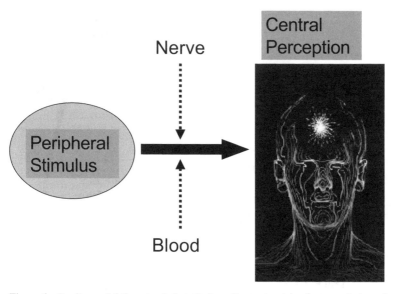

Figure 1 Pruritus and fatigue in cholestatic liver disease involves the transmission of peripheral stimuli or signals, either through nerves or by substances carried in the blood, to the brain. These signals ultimately stimulate areas of the brain which are ultimately responsible for the conscious perception of symptoms such as pruritus and fatigue

affecting the majority of patients. Specifically, pruritus occurs in up to 65% of patients with PBC and up to 61% of patients with PSC[1–3]. Moreover, pruritus is directly correlated with decreases in health-related quality of life in cholestatic patients[2]. Pruritus can be so severe and refractory that it can be an indication for liver transplantation[4]. The presence or degree of pruritus does not correlate with cholestatic disease severity, although interestingly pruritus has been reported to disappear in some patients with end-stage PBC despite the persistence of profound cholestasis.

Pathogenesis

The pathogenesis of pruritus in cholestasis remains unknown; however, any theory put forward to explain the development of cholestasis-related itch must incorporate a peripheral pruritogen(s), possible peripheral itch-augmenting substances, neural itch pathways, and central itch modulators (Figure 2). Traditionally, cholestasis-associated itch has been postulated as resulting from the interaction of free unmyelinated cutaneous nerve endings with a substance(s) retained in the circulation as part of the cholestatic syndrome. The likely nerve involved in this process is the recently defined unmyelinated 'itch' C-fibre, which appears to specifically carry itch impulses from the skin to the dorsal horn of the spinal cord[5,6]. Spinal projections then carry the itch signals in the contralateral spinothalamic tract to the thalamus and ultimately to the somatosensory cortex[7]. These central neural connections in pruritus allow for the

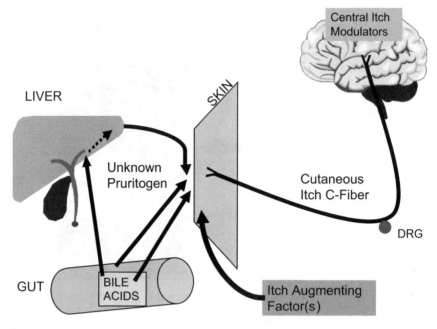

Figure 2 In cholestatic pruritus a peripheral pruritogen stimulates cutaneous C fibres which transmit itch signals. The peripheral pruritogen is unknown, but may be bile acids retained in cholestasis, a pruritogen released from liver cells by the detergent action of bile acids on liver cells, or an as-yet-unrecognized pruritogenic substance. In addition, a number of circulating or cutaneous factors may act to augment the action of the cholestatic pruritogen by enhancing the stimulation of cutaneous itch C fibres. Ultimately the 'itch nerves' carry the itch signal from the skin to the brain where the sensation of itch is ultimately perceived by the individual. However, in the brain other factors may act as itch modulators (e.g. endogenous opioids) by altering the perception or appreciation of the itch sensation

central modulation of the itch sensation, as well as the potential for pruritus caused *de novo* by a central (i.e. not peripheral) stimulus[7,8].

Peripheral itch inducers

Bile acids

Traditionally bile acids retained in the body in cholestatic liver disease and interacting with cutaneous nerve endings have been directly implicated in the genesis of cholestasis-associated itch (Figure 2). A role of bile acids in this light has significant clinical support. Specifically, pruritus is typically relieved or significantly reduced in the majority of cholestatic patients given the non-absorbable anion-binding resin cholestyramine (which binds bile salts in the gut lumen and prevents their resorption). In addition, bile acids accumulate in the skin of cholestatic patients and bile acids can induce pruritus when administered to healthy volunteers[11-13]. Moreover, biliary drainage and biliary diversion can ameliorate cholestasis-associated pruritus[14].

Other clinical observations have cast doubt on skin bile acids being the sole pruritogen in cholestasis. Specifically, skin bile acid levels do not appear to correlate with the presence or absence of pruritus in cholestatic patients[15]. In addition, pruritus can disappear rarely in patients with end-stage PBC despite the presence of very high serum bile acid levels, and non-pruritic cholestatic patients may have high serum bile acid levels[16].

More recently Cam Ghent has proposed that bile acids do not act directly as pruritogens, but act at the level of the hepatocyte membrane to release a substance(s) which is the true pruritogen in cholestasis[17] (Figure 2).

Histamine

Histamine is a classical pruritogen, being first recognized as such in the 1920s. Histamine is released from activated mast cells, and cholestatic patients have elevated circulating histamine levels[18], in addition to evidence of increased cutaneous mast cell numbers associated with degranulation in cholestatic rats[19]. Typically histamine-induced itch is associated with a cutaneous wheal-and-flare response; a response conspicuously absent in pruritic cholestatic patients. Moreover antihistamines, although widely used clinically to treat cholestatic pruritus, are poorly efficacious in relieving itch, and any clinical effectiveness they exhibit has been attributed by some as being due solely to their sedative effects[20]. These observations suggest that histamine is unlikely to act as a direct pruritogen in cholestatic patients. Interestingly, bile acids can induce histamine release from mast cells[21].

Peripheral itch augmentors

Mast cell products

Mast cells accumulate in the skin[19] and liver[22,23] during cholestatic liver disease. In addition, elevated serum histamine levels and evidence of cutaneous mast cell degranulation have been reported in PBC patients and in experimental cholestasis[18,19]. Bile acids can also directly induce mast cell degranulation[21]. These observations all support the suggestion that cholestasis is associated with mast cell activation and degranulation. Mast cells produce and release a number of substances which are known to act as itch 'augmentors', instead of being directly pruritogenic (Figure 2).

1. Histamine: histamine acts as a direct pruritogen, associated with a cutaneous wheal-and-flare reaction; however, histamine may also act in a facilitatory fashion with regard to other pruritic stimuli[24,25].
2. Tryptase: mast cells can release tryptase which is capable of activating proteinase-activated receptor 2 (PAR2)[26,27]; moreover, PAR2 is present on C-fibre terminals, and stimulation of PAR2 has been shown to excite afferent C fibres[26,27]. Therefore, mast cell tryptase may facilitate C-fibre activation produced by other direct pruritogens.
3. Prostaglandins: mast cells represent a rich source of prostaglandins; moreover, prostaglandins of the E series have been shown to potentiate histamine-induced itch[28,29]. In addition, PBC is associated with enhanced PGE2 production[30], suggesting a potential role of prostaglandins as itch 'augmentors' in cholestatic patients.
4. Tumour necrosis factor (TNF)-α: mast cells, in addition to other immune cell populations, produce and secrete TNF-α; moreover, serum TNF-α levels are

elevated in PBC patients[31,32]. Although it has not been studied with regard to pruritus, TNF-α has been shown to sensitize nerve endings of nociceptive C fibres in the skin[7]; therefore, if TNF-α had similar effects on 'itch' C fibres it could potentially act as a peripheral itch-augmenting factor.

Opioids

Circulating levels of endogenous opioids are elevated in patients with cholestasis, as well as in experimental models of cholestatic liver injury[33,34]; however, pruritus in cholestatic patients does not appear to directly correlate with circulating endogenous opioid levels[35]. Opioids can activate mast cells, and in this fashion potentially augment other pruritogenic stimuli such as histamine[36]; however, opioid receptors have been documented on nerve endings of nociceptive C fibres[37], as well as on nerve cell bodies in the dorsal root ganglion[38]. Opioids can act on these peripheral neuronal receptors to directly modulate nociception[37,38]; therefore one might speculate that raised levels of circulating opioids in cholestasis may act peripherally to augment itch. Interestingly, histamine-induced cutaneous itch is significantly enhanced by the intradermal injection of a stable met-enkephalin analogue, although this effect was not abolished by pretreatment with the opioid receptor blocker naloxone[39].

Central itch modulators

The perception of itch in pruritic cholestatic patients can be modulated by input from higher centres within the CNS (Figure 2). Clinically this is evidenced in cholestatic patients as alterations in itch perception depending on the time of day or how occupied a patient's mind is. Specifically, cholestatic patients often describe their itch as being worse at night when their minds are clear, just before sleep. During the day, when their minds are distracted, their itch is less. Scratching activity in pruritic cholestatic patients appears to follow a diurnal rhythm[40]; therefore there must be neural pathways within the CNS which subserve a central itch-modulatory role. Endogenous opioids have been postulated as playing a major role as central itch modulators, and a significant body of research has provided evidence of enhanced opioidergic tone within the CNS of cholestatic patients. Specifically, the administration of the opioid receptor blockers naloxone and naltrexone to pruritic cholestatic patients results in the significant amelioration of pruritus, as well as the development of an opiate withdrawal-like syndrome in some patients[40,41]. Experimental cholestasis in the rat is associated with naloxone-reversible analgesia coupled with a down-regulation of central μ opioid receptor expression[42,43]. These findings are consistent with enhanced opioid peptide release within the brain in cholestasis.

The question which arises from the above observations is: how do opioids released within the CNS modulate itch? Certainly the induction of itch by centrally administered opiates, such as morphine, is widely recognized, as is the naloxone reversibility of this effect[44]; therefore, is the pruritus observed in cholestatic patients due to a direct central opioid-driven pruritic effect analogous to that observed with spinal opiates? This seems unlikely. With opiate-induced pruritus (e.g. spinal morphine) the facial areas innervated by the trigeminal nerve are predominantly affected[45]; however, in cholestatic patients this distribution of pruritus is uncommon. Typically, cholestatic pruritus is more generalized and often felt initially on the palms of the hands and soles of the feet. In addition, opioid receptor blockade is not effective in ameliorating pruritus in all cholestatic pruritic patients, suggesting that other factors are involved. Finally, pruritus induced by the intravenous injection of morphine is reduced by an opioid receptor blocker which does not penetrate the CNS[45].

Endogenous opioids released within the brain in cholestatic patients therefore probably play a modulating role with respect to pruritus. It is known that centrally acting pain inhibiting opioids enhance itch by disinhibition[7,44,46]; therefore scratching in pruritic cholestatic patients would activate pain receptors and related neural pathways. Activation of pain pathways is known to inhibit itch; therefore the inhibition of pain processing by central opioid release may decrease the inhibitory effect of pain on neural itch pathways, and subsequently increase the perception of itch[7,47]. This hypothesis could account for the positive ameliorating effect of opioid receptor blockers on cholestatic itch.

Pruritus summary

Pruritus in cholestatic patients is a common problem significantly affecting a patient's quality of life. Although the exact aetiology of pruritus in cholestasis is still unclear, progress is being made in our understanding of this distressing symptom. It appears that pruritus results from a peripheral pruritogen, potentially bile acids, activating cutaneous itch C fibres possibly in conjunction with other substances which accumulate in cholestasis and which augment the itch response. These activated itch fibres transmit pruritic signals to the brain, where their perception is altered by itch modulators such as endogenous opioids. Targeting these abnormalities will provide improved therapeutic approaches to pruritus in cholestatic patients.

FATIGUE IN CHOLESTATIC LIVER DISEASE

Clinical setting

Fatigue is a symptom which may be described by patients as lethargy, malaise, lassitude, or exhaustion. Given its subjective nature, fatigue is difficult to quantify and is therefore often overlooked or minimized by physicians treating cholestatic patients. Moreover, fatigue is the most commonly encountered symptom in patients with cholestatic liver diseases[1–3,47]. Fatigue can be minimal or so severe as to significantly impair a patient's quality of life. In patients with PBC, fatigue constitutes the worst symptom in about 50% of patients, and in 25% of patients it is felt to be severely disabling[2,48]. Fatigue scores in PBC patients, as determined by questionnaires, are similar to those encountered in patients with multiple sclerosis and lupus[48]. In cholestatic patients the fatigue does not correlate with disease stage or liver biochemistries and does not improve with ursodeoxycholic acid therapy[48,49].

When discussing fatigue it is important to differentiate central from peripheral fatigue, although the two forms of fatigue can coexist. Peripheral fatigue relates to neuromuscular dysfunction (i.e. outside the CNS) and can result from overutilization of muscles or disease. Central fatigue, on the other hand, is due to altered neurotransmitter pathways within the CNS (reviewed in ref. 45). Patients with cholestatic liver disease often describe problems initiating exertion or activity, despite their desire to be active. Moreover, electromyography (EMG) studies in PBC patients are normal[51]. These observations are consistent with fatigue in cholestatic liver disease as being central in origin. In addition, fatigue in cholestatic patients correlates closely with other complaints typically associated with altered neurotransmission, namely depression and anxiety[48,49].

A recent report suggests that fatigued PBC patients exhibit diminished grip strength compared to non-fatigued PBC patients and normal controls[52]. Although baseline grip strength was similar in all three groups, the grip strength in fatigued PBC patients decreased to a greater extent upon repeated testing than it did in the other two groups[52]. In addition, grip strength reduction per test repeat correlated significantly with patient fatigue scores obtained on questionnaire. In light of the previous report of normal EMG studies in PBC patients, the observation of reduced grip strength with repeated testing probably reflects a failure in the central neural drive which is required for sustained or repeated muscle contraction[53]; however, these findings are of interest and warrant further exploration.

Pathogenesis

The pathogenesis of fatigue, in general, is poorly understood, and this holds true for fatigue in cholestatic patients. However, in cholestatic liver disease fatigue appears to be the result of altered central neurotransmission; therefore any discussion of the pathogenesis of cholestasis-related fatigue needs to incorporate two main concepts: first, how does the retention of substances normally secreted in bile, in addition to associated liver damage, signal the brain to cause changes in central neurotransmission? Secondly, what changes in central neurotransmission occur in the context of cholestatic liver disease and how do these changes give rise to fatigue?

Liver-to-brain signalling

Communication between the periphery and the CNS traditionally has been considered to involve neural (i.e. nerve projections) and/or humoral (i.e. substances within the circulation) pathways[54]. In the setting of cholestatic liver disease, either or both pathways may be involved.

Neural pathways. The liver is a richly innervated organ, with afferent signals being carried from the liver to the brain in the vagus nerve as well as in spinal nerve projections[55,56]. Intraperitoneal inflammation induces the expression of FOS (a neuronal activation marker) in the brain of rodents, in conjunction with the development of behaviours consistent with fatigue[57,58]; however, these effects are abolished by subdiaphragmatic vagotomy[58]. FOS expression induced within the brain by intraperitoneal inflammation initially occurs in the nucleus tractus solitarius (NTS), the main relay centre for nerve impulses travelling from the periphery to the brain via the vagus nerve[60].

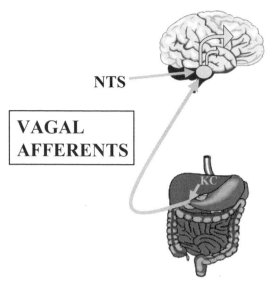

NTS

VAGAL AFFERENTS

Figure 3 Fatigue in cholestatic liver disease may result from the activation of Kupffer cells (KC) within the liver and subsequent release of inflammatory mediators (e.g. IL-1β) which stimulate vagus nerve endings within the liver. The vagus nerve then transmits these signals to the nucleus tractus solitarius (NTS; the midbrain vagal nerve relay centre) and ultimately the signals are carried to higher centres within the brain. Ultimately, these signals alter central neurotransmission to give rise to fatigue or lethargy

Cholestatic liver injury is associated with the increased production of a number of inflammatory mediators, including the cytokines IL-1β, TNF-α, and IL-6[61]. Infusion of IL-1β into the portal vein of rats results in increased electrical activity in the hepatic branch of the vagus nerve[62]. In addition, the intraperitoneal injection of endotoxin or IL-1β in rodents causes changes in neurotransmitter levels within the brain which have been implicated in the genesis of fatigue (i.e. CRH, see below); an effect blocked by subdiaphragmatic vagotomy[63,64].

These observations implicate neural pathways in the communication between the liver and the brain to produce fatigue in cholestatic patients (Figure 3); however, patients with end-stage primary biliary cirrhosis who undergo liver transplantation can exhibit fatigue levels similar to those documented pre-transplant[65]. Given that liver transplantation results in complete denervation of the liver, this observation suggests that neural pathways may not play a major role in the genesis of cholestasis-associated fatigue; however, cytokine receptors (i.e. for IL-1β) exist on hepatic vagal nerves themselves, and these may still be stimulated[66]. In addition, patients who are post-transplant have a number of ongoing, often significant, psychological issues, in addition to their need to ingest a large number of medications, all of which may contribute to fatigue.

Humoral Pathways. Liver-to-brain signalling may occur via mediators released into the circulation from the damaged liver (e.g. cytokines) or retained in the

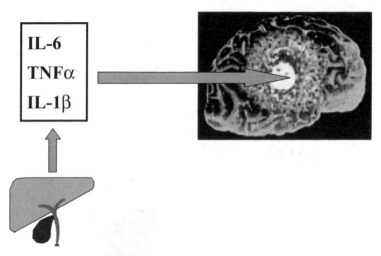

Figure 4 Fatigue in cholestatic liver disease may result from the release of substances into the circulation (e.g. cytokines such as IL-1β, TNF-α, IL-6) from the diseased liver. These circulating substances would interact with cerebral endothelial cells to induce the release of secondary messengers (e.g. PGE$_2$ or nitric oxide), which then would cause alterations in neurotransmission within the brain to ultimately give rise to fatigue

circulation as part of the cholestatic syndrome (e.g. manganese). With regard to the mediators of humoral signalling of damaged tissues to the brain, cytokines have received the greatest attention[67,68]; moreover, the liver contains the largest fixed macrophage population in the body, which represents a rich source of inflammatory mediators, including cytokines. The cytokines which have received the greatest scientific attention in relation to periphery-to-brain signalling include IL-1β, IL-6 and TNF-α[67,68] (Figure 4). In patients and rodents with cholestatic liver injury circulating IL-6 and TNF-α levels are increased[61,69,70]; moreover, plasma endotoxin levels are elevated in PBC patients[71] and rodents with experimental cholestasis[72]. In addition, the intravenous administration of endotoxin and cytokines produces fatigue-like behaviours (e.g. decreased locomotion, lethargy, decreased social exploration) in rodents (reviewed in ref. 73); furthermore, intravenous cytokine or endotoxin administration in rodents results in altered central neurotransmitter levels (e.g. CRH, serotonin) which have been implicated in fatigue[63,64,74].

The blood–brain barrier represents a significant barrier to cytokine and/or endotoxin entrance into the brain; moreover, in rats with experimental cholestatic liver disease blood–brain barrier permeability is decreased[75], making the direct penetration of the brain by circulating substances appear even less likely in cholestasis. However, there are well-recognized areas of the brain which are devoid of an intact blood–brain barrier[76], and these areas could represent potential areas for cytokines to enter the brain. In addition, cerebral endothelial cells and perivascular cells express receptors for a number of inflammatory mediators, and can be activated by cytokines and endotoxin to produce a variety of secondary messengers[67,68,77–79]. These secondary messengers include PGE$_2$ and nitric oxide, both of which are capable of inducing changes in central neurotransmission[67,68]. In addition, circulating cytokines and endotoxin can induce the *de-novo* synthesis and release of cytokines within the brain[67,68,73]. Interestingly, cholestatic rats exhibit an enhanced sensitivity to behavioural depression induced by the central administration of IL-1β compared to non-cholestatic controls[80]. These observations support the existence of a humoral–immune communication pathway between the liver and the brain in cholestatic liver disease as potentially contributing to cholestasis-associated fatigue.

Interestingly, a recent report has implicated manganese (normally secreted in bile) retention and accumulation in the globus pallidus of the brain in the genesis of fatigue in PBC patients[81]. These investigators found that fatigue scores in their patients correlated with blood manganese levels, as well as with a reduction in globus pallidus magnetization transfer ratios on brain scanning[81]. Given that manganese toxicity is associated with lethargy, these findings are provocative and warrant further exploration.

Central neurotransmitter changes

Whatever mediators or pathways drive altered liver-to-brain signalling in cholestasis, the ultimate cause of central fatigue in cholestatic liver disease must entail alterations in neurotransmitter systems within the brain which underlie behavioural activation. A number of neurotransmitter systems have been directly linked to behavioural activation, and defects in these systems to fatigue states. The neurotransmitter systems which have received the greatest attention with regard to central fatigue are the corticotropin-releasing hormone (CRH) and serotonin systems (reviewed in ref. 82).

CRH system and central fatigue

CRH was identified initially as the most potent activator on the hypothalamic–pituitary–adrenal (HPA) axis; however, later it became apparent that CRH-containing nerve fibres project throughout the brain and are intimately involved in the coordination of a number of behaviours, including behavioural activation[83,84]. Specifically, the central infusion of CRH in rodents induces increased arousal and locomotor activity[85]. These observations led to the hypothesis that defective central CRH release could lead to fatigue; a hypothesis supported by clinical observation in patients with chronic fatigue syndrome and atypical depression[86,87]; moreover, defective central CRH release may occur in patients with PBC. Specifically, PBC patients demonstrate enhanced pituitary ACTH release when CRH is administered intravenously; a finding consistent with decreased central CRH stimulation of the anterior pituitary leading to increased pituitary sensitivity to exogenous CRH stimulation[88]. These clinical observations in PBC patients have been supported by data from rodent models of cholestatic liver injury. Cholestatic rats exhibit decreased brain CRH protein and mRNA levels[89], behaviours which are consistent with decreased central CRH release[90], and increased sensitivity to the behavioural activating effects of centrally infused CRH coupled to increased levels of CRH type 1 receptors, the CRH receptor type mediating behavioural activation induced by CRH in their brains[91]. These observations implicate defective CRH-mediated behavioural activation in the genesis of cholestasis-associated fatigue; moreover, peripheral administration of cytokines and endotoxin in rodents directly impacts central CRH levels[59,63,64], suggesting that a similar effect may occur in the setting of cholestatic liver disease.

Serotonergic system and central fatigue

Altered central serotonergic neurotransmission has also been linked to the genesis of central fatigue[92]. Interestingly, the CRH and serotonergic neurotransmitter systems are intimately interrelated within the brain[59,60]. Serotonergic nerve fibres in the brain originate mainly from the midbrain dorsal raphe nucleus and project widely throughout the brain. These serotonin-containing nerve fibres directly innervate CRH-containing neurons within the hypothalamus and activation of these CRH neurons involves, at least in part, stimulation by these serotonergic neurons[93].

The role played by serotonin in the genesis of central fatigue in unclear. Both increased and decreased central serotonergic neurotransmission have been implicated in fatigue states. Specifically, rodents exercised to exhaustion exhibit increased central serotonin levels[94]. In addition, athletes given serotonin re-uptake inhibitors (i.e. increase central serotonin levels) have diminished exercise capacity[95]. These findings suggest that increased central serotonin release may contribute to fatigue. In contrast, patients with chronic fatigue syndrome exhibit enhanced central responses to serotonin receptor agonists, suggesting increased central serotonin sensitivity in these patients secondary to decreased serotonin release in the brain[96]; moreover, serotonin re-uptake inhibitors have been used clinically to treat patients with fatigue states, albeit with mixed results[97].

Serotonin produces its biological effects by interacting with numerous different receptor subtypes[98]. The serotonin receptor subtype involved in central serotonin–fatigue pathway(s) is at present unclear. 5-HT$_{1A}$ receptors exist on serotonin nerve cell bodies in the midbrain dorsal raphe nucleus, and stimulation of these receptors decreases serotonin release within the brain[98]; however, with repeated stimulation these receptors are rapidly desensitized[99]. Rats with experimental cholestasis demonstrate increased midbrain 5-HT$_{1A}$ receptor number and responsiveness[100]. In addition, repeated administration of a 5-HT$_{1A}$ agonist to cholestatic rats (desensitizes midbrain 5-HT$_{1A}$ receptors and thereby increases central serotonin release) ameliorates fatigue-like behaviours in these animals[101]. These observations highlight the potential importance of serotonergic neurotransmission, and the 5-HT$_{1A}$ receptor subtype, in the genesis of cholestasis-associated fatigue.

Recently the 5-HT$_3$ receptor antagonist ondansetron was reported as improving fatigue in a hepatitis C patient with cirrhosis[102]. Similar findings have been reported in fatigued PBC patients[103]. The precise role played by 5-HT$_3$ receptors in the brain is unclear, but these results suggest that 5-HT$_3$ receptor activation contributes to liver disease-associated fatigue and warrants further exploration.

Other neurotransmitter systems

A number of other central neurotransmitter systems have been implicated in behavioural activation, locomotion and fatigue; including the norepinephrine and dopamine systems[104,105]; however, these systems have not been examined with regard to the development of central fatigue in general, and cholestasis-associated fatigue in particular, but warrant further investigation.

Fatigue summary

Fatigue is a common and often disabling symptom in patients with cholestatic liver disease. Although the cause of fatigue in these patients remains unclear, it seems apparent that it involves a complex interplay between signals generated from the diseased liver (and/or via substances retained in the blood) in cholestasis and brain neurotransmitter pathways which are important in behavioural activation. By better defining these signalling and neurotransmitter pathways, novel and effective therapies may be developed to treat fatigue in the setting of cholestatic liver disease.

References

1. Witt-Sullivan M, Heathcote J, Cauch K et al. The demography of primary biliary cirrhosis in Ontario, Canada. Hepatology. 1990;12:98–105.
2. Younossi ZM, Kiwi ML, Bopari N, Price LL, Guyatt G. Cholestatic liver diseases and health-related quality of life. Am J Gastroenterol. 2000;95:497–502.
3. van Hoogstraten MJF, Vleggar FP, Boland GJ et al. Budesonide or prednisone in combination with ursodeoxycholic acid in primary sclerosing cholangitis: a randomized double blind pilot study. Am J Gastroenterol. 2000;95:2015–22.
4. Neuberger J, Jones EA. Liver transplantation for intractable pruritus is contraindicated before an adequate trial of opiate antagonist therapy. Eur J Gastroenterol Hepatol. 2001;13:1393–4.
5. Schmelz M, Schmidt R, Bickel A, Handwerker HO, Torebjork HE. Specific C-receptors for itch in human skin. J Neurosci. 1997;17:8003–8.
6. Andrew D, Craig AD. Spinothalamic lamina 1 neurons selectively sensitize to histamine: a central neural pathway for itch. Nat Neurosci. 2001;4:72–7.
7. Yosipovitch G, Greaves MW, Schmelz J. Itch. Lancet. 2003;361:690–4.
8. Twycross R, Greaves MW, Handwerker H et al. Itch: scratching more than the surface. Q J Med. 2003;96:7–26.
9. Mela M, Mancuso A, Burroughs AB. Review article: Pruritus in cholestatic and other liver diseases. Aliment Pharmacol Ther. 2003;17:857–70.
10. Datta DV, Sherlock S. Cholestyramine for long term relief of the pruritus complicating intra-hepatic cholestasis. Gastroenterology. 1966;50:323–32.
11. Schoenfield LJ, Sjovall J, Perman E. Bile acids on the skin of patients with pruritic hepatobiliary disease. Nature. 1967;213:93–4.
12. Stiehl A. Bile acids and bile acid sulfates in the skin of patients with cholestasis and pruritus. Z Gastroeneterol. 1974;12:121–4.
13. Kirby J, Heaton KW, Button JL. Pruritic effect of bile salts. Br Med J. 1974;4:693–5.
14. Whitington PF, Whitington GL. Partial external diversion of bile for the treatment of intractable pruritus associated with intrahepatic cholestasis. Gastroenterology. 1988;95:130–6.
15. Bartholomew TC, Summerfield JA, Billing BH, Lawson AM, Setchell KD. Bile acid profiles of human serum and skin interstitial fluid and their relationship to pruritus studied by gas chromatography–mass spectrometry. Clin Sci. 1982;63:65–73.
16. Murphy GM, Ross A, Billing BH. Serum bile acids in primary biliary cirrhosis. Gut. 1972;13:201–6.
17. Ghent CN. Pruritus of cholestasis is related to effects of bile salts on the liver, not the skin. Am J Gastroenterol. 1987;82:117–18.
18. Gittlen SC, Schulman ES, Maddrey WV. Raised histamine concentrations in chronic cholestatic liver disease. Gut. 1990;31:96–9.
19. Clements WD, O'Rourke DM, Rolands BJ, Ennis M. The role of mast cell activation in cholestatic pruritus. Agents Actions. 1994;41:C30–1.

20. Simons FE, Watson WT, Chen XY, Minuk GY, Simons KJ. The pharmacokinetics and pharmacodynamics of hydroxyzine in patients with primary biliary cirrhosis. J Clin Pharmacol. 1989;29:809–15.

21. Quist RG, Ton-Nu HT, Lillienau J, Hormann AF, Barrett KE. Activation of mast cells by bile acids. Gastroenterology. 1991;101:446–56.

22. Farrell DJ, Hines JE, Walls AF, Kelly PJ, Bennett MK, Burt AD. Intrahepatic mast cells in chronic liver diseases. Hepatology. 1995;22:1175–81.

23. Rioux KP, Sharkey KA, Wallace JL, Swain MG. Hepatic mucosal mast cell hyperplasia in rats with secondary biliary cirrhosis. Hepatology. 1996;23:888–95.

24. Jinks SL, Carstens E. Spiral NMDA receptor involvement in expansion of dorsal horn neuronal receptive field area produced by intracutaneous histamine. J Neurophysiol. 1998;79:1613–18.

25. Carstens E. Responses of rat spiral dorsal horn neurons to intracutaneous microinjection of histamine, capsaicin and other irritants. J Neurophysiol. 1997;77:2499–514.

26. Kirkup AJ, Jiang W, Bunnett NW, Grundy D. Stimulation of the proteinase-activated receptor 2 excites jejunal afferent nerves in anaesthetized rats. J Physiol. 2003 (In press).

27. Steinhoff M, Neisius U, Ikoma A et al. Proteinase-activated receptor 2 mediates itch: a novel pathway for pruritus in human skin. J Neurosci. 2003;23:6176–80.

28. Lovell CR, Burton PA, Duncan EH, Burton JC. Prostaglandins and pruritus. Br J Dermatol. 1976;94:273–5.

29. Hagermark O, Strandberg K. Pruritogenic activity of prostaglandin E2. Acta Derm Venereol. 1977;57:37–43.

30. Chiricolo M, Lenzi M, Bianchi F et al. Immune dysfunction in primary biliary cirrhosis. II. Increased production of prostaglandin E. Scand J Immunol. 1989;30:363–7.

31. Hokari A, Zeniya M, Esumi H, Kawabe T, Gershwin ME, Toda G. Detection of serum nitrite and nitrate in primary biliary cirrhosis; possible role of nitric oxide in bile duct injury. J Gastroenterol Hepatol. 2002;17:308–15.

32. Neuman M, Angulo P, Malkiewicz I et al. Tumor necrosis factor-alpha and transforming growth factor-beta reflect severity of liver damage in primary biliary chirrhosis. J Gastroenterol Hepatol. 2002;17:196–202.

33. Thornton JR, Lasowsky MS. Plasma methionine enkephalin concentration and prognosis in primary biliary cirrhosis. Br Med J. 1988;297:1241–2.

34. Swain MG, Rothman RB, Xu H, Vergalla J, Bergasa NW, Jones EA. Endogenous opioids accumulate in plasma in a rat model of acute cholestasis. Gastroenterology. 1992;103:630–5.

35. Spivey JR, Jorgensen RA, Gores GJ, Lindor KD. Methionine–enkephalin concentration correlate with stage of disease but not pruritus in patients with primary biliary cirrhosis. Am J Gastroenterol. 1994;89:2028–32.

36. Barke KE, Hough LB. Opiates, mast cells and histamine release. Life Sci. 1993;53:1391–9.

37. Machelska H, Stein C. Pain control by immune-derived opioids. Clin Exp Pharmacol Physiol. 2000;27:533–6.

38. Stein C, Schafer M, Hassan AH. Peripheral opioid receptors. Ann Med. 1995;27:219–21.

39. Fjellner B, Hagermark O. Potentiation of histamine-induced itch and flare responses in human skin by the enkephalin analogue FK-33-824, beta endorphin and morphine. Arch Dermatol Res. 1982;274:29–37.

40. Bergasa NV, Alling DW, Talbot TL et al. Effects of naloxone infusions in patients with the pruritus of cholestasis. A double-blind, randomized, controlled trial. Ann Intern Med. 1995; 123:161–7.

41. Wolfhagen FH, Sternieri E, Hop WC et al. Oral naltrexone treatment of cholestatic pruritus: a double-blind, placebo controlled study. Gastroenterology. 1997;113:1264–9.

42. Bergasa NV, Alling DW, Vergalla J, Jones EA. Cholestasis in the male rat is associated with raloxone-reversible antinociception. J Hepatol. 1994;20:85–90.

43. Bergasa NV, Rothman RB, Vergalla J, Xu H, Swain MG, Jones EA. Central mu-opioid receptors are down-regulated in a rat model of acute cholestases. J Hepatol. 1992;15:220–4.

44. Szarvas S, Harmon D, Murphy D. Neuraxial opioid-induced pruritus: a review. J Clin Anesth. 2003;15:234–9.

45. Yuan C-S, Foss JF, O'Connor M, Osinski J, Roizen M, Moss J. Efficacy of orally administered methylvathexone in decreasing subjective effects after intravenous morphine. Drug Alcohol Dep. 1998;52:161–5.

46. Schmelz M. Itch-mediators and mechanisms. J Dermatol Sci. 2002;28:91–6.

47. Angulo P, Lindor KD. Primary sclerosing cholangitis. Hepatology. 1999;30:325–32.
48. Huet PM, Deslauriers J, Tran A, Faucher C, Charbonneau J. Impact of fatigue on the quality of life in patients with primary biliary cirrhosis. Am J Gastroenterol. 2000;95:760–7.
49. Cauch-Dudek K, Abbey S, Stewart DE, Heathcote EJ. Fatigue in primary biliary cirrhosis. Gut. 1998;43:705–10.
50. Swain, MG. Fatigue in chronic disease. Clin Sci. 2000;99:1–8.
51. Jalan R, Gibson H, Lombard MG. Patients with PBC have central but no peripheral fatigue. Hepatology. 1996;24:A162.
52. Goldblatt J, James OFW, Jones DEJ. Grip strength and subjective fatigue in patients with primary biliary cirrhosis. J Am Med Assoc. 2001;285:2196–7.
53. Enoka RM, Stuart DG. Neurobiology of muscle fatigue. J Appl Physiol. 1992;72:1631–48.
54. Blatteis CM. The afferent signalling of fever. J Physiol. 2000;526:653–61.
55. Adachi A. Projection of the hepatic vagal nerve in the medulla oblongata. J Auton Nerv Syst. 1984;10:287–93.
56. Magni F, Carobi C. The afferent and preganglionic parasympathetic innervation of the rat liver, demonstrated by the retrograde transport of horseradish peroxidase. J Auton Nerv Syst. 1983;8:237–60.
57. Wan W, Wetmore L, Sorensen CM, Greenberg AH, Nance DM. Neural and biochemical mediators of endotoxin and stress-induced c-fos expression in the rat brain. Brain Res Bull. 1994;34:7–14.
58. Konsman JP, Lubeshi GN, Bluthe RM, Dantzer R. The vagus nerve mediates behavioural depression, but not fever, in response to peripheral immune signals: a functional anatomical analysis. Eur J Neurosci. 2000;12:4434–46.
59. Molina-Holgado F, Guaza C. Endotoxin administration induced differential neurochemical activation of the rat brain stem nuclei. Brain Res Bull. 1996;40:151–6.
60. Buller KM. Neuroimmune stress response: reciprocal connections between the hypothalamus and the brainstem. Stress. 2003;6:11–17.
61. Tilg H, Wilmer A, Vogel W, Herold M, Nolchen B, Judmaier G, Huber C. Serum levels of cytokines in chronic liver diseases. Gastroenterology. 1992;103:264–74.
62. Niijma A. The afferent discharges from sensors for interleuken-1 beta in the hepatoportal system in the anaesthetized rat. J Auton Nerv Syst. 1996;61:287–91.
63. Suda T, Tozawa F, Ushiyama T, Sumimoto T, Yamada M, Demura H. Interleukin-1 stimulates corticotropin-releasing factor gene expression in rat hypothalamus. Endocrinology. 1990;126:1223–8.
64. Gaykema RP, Dijkstra I, Tilder FJ. Subdiaphragmatic vagotomy suppresses endotoxin-induced activation of the hypothalamic corticotropin-releasing hormone neurons and ACTH secretion. Endocrinology. 1995;136:4717–29.
65. Goldblatt J, Taylor PJ, Lipman T et al. The true impact of fatigue in primary biliary cirrhosis: a population study. Gastroenterology. 2002;122:1235–41.
66. Goehler LE, Relton JK, Dripps D et al. Vagal paraganglia bind biotinylated interleukin-1 receptor agonist: a possible mechanism for immune-to-brain communication. Brain Res Bull. 1997;43:357–64.
67. Turnbull AV, Rivier CL. Regulation of the hypothalamic–pituitary axis by cytokines: actions and mechanisms of action. Physiol Rev. 1999;79:1–71.
68. Licinio J, Wong M-L. Cytokines and the brain: pathways and mechanisms for cytokine signalling of the central nervous system. J Clin Invest. 1997;100:2941–7.
69. Bemelmans MH, Gouma DJ, Greve JW, Buurman WA. Cytokines tumour necrosis factor and interleukin-6 in experimental biliary obstruction in mice. Hepatology. 1992;15:1132–6.
70. Swain MG, Appleyard CB, Wallace JL, Maric M. TNFα facilitates inflammation-induced glucocorticoid secretion in rats with biliary obstruction. J Hepatol. 1997;26:361–8.
71. Yamamoto Y, Sezai S, Sakurabayashi S, Hirano M, Kamisaka K, Oka H. A study of endotoxemia in patients with primary biliary cirrhosis. J Intern Med Res. 1994;22:95–9.
72. Clements WD, Erwin P, McCaigue MD, Halliday I, Barclay GR, Rowlands BJ. Conclusive evidence of endotoxemia in biliary obstruction. Gut. 1998;42:293–9.
73. Dantzer R. Cytokine-induced sickness behaviour: where do we stand? Brain Behav Immun. 2001;15:7–24.
74. Linthorst AC, Reul JM. Brain neurotransmission during peripheral inflammation. Ann NY Acad Sci. 1998;840:139–52.

75. Wahler JB, Swain MG, Carson R, Bergasa NV, Jones EA. Blood–brain permeability is markedly decreased in cholestasis in the rat. Hepatology. 1993;17:1103–8.
76. McKinley MJ, McAllen RM, Davern P et al. The sensory circumventricular organs of the mammalian brain. Adv Anat Embryol Cell Biol. 2003;172:1–122.
77. Vallieres L, Rivest S. Regulation of the genes encoding interleukin-6, its receptor, and gp130 in the rat brain in response to the immune activation lipopolysaccharide and the proinflammatory cytokine interleukin-1 beta. J Neurochem. 1997;69:1668–83.
78. Van Dam AM, De Vries HE, Kniper J et al. Interleukin-1 receptors on rat brain endothelial cells: a role in neuroimmune interaction? FASEB J. 1996;10:351–6.
79. Nadeau S, Rivest S. Effects of circulatory tumor necrosis factor on the neuronal activity and expression of the genes encoding the tumor necrosis factor receptors (p55 and p75) in the rat brain: a view from the blood brain barrier. Neuroscience. 1999;93:1449–64.
80. Swain MG, Beck P, Rioux K, Le T. Augmented interleukin-1 beta induced depression of locomotor activity in cholestatic rats. Hepatology. 1998;28:1561–5.
81. Forton DM, Patel N, Prince M et al. Fatigue and primary biliary cirrhosis: association of globus pallidus magnetization transfer ratio measurements with fatigue severity and blood manganese levels. Gut. 2004;53:587–92.
82. Beam J, Wessely S. Neurobiological aspects of the chronic fatigue syndrome. Eur J Clin Invest. 1994;24:79–90.
83. Swanson LW, Sawchenko PE, Rivier J, Vale WW. Organization of ovine corticotropin-releasing factor immunoreactive cells and fibres in the rat brain: an immunohistological study. Neuroendocrinology. 1983;36:165–86.
84. Koob GF, Henrichs SC, Pich EM et al. The role of corticotropin-releasing factor in behavioural responses to stress. Ciba Found Symp. 1993;172:277–89.
85. Sutton RE, Koob GF, LeMoal M, Rivier J, Vale W. Corticoptropin-releasing factor produces behavioural activation in rats. Nature. 1982;297:331–3.
86. Gold PW, Chrousos GP. The endocrinology of melancholic and atypical depression: relation to neurocircuitry and somatic consequences. Proc Assoc Am Phys. 1998;111:22–34.
87. Clauw DJ, Chrousos GP. Chronic pain and fatigue syndromes: overlapping clinical and neuroendocrine features and potential pathogenic mechanisms. Neuroimmunomodulation. 1997;4:134–53.
88. Swain MG, Mogiaku MA, Bergasa NV, Chrousos GP. Facilitation of ACTH and cortisol responses to corticotropin-releasing hormone (CRH) in patients with primary biliary cirrhosis. Hepatology. 1994;20:A197.
89. Swain MG, Patchev V, Vergalla J, Chrousos G, Jones EA. Suppression of hypothalamic–pituitary–adrenal axis responsiveness to stress in a rat model of acute cholestasis. J Clin Invest. 1993;91:1903–8.
90. Swain MG, Maric M. Defective corticotropin-releasing hormone mediated neuroendocrine and behavioural responses in cholestatic rats: implications for cholestatic liver disease related sickness behaviours. Hepatology. 1995;22:1560–4.
91. Burak KW, Le T, Swain MG. Increased sensitivity to the locomotor-activating effects of corticoptropin-releasing hormone in cholestatic rats. Gastroeneterology. 2002;122:681–8.
92. Neeck G, Crofford LJ. Neuroendocrine perturbations in fibromyalgia and chronic fatigue syndrome. Rheum Dis Clin N Am. 2000;26:989–1002.
93. Liposizs Z, Phelix C, Paull W. Synaptic interaction of serotonergic axons and corticotropin-releasing factor (CRF) synthesizing neurons in the hypothalamic paraventricular nucleus of the rat. Histochemistry. 1987;86:541–9.
94. Bailey SP, Davis JM, Ahlborn EN. Neuroendocrine and substrate responses to altered brain 5HT activity during prolonged exercise to fatigue. J Appl Physiol. 1993;7U:3006–12.
95. Wilson WM, Maughan RJ. Evidence for a possible role of 5-hydroxytryptamine in the genesis of fatigue in man: administration of paroxetine, a 5HT reuptake inhibitor reduces the capacity to perform prolonged exercise. Exp Physiol. 1992;77:921–4.
96. Bakheit AMO, Behan PO, Dinan TG, Gray CE, O'Keane V. Possible upregulation of hypothalamic 5-hydroxytryptamine receptors in patients with postural fatigue syndrome. Br Med J. 1992;304:1010–12.
97. Goldenberg D, Mayskiy M, Mossey C, Ruthazer R, Schmid C. A randomized double-blind, crossover trial of fluoxetine and amitryptilline in the treatment of fibromyalgia. Arthritis Rheum. 1996;39:1852–9.

98. Roth BL. Multiple serotonin receptors: clinical experimental aspects. Am Clin Psychiatry. 1994;6:67–78.

99. Riad M, Watkins KC, Doucet E, Hamon M, Descarries L. Agonist-induced internalization of serotonin-1a receptors in the dorsal raphe nucleus (autoreceptors) but not hippocampus (heteroreceptors). J Neurosci. 2001;21:8378–86.

100. Burak K, Le T, Swain MG. Increased midbrain 5-HT 1a receptor number and responsiveness in cholestatic rats. Brain Res. 2001;892:376–9.

101. Swain MG, Maric M. Improvement in cholestasis-associated fatigue with a serotonin receptor agonist using a novel rat model of fatigue assessment. Hepatology. 1997;25:291–4.

102. Jones EA. Relief from profound fatigue associated with chronic liver disease by long term ondansetron therapy. Lancet. 1999;357–8.

103. Theal JL, Toosi MN, Girlan LM et al. Ondansetron ameliorates fatigue in patients with primary biliary cirrhosis (PBC). Hepatology. 2002;36:A533.

104. Berridge CW, Waterhouse BD. The locus coeruleus–noradrenergic system: modulation of behavioural state and state-dependent cognitive processes. Brain Res Rev. 2003;42:33–84.

105. Tzschentke TM. Pharmacology and behavioural pharmacology of the mesocortical dopamine system. Prog Neurobiol. 2001;63:241–320.

10
Is osteoporosis a specific complication of primary biliary cirrhosis?

J. L. NEWTON and D. JONES

INTRODUCTION

Primary biliary cirrhosis (PBC) is typically progressive, with a significant proportion of patients going on to develop cirrhosis. However, the rate of progression to cirrhosis differs between patients[1]. Recent studies have shown that PBC is typically a disease of postmenopausal females that develops in middle age[2]. In most centres the median age for presentation is in the range 55–60 years, and in our well-characterized series[3], 39% presented for the first time over the age of 65.

The demographics of the PBC population have changed. Historically, PBC was a rare disease characterized by the complications of decompensated liver disease such as hepatocellular failure and portal hypertension. PBC is now regarded as a significantly commoner disease, affecting up to 1 in 700 women over the age of 40, that presents asymptomatically, or with symptoms typical of early disease, e.g. fatigue and pruritus. This change is in part due to increased awareness of the disease, but also to the availability of powerful and sensitive diagnostic tools for the disease[4]. The presence of circulating antimitochondrial antibodies (AMA) is highly specific for PBC, and availability of this diagnostic tool has resulted in a tendency to diagnose the disease at earlier stages than was previously the case[1].

With this shift in the spectrum of PBC from a rare, advanced disease to a commoner, milder disease it is important to question whether previously accepted associations continue to hold true. In this context it is vital to revisit the relationship between PBC and osteoporosis.

THE PREVALENCE OF OSTEOPOROSIS IN PBC

Osteoporosis is a progressive systemic skeletal disease characterized by low bone mass and micro-architectural deterioration of bone tissue with a consequent increase in bone fragility and susceptibility to fracture[5]. Bone loss increases with advancing age and hence osteoporosis is more prevalent in older people[6]. Unlike in osteomalacia, there is no impairment of bone mineralization or accumulation of osteoid.

Osteoporosis is diagnosed by bone mineral density assessment. Radiological measurement generates data of absolute bone density (g/m^2); this is then compared to international norms to provide data relating this value to expected peak lifetime density for individuals of the same gender. This comparison provides a 'T score', which represents the number of standard deviations difference between the observed value and peak lifetime density. A further comparison with individuals of the same gender and age provides the 'Z score' (number of standard deviations difference between the observed value and the expected density for age- and sex-matched individuals).

Osteoporosis has been defined by the WHO[7] as being present when an individual's T score is less than -2.5. The Z score does not contribute to the diagnosis of osteoporosis, but does provide insight into whether T score abnormalities in a patient group are truly a reflection of increased prevalence of osteoporosis in that group, or whether they result from the condition occurring in an older demographic group who would be intrinsically at risk of osteoporosis by virtue of advancing age. Considering the propensity for PBC to affect women over the age of 50 this is a critical distinction. Whether bone disease is a specific complication of PBC has proved controversial. The question is whether PBC itself conveys increased risk of osteoporosis, or whether osteoporosis is seen in those with PBC as it is predominantly a disease of postmenopausal women.

It had become accepted wisdom that PBC patients have an increased incidence of osteoporosis and its complications. This view arose from the early descriptions of the disease and its associations that emphasized the frequency of metabolic bone disease[8,9]. Subsequent small studies appeared to confirm that PBC patients were at high risk of the development of osteoporosis and its complications, in particular fracture[10-12]. Suggested mechanisms for osteoporosis development in PBC include impaired calcium and vitamin D absorption resulting from profound cholestasis and hyperbilirubinaemia impairing osteoblast proliferative capacity[13] (Table 1). Other contemporary studies suggested no increased risk of osteoporosis[14]; however, the dogma has remained until the more recent publication of four large clinical series[15-18].

Table 1 Potential risk factors for osteoporosis in liver disease

Risk factors common to all	Cholestatic-related risk factors
Advancing age	Calcium malabsorption
Female sex	Vitamin D malabsorption
Alcohol consumption	Cholestyramine therapy
Hypogonadism	Hyperbilirubinaemia
Steroid therapy	Cirrhosis
Low body mass index	
Vitamin D receptor polymorphisms	
Impaired conversion of vitamin D	
Reduced osteocalcin activity	

Perhaps what is most striking about the historical landmark studies linking PBC and osteoporosis[8–11] is the difference between the PBC disease phenotype described in these studies and that typically seen in modern clinics. The four historical cohorts were also small, and used varying diagnostic criteria for both PBC and osteoporosis. Despite this they concluded that between 13% and 35% of PBC patients were osteoporotic; however, 81% of these patients were cholestatic and would be regarded as having advanced disease, which is in sharp contrast with recent observations from a geographically based patient cohort of 136 PBC patients which demonstrated elevated serum bilirubin levels in only 10%[19].

The debate has been further fuelled by four more recent prevalence studies from the UK[17], Canada[15], the USA[16], and Germany[18]. These studies have been significantly larger, with a total of 635 patients, used whole clinic cohorts and were therefore, within the constraints of local referral patterns, comprehensive. The three published series show remarkable consistency, with osteoporosis prevalences of 31%, 35%, and 24% for the UK, Canadian and USA series respectively (defined using the WHO criteria as $T < -2.5$ at the hip and/or neck of femur). Therefore it is reasonable to conclude, from these recent studies and earlier work, that approximately one-third of all PBC patients are osteoporotic at any one time. This suggests that screening PBC patients for osteoporosis and instigation of appropriate therapy will be of benefit, and is to be recommended.

THE RISK OF OSTEOPOROSIS IN PBC

PBC patients could develop osteoporosis with such apparent frequency because the disease process in PBC promotes the development of osteoporosis or, alternatively, because the typical PBC patient in modern practice is a postmenopausal female who would be at risk of osteoporosis for reasons entirely unrelated to PBC.

The UK series is approximately twice the size of any prior or subsequent study of osteoporosis in PBC with 272 patients, and suggests that the high prevalence of osteoporosis in PBC is simply due to the demographics of the population[17]. When comparing absolute bone density values to age- and sex-matched non-PBC norms to provide a Z score the degree of bone loss is no less than would be expected across the population as a whole (-0.1 at the neck of femur and 0.1 at the lumbar spine). The smaller German series has subsequently confirmed these findings[18].

However, even in the UK series, 7% of individuals had significantly lower bone density than age and sex norms predicted ($Z < -2.0$ at neck of femur and/or lumbar spine). Interestingly, the proportion of patients with $Z < -2.0$ was significantly higher in both the Canadian and USA series (18% and 12%, respectively)[15,16]. These findings may be explained by differences in case acquisition between the UK and the Canadian and USA series. The patients in the UK series are older (mean age 62 vs 55 and 53 years) and typically have milder disease compared to the other series, suggesting a fundamental difference in the PBC population studied. Potentially a large number of early disease patients in the cohort could 'dilute' the effect of patients with more aggressive disease which could be associated with osteoporosis. This scenario would be supported by the findings of Narayanan Menon et al., who demonstrated, using univariate

Table 2 Summary of conclusions

---

1. PBC patients are, whether for PBC or non-PBC related reasons, at risk of osteoporosis development.
2. Milder forms of disease change the risk either through accelerating development of osteoporosis in individuals 'at-risk' for non-PBC-related reasons or through increasing, to a limited extent, the overall risk. Long-term prospective studies based on the USA and Canadian series will hopefully help us to distinguish between these possibilities.
3. Advanced cholestatic PBC is a risk factor for osteoporosis.
4. Liver transplantation is associated with improvements in bone density.

---

analysis[16], that PBC histological stage is a risk factor for the development of osteoporosis and would be compatible with a causal association between osteoporosis and PBC stage. It is not clear whether this is specific to PBC, or more to the cholestasis of advanced liver disease of all causes.

Alternatively the contradictory Z score data and complementary T score data in populations with different ages could be explained by the fact that PBC accelerates the development of osteoporosis, without increasing the absolute risk. In this model the younger USA and Canadian series have an absolute prevalence of 25–35%, which is higher than predicted. In the older UK series the absolute prevalence remains the same; however, this is no longer significantly higher than predicted as the matched normal population has 'caught up'. Evidence for this hypothesis comes from the follow-up arm of the UK study in which the mean number of bone density assessments was five per patient. No patient who did not have osteoporosis detected on the index scan went on to develop it during follow-up, suggesting that 'at-risk' patients always appeared to have developed their osteoporosis by the time they were first assessed whilst not 'at-risk' patients remained not 'at-risk' during follow-up.

A reasonable consensus from the early and late studies of prevalence of osteoporosis is shown in Table 2.

HOW FREQUENTLY SHOULD PBC PATIENTS BE ASSESSED FOR OSTEOPOROSIS?

The goal of all approaches to therapy in osteoporosis is to prevent, or at least lower, the risk of fracture, by identifying at-risk individuals before their first fracture, in order to allow intervention. In current clinical practice monitoring is performed by bone mineral densitometry.

Identifying who should be screened, and how frequently, is controversial. The British Society of Gastroenterology has produced consensus guidelines for the management of osteoporosis which predate the publication of the recent prevalence studies[20]. The guidelines recommend that bone mineral density studies be carried out in those with cirrhosis or severe cholestasis, and in those who have non-cirrhotic disease and other risk factors for osteoporosis. The UK cohort study[17] suggested that the presence of osteoporosis at initial bone density assessment was poorly predicted by clinical and biochemical parameters and, contrary to the guidelines, would support screening of all patients diagnosed with PBC irrespective of stage.

The guidelines also suggest repeat assessments every 2 years; however, the follow-up arm of the UK study showed that the pick-up rate for newly developed osteoporosis on repeat bone density assessment, in patients who did not have osteoporosis on their initial assessment, was very low. If scans were performed every 5 years then no new cases of osteoporosis would have been missed. Reviewing the UK data, repeat assessment of PBC patients every 5 years would have avoided 628 assessments without missing one case of osteoporosis. This has massive implications for the provision of bone density measurement.

TREATMENT OF OSTEOPOROSIS IN PBC

The guidelines suggest that treatment should be initiated with the same thresholds as in non-liver disease groups (i.e. T score is > -2.5 – no treatment, with T score < -2.5 – treatment). Evidence specific for the management of osteoporosis specific to patients with PBC is weak and, with respect to the effects on actual fracture rate, almost non-existent. If a substantial component of osteoporosis susceptibility in PBC results from non-PBC-related factors then conventional approaches used for the treatment of non-PBC osteoporosis are applicable in the context of PBC.

Common sense suggests that patients should be advised regarding adequate diet (in particular calcium intake), adequate exercise and smoking. Several studies have suggested that vitamin D supplementation is unhelpful, although clearly normalization of vitamin D and calcium levels is desirable to prevent the rare complication of osteomalacia[9,12,21,22]. The strongest evidence is in support of the use of bisphosphates in PBC osteoporosis. Published trial data support the use of cyclical etidronate[23]. A further study, as yet published only in abstract form, has suggested that alendronate may be more efficacious than etidronate in PBC patients, in the absence of unacceptable side-effects[24]. Hormone replacement therapy also appears to be safe and effective in PBC patients with osteoporosis[25].

OSTEOPOROSIS AND TRANSPLANTATION

Liver transplantation has been associated with an acute, short-term worsening of bone density with consequent increase in fracture rate[26,27]. This acute deterioration probably results from the effects of the immobility and steroid therapy associated with the early post-transplant period, superimposed on the pro-osteoporotic effects of the advanced liver disease for which transplantation is indicated. Aggressive pre-transplant treatment with the intravenous bisphosphonate pamidronate reduces the risk of fracture post-transplant[28]. Given the risks associated with osteoporosis in the peri-transplant period, and the apparent benefits of treatment, all patients approaching liver transplantation for PBC should undergo screening for osteoporosis and appropriate remedial therapy prior to surgery.

Following the early deterioration in bone density, transplantation is associated with a long-term improvement in bone density and a reduction in fracture rate, presumably as a result of correction of the pro-osteoporotic effects of advanced disease[26]. Given the potentially beneficial long-term effects, therefore, osteoporosis should not be regarded as a contraindication to transplantation in PBC.

CONCLUSIONS

When assessing the true extent of the association between osteoporosis and PBC, it is critical that conclusions be drawn from large populations. In addition, in a disease such as osteoporosis that is common in older people, age-matched values should be used to draw any conclusions. PBC is a disease that often presents for the first time over the age of 65. It is therefore not surprising that osteoporosis is a common problem in a disease predominantly affecting peri-menopausal or postmenopausal women. It seems that the apparent risk of osteo-porosis in PBC reflects, to a significant although not exclusive extent, the demographics of the disease population rather than a specific disease process.

Given the very real problems experienced by some PBC patients as a result of osteoporotic fracture, particularly in the early post-transplant period, further study of aetiology is appropriate. We suggest that the search for risk factors for osteoporosis in PBC not be focused exclusively on liver specific factors, but could more usefully be directed at more generalized population risk factors.

References

1. Prince MI, Jones DEJ. Primary biliary cirrhosis: new perspectives in diagnosis and treatment. Postgrad Med J. 2000;76:199–206.
2. Sherlock S, Scheuer PJ. The presentation and diagnosis of 100 patients with primary biliary cirrhosis. N Engl J Med. 1973;289:674–8.
3. Newton JL, Jones DEJ, Metcalf JV et al. The presentation and mortality of primary biliary cirrhosis in older patients. Age Ageing. 2000;29:305–9.
4. Jones DEJ. Autoantigens in primary biliary cirrhosis. J Clin Pathol. 2000;53:1–8.
5. Consensus Development Conference. Diagnosis, prophylaxis and treatment of osteoporosis. Am J Med. 1991;90:107–10.
6. Sutcliffe AM, Francis RM. Osteoporosis: treatment options in elderly patients. Prescriber. 1998;9:91–4.
7. WHO Study Group. Assessment of fracture risk and its application to screening for post-menopausal osteoporosis. report of a WHO study group. Geneva: World Health Organization, 1994.
8. Atkinson M, Nordin BEC, Sherlock S. Bone disease in obstructive jaundice. Q J Med. 1956;25:299–312.
9. Kehayoglou AK, Holdsworth CD, Agnew JE, Whelton MJ, Sherlock S. Bone disease and calcium absorption in primary biliary cirrosis with special reference to vitamin-D therapy. Lancet. 1968;1:715–18.
10. Guanabens N, Pares A, Marasino L et al. Factors influencing the development of metabolic bone disease in primary bilary cirrhosis. Am J Gastroenterol. 1990;85:1356–62.
11. Hodgson SF, Rolland-Dickson E, Wahner HW, Johnson KA, Mann KG, Riggs BL. Bone loss and reduced osteoblast function in primary biliary cirrhosis. Ann Intern Med. 1985;103: 855–60.
12. Matloff DS, Kaplan MM, Neer RM, Goldberg MJ, Bitman W, Wolfe HJ. Osteoporosis in primary biliary cirrhosis: effects of 25-hydroxyvitamin D3 treatment. Gastroenterology. 1982; 83:97–102.
13. Janes CH, Rolland-Dickson E, Okazaki R, Bonde S, McDonagh AF, Lawrence-Riggs B. Role of hyperbilirubinaemia in the impairment of osteoblast proliferation associated with cholestatic jaundice. J Clin Invest. 1995;95:2581–6.
14. Almdal T, Schaadt O, Veaterdal-Jorgensen J, Lindgreen P, Ranek L. Vitamin D, parathyroid hormone and bone mineral content of lumbar spine and femur in primary biliary cirrhosis. J Intern Med. 1989;225:207–13.
15. Springer JE, Cole DEC, Rubin LA et al. Vitamin D-receptor genotypes as independent genetic predictors of decreased bone mineral density in primary biliary cirrhosis. Gastroenterology. 2000;118:145–51.

16. Narayanan Menon KV, Angulo P, Weston S, Dickson ER, Lindor KD. Bone disease in primary biliary cirrhosis: independent indicators and rate of progression. J Hepatol. 2001;35:316–23.
17. Newton JL, Francis R, Prince M et al. Osteoporosis in primary biliary cirrhosis revisited. Gut. 2001;49:282–7.
18. Lindenthal B, Leuschner MS, Ackermann H, Happ J, Leuschner UF. Is primary biliary cirrhosis (PBC) in itself a risk factor for osteoporosis? Hepatology. 2000;32:168A.
19. Goldblatt J, Taylor PJS, Lipman T, James OFW, Jones DEJ. Prevalence of fatigue in a geographically based primary biliary cirrhosis population: comparison with community controls. Hepatology. 2000;32:28.
20. BSG guidelines. British Society of Gastroenterology, <http://www.bsg.org.uk/pdf_word_docs/clinguideostcld.pdf>.
21. Herlong HF, Recker RR, Maddrey WC. Bone disease in primary biliary cirrhosis: histologic features and response to 25-hydroxyvitamin D. Gastroenterology. 1982;83:103–8.
22. Floreani A, Azappala F, Fries W et al. A 3-year pilot study with 1,25-dihydroxyvitamin D, calcium and calcitonin for severe osteodystrophy in primary biliary cirrhosis. J Clin Gastroenterol. 1997;24:239–44.
23. Lindor KD, Jorgensen RA, Tiegs RD, Khosla S, Dickson ER. Etidronate for osteoporosis in primary biliary cirrhosis: a randomised trial. J Hepatol. 2000;33:878–82.
24. Pares A, Guanabens N, Ros I et al. Alendronate is more effective than etidronate for increasing bone mass in osteopenic patients with primary biliary cirrhosis. Hepatology. 1999;30:472A.
25. Olsson R, Mattsson LA, Obrant K, Mellstrom D. Estrogen–progestegen therapy for low bone mineral density in primary biliary cirrhosis. Liver. 1999;19:188–92.
26. Eastell R, Rolland-Dickson E, Hodgson SF et al. Rates of vertebral bone loss before and after liver transplantation in women with primary biliary cirrhosis. Hepatology. 1991;14:296–300.
27. Ninkovic M, Skingle SJ, Bearcroft PW, Bishop N, Alexander GJ, Compston JE. Incidence of vertebral fractures in the first three months after orthotopic liver transplantation. Eur J Gastroenterol Hepatol. 2000;12:931–5.
28. Reeves HL, Francis RM, Manas DM, Hudson M, Day CP. Intravenous bisphosphonate prevents symptomatic osteoporotic vertebral collapse in patients after liver transplantation. Liver Trans Surg. 1998;4:404–9.

11
Diseases associated with primary biliary cirrhosis

P. C. J. ter BORG, H. R. VAN BUUREN,
K. M. J. van NIEUWKERK, E. B. HAAGSMA,
J. W. DEN OUDEN, M. H. M. G. HOUBEN,
R. W. de KONING, E. W. van der HOEK, R. ADANG and
G. P. van BERGE HENEGOUWEN*

INTRODUCTION

Primary biliary cirrhosis (PBC) is a chronic cholestatic liver disease with a presumed autoimmune aetiology[1]. Associations with many autoimmune and non-autoimmune conditions have been reported, and some disorders appear to occur with increased frequency in patients with PBC. Several previous studies aimed to quantify the occurrence of some of these associated disorders in series of PBC patients, and some previous reports on series of PBC patients have included data on coexisting diseases. In previous studies, data on the following disorders have been reported: thyroid disorders[2], rheumatic disorders[3–5], Sjögren's syndrome[6,7], systemic lupus erythematosus[8], systemic sclerosis[9,10], renal tubular acidosis[11], bacteriuria[12], coeliac disease[13–22], ulcerative colitis[23] and malignant diseases[24–29]. All these studies aimed to quantify the occurrence of individual diseases or groups of related diseases. Since these studies may have been initiated because an association was suspected after some cases were observed, significant bias may have been introduced. This is illustrated by the finding of an increased risk of carcinoma of the breast in two early studies[24,25], which could not be confirmed in a number of subsequent reports on the occurrence of malignant diseases in PBC[26–30].

For the sake of clarity one should differentiate symptoms and signs of PBC which are specifically liver-related from those that are due to associated disorders,

* For the Dutch Multicentre Primary Biliary Cirrhosis Study Group.

Table 1 Manifestations of PBC[38]

Specific to PBC	Reported associated disorders
Fatigue	Thyroid dysfunction
Pruritus	Sicca syndrome
Portal hypertension	CREST
Metabolic bone disease	Raynaud's syndrome
Xanthomata	Rheumatoid arthritis
Fat-soluble vitamin malabsorption	Coeliac disease
Urinary tract infection	Inflammatory bowel disease
Malignancy	Depression

which usually have a common autoimmune pathogenesis. Specific symptoms and signs, as well as associated disorders, are presented in Table 1. In order to avoid bias in selection we recently performed a multicentre study aiming to quantify the prevalence of all previously reported associated conditions. Although in this study many of the previously reported diseases also occurred, the prevalence of most of the individual diseases was low. In addition to previously reported data, some results from this study will be presented.

STUDIES OF ASSOCIATED DISEASES IN PATIENTS FROM THE DUTCH MULTICENTRE PBC STUDY GROUP

The most extensively studied disorder associated with PBC is coeliac disease, with varying results. Previous studies reported prevalences of coeliac disease between 0% and 30%, while the median prevalence in these studies was only 3.4%. We found no cases of coeliac disease in our series of 237 patients with PBC; however, in our study no systematic screening for coeliac disease has been performed, in contrast to some of the other studies. As a result, testing for coeliac disease in our study may have been performed more frequently in patients in whom coeliac disease was clinically suspected. Since coeliac disease can occur with minimal or no symptoms, the true prevalence of coeliac disease was possibly underestimated. However, altogether the lack of any cases of coeliac disease suggests that its prevalence in PBC is indeed low, especially since in none of the 22 patients in whom duodenal tissue was obtained was the diagnosis made. Besides selection bias, another explanation for the differences between the various studies may be regional differences in the occurrence of coeliac disease.

The single most prevalent disorder in our study was cholelithiasis, which occurred in 21% of patients. However, since most patients were females in a high-risk age group, a high prevalence was expected. The proportion is comparable to previously reported data on cholelithiasis in patients with cirrhosis[31–33], and in several population studies the prevalence of cholelithiasis in females over 50 years of age was comparable to the prevalence found in our study[34–36]. Altogether, although cholelithiasis frequently occurs in patients with PBC, its prevalence might not be markedly increased compared to the general population and patients with other hepatic conditions.

Two previous studies reported an increased risk of breast cancer in patients with PBC[24,25]; however, subsequent studies could not confirm this finding[26–28,30]. We found that breast cancer at any time before or during follow-up occurred in eight (4%) patients. However, in only three of these patients did breast cancer occur after the diagnosis of PBC had been made. In the general population the lifetime risk of breast cancer is approximately 12.5%, and the 4% risk of breast cancer in our series might well be comparable to the normal prevalence occurring in any series of females[37].

Previous studies reported prevalences of thyroid disease of 14% and 19%, whereas this diagnosis had been made in 7% of patients in our study[2,3]. Scleroderma (including CREST) was previously found in 0%, 10%, 12% and 22% of patients, and we found a prevalence of 0.9%[3,5,8,10]. Rheumatoid arthritis was previously reported in 2%, 10% and 27% of patients, compared to 4% in our study[3–5]. Finally, Sjögren's syndrome was previously diagnosed in 27% of patients, and another study reported histological changes compatible with Sjögren's syndrome in 26% of tested patients[6,7], while in our series of Dutch patients this diagnosis was made in only 2% of patients. Overall, the prevalence of other autoimmune and rheumatic diseases was low when compared to previous studies.

CONCLUSIONS

The prevalence of most of the previously reported associated diseases, especially coeliac disease, breast cancer and rheumatoid diseases, was low in our series of unselected PBC patients. Some of the previously reported data may have been influenced by selection bias. There seem to be only a few truly associated disorders with PBC, such as Raynaud's syndrome and thyroid disease (thyroiditis and hypothyroidism). We could not confirm the described association with coeliac disease or with malignant disease with the exception of hepatocellular carcinoma.

References

1. Kaplan MM. Primary biliary cirrhosis. N Engl J Med. 1996;335:1570–80.
2. Crowe JP, Christensen E, Butler J et al. Primary biliary cirrhosis: the prevalence of hypothyroidism and its relationship to thyroid autoantibodies and sicca syndrome. Gastroenterology. 1980;78:1437–41.
3. Culp KS, Fleming CR, Duffy J, Baldus WP, Dickson ER. Autoimmune associations in primary biliary cirrhosis. Mayo Clin Proc. 1982;57:365–70.
4. Uddenfeldt P, Danielsson A. Evaluation of rheumatic disorders in patients with primary biliary cirrhosis. Ann Clin Res. 1986;18:148–53.
5. Marasini B, Gagetta M, Rossi V, Ferrari P. Rheumatic disorders and primary biliary cirrhosis: an appraisal of 170 Italian patients. Ann Rheum Dis. 2001;60:1046–9.
6. Uddenfeldt P, Danielsson A, Forssell A, Holm M, Ostberg Y. Features of Sjögren's syndrome in patients with primary biliary cirrhosis. J Intern Med. 1991;230:443–8.
7. Tsianos EV, Hoofnagle JH, Fox PC et al. Sjögren's syndrome in patients with primary biliary cirrhosis. Hepatology. 1990;11:730–4.
8. Fonollosa V, Simeon CP, Castells L et al. Morphologic capillary changes and manifestations of connective tissue diseases in patients with primary biliary cirrhosis. Lupus. 2001;10:628–31.

9. Powell FC, Schroeter AL, Dickson ER. Primary biliary cirrhosis and the CREST syndrome: a report of 22 cases. Q J Med. 1987;62:75–82.
10. Pares A, Grande L, Bruix J, Pera C, Rodes J. Esophageal dysfunction in primary biliary cirrhosis. J Hepatol. 1988;7:362–7.
11. Pares A, Rimola A, Bruguera M, Mas E, Rodes J. Renal tubular acidosis in primary biliary cirrhosis. Gastroenterology. 1981;80:681–6.
12. Burroughs AK, Rosenstein IJ, Epstein O, Hamilton-Miller JM, Brumfitt W, Sherlock S. Bacteriuria and primary biliary cirrhosis. Gut. 1984;25:133–7.
13. Bardella MT, Quatrini M, Zuin M et al. Screening patients with coeliac disease for primary biliary cirrhosis and vice versa. Am J Gastroenterol. 1997;92:1524–6.
14. Dickey W, McMillan SA, Callender ME. High prevalence of celiac sprue among patients with primary biliary cirrhosis. J Clin Gastroenterol. 1997;25:328–9.
15. Kingham JG, Parker DR. The association between primary biliary cirrhosis and coeliac disease: a study of relative prevalences. Gut. 1998;42:120–2.
16. Niveloni S, Dezi R, Pedreira S et al. Gluten sensitivity in patients with primary biliary cirrhosis. Am J Gastroenterol. 1998;93:404–8.
17. Sorensen HT, Thulstrup AM, Blomqvist P, Norgaard B, Fonager K, Ekbom A. Risk of primary biliary liver cirrhosis in patients with coeliac disease: Danish and Swedish cohort data. Gut. 1999;44:736–8.
18. Gillett HR, Cauch-Dudek K, Jenny E, Heathcote EJ, Freeman HJ. Prevalence of IgA antibodies to endomysium and tissue transglutaminase in primary biliary cirrhosis. Can J Gastroenterol. 2000;14:672–5.
19. Chatzicostas C, Roussomoustakaki M, Drygiannakis D et al. Primary biliary cirrhosis and autoimmune cholangitis are not associated with coeliac disease in Crete. BMC Gastroenterol. 2002;2:5.
20. Floreani A, Betterle C, Baragiotta A et al. Prevalence of coeliac disease in primary biliary cirrhosis and of antimitochondrial antibodies in adult coeliac disease patients in Italy. Dig Liver Dis. 2002;34:258–61.
21. Volta U, Rodrigo L, Granito A et al. Celiac disease in autoimmune cholestatic liver disorders. Am J Gastroenterol. 2002;97:2609–13.
22. Habior A, Lewartowska A, Orlowska J et al. Association of coeliac disease with primary biliary cirrhosis in Poland. Eur J Gastroenterol Hepatol. 2003;15:159–64.
23. Koulentaki M, Koutroubakis IE, Petinaki E et al. Ulcerative colitis associated with primary biliary cirrhosis. Dig Dis Sci. 1999;44:1953–6.
24. Wolke AM, Schaffner F, Kapelman B, Sacks HS. Malignancy in primary biliary cirrhosis. High incidence of breast cancer in affected women. Am J Med. 1984;76:1075–8.
25. Goudie BM, Burt AD, Boyle P et al. Breast cancer in women with primary biliary cirrhosis. Br Med J (Clin Res Ed). 1985;291:1597–8.
26. Loof L, Adami HO, Sparen P et al. Cancer risk in primary biliary cirrhosis: a population-based study from Sweden. Hepatology. 1994;20:101–4.
27. Floreani A, Biagini MR, Chiaramonte M, Milani S, Surrenti C, Naccarato R. Incidence of hepatic and extra-hepatic malignancies in primary biliary cirrhosis (PBC). Ital J Gastroenterol. 1993;25:473–6.
28. Howel D, Metcalf JV, Gray J, Newman WL, Jones DE, James OF. Cancer risk in primary biliary cirrhosis: a study in northern England. Gut. 1999;45:756–60.
29. Nijhawan PK, Therneau TM, Dickson ER, Boynton J, Lindor KD. Incidence of cancer in primary biliary cirrhosis: the Mayo experience. Hepatology. 1999;29:1396–8.
30. Floreani A, Baragiotta A, Baldo V, Menegon T, Farinati F, Naccarato R. Hepatic and extrahepatic malignancies in primary biliary cirrhosis. Hepatology. 1999;29:1425–8.
31. Conte D, Barisani D, Mandelli C et al. Cholelithiasis in cirrhosis: analysis of 500 cases. Am J Gastroenterol. 1991;86:1629–32.
32. Elzouki AN, Nilsson S, Nilsson P, Verbaan H, Simanaitis M, Lindgren S. The prevalence of gallstones in chronic liver disease is related to degree of liver dysfunction. Hepatogastroenterology. 1999;46:2946–50.
33. Del Olmo JA, Garcia F, Serra MA, Maldonado L, Rodrigo JM. Prevalence and incidence of gallstones in liver cirrhosis. Scand J Gastroenterol. 1997;32:1061–5.
34. Barbara L, Sama C, Morselli Labate AM et al. A population study on the prevalence of gallstone disease: the Sirmione Study. Hepatology. 1987;7:913–17.

35. Caroli-Bosc FX, Deveau C, Harris A et al. Prevalence of cholelithiasis: results of an epidemio-logic investigation in Vidauban, southeast France. General Practitioner's Group of Vidauban. Dig Dis Sci. 1999;44:1322–9.
36. Jorgensen T. Prevalence of gallstones in a Danish population. Am J Epidemiol. 1987; 126:912–21.
37. Feuer EJ, Wun LM, Boring CC, Flanders WD, Timmel MJ, Tong T. The lifetime risk of develop-ing breast cancer. J Natl Cancer Inst. 1993;85:892–7.
38. Heathcote EJ. Management of primary biliary cirrhosis. Hepatology. 2000;31:1005–13.

Section IV
Overlap syndromes

12
Overlap syndromes, outlier syndromes and changing diagnoses

J. HEATHCOTE

INTRODUCTION

This chapter will discuss a variety of presumed autoimmune liver diseases which may not necessarily fit into the textbook description of either autoimmune hepatitis (AIH), primary biliary cirrhosis (PBC), or primary sclerosing cholangitis (PSC). The pathogeneses of these three conditions remain elusive. It is anticipated that molecular techniques currently being explored will help to lead to the identification of factors which provoke the mediators of hepatocyte and/or bile duct change. Only then will we be able to more definitively clarify overlap syndromes, outlier syndromes and changing diagnosis.

OVERLAP SYNDROMES

This term has been used to describe cases in individuals who appear to have two autoimmune liver diseases which present simultaneously or, as is more often the case, individuals with one overt autoimmune liver disease who have additional features of another. Much less common is presentation with one autoimmune disease which, after several months or years, changes to an entirely different one.

TWO AUTOIMMUNE LIVER DISEASES WHICH PRESENT SIMULTANEOUSLY

This has best been described in the paediatric population. Gregorio et al.[1] recently published a prospective study of 76 children who presented between 1984 and 1997 with a liver disease thought to be autoimmune hepatitis; 55 of these 76 children underwent cholangiographic examination of their biliary tree at the time of their initial diagnosis (21 were too ill). Twenty-three were found to have abnormalities of the common bile duct which the authors describe as autoimmune sclerosing cholangitis (ASC). There was no difference in the pattern of presentation in terms of symptoms, in particular pruritus, in those with or without ASC. Inflammatory bowel disease (IBD) was more common in the children with AIH + ASC, but IBD was by no means confined to the children found to have a cholangitis. The cholangiographic findings included stricturing of the common bile duct in a few (9%), but more often the radiological picture was of mucosal irregularity without strictures. Calculi were seen in 9%, and 13% had an abnormal pancreatic duct. There were some differences in the biochemical features of those with and without biliary lesions but they were not as one would expect, in that the heights of the serum alkaline phosphatase or gamma-glutamyl transpeptidase were not distinguishing features; rather the height of the serum aminotransferases (significantly higher in those with uncomplicated AIH). The distribution of non-organ-specific antibodies was also different in that pANCA was detected in 74% of the children with ASC, but in only 36% of the children with only AIH. There was no difference in the distribution of antinuclear antibody (ANA) and smooth muscle antibody (SMA) between the two groups.

The overall histological assessment did identify some differences when the group was examined as a whole; for example, in the height of the HAI score (greater in those with simple AIH) and in the pattern of the periportal hepatitis (being more often biliary in those with ASC and more often lymphocytic in those with AIH). But none of these histological findings was sensitive enough to confidently differentiate on an individual basis, without the benefit of cholangiography, whether these children did or did not have large duct disease in addition to their autoimmune hepatitis.

A scoring system first developed in 1993, to more accurately diagnose AIH, was revised in 1999[2]. When this latter score was applied to these children, all of those given a diagnosis of simple AIH could be classified as 'definite' cases of AIH, whereas only 15 of the 25 children who were thought to have both AIH and ASC had a 'definite' AIH score. Wilshanski et al.[3] approached the issue of an overlap between AIH and PSC in children from the opposite angle, i.e. by looking for features of AIH in children given a primary diagnosis of PSC on cholangiography. Their study, which was a retrospective rather than prospective study, published somewhat prior to those of Gregorio, concurs with the findings of Gregorio. Of concern is that, in both studies, the children who developed liver failure and needed a liver transplant were much more likely to have had the PSC/AIH overlap, suggesting that the outcome is less good in children when these two autoimmune liver diseases present simultaneously.

There have been three reports examining the coexistence of AIH in PSC as judged by applying both the old and the new AIH score in affected adults[4–6]. Whereas the chance of an AIH score in the 'definite' range did not vary between the old score and the 1999 revised score, there was a big fall in the number given a 'probable' score for AIH when employing the revised version. In the study from the Netherlands[6] in which the patients were much younger than in the other two studies (one from Scandinavia and one from the United States), 7% rather than 2% appeared to have both PSC and 'definite' AIH. Thus it appears that the coexistence of PSC and AIH is most often seen in children and young adults.

The real challenge in individuals with both PSC and AIH is to decide the appropriate therapy. It is unlikely that there will ever be a sufficient sample size which will allow therapy to be assessed in a randomized manner, even with a multicentre study. It is generally advised that, in those individuals thought to have both AIH and PSC, dual therapy with immunosuppressives and a bile acid, namely ursodeoxycholic acid (UDCA), is appropriate. However, the value of UDCA in PSC remains debatable. It is probable that those with both diseases will have more frequent and more severe metabolic bone disease, namely osteoporosis; thus preventive strategies, e.g. calcium, vitamin D and bisphosphonates, particularly if corticosteroids are being used, should probably be initiated early.

OVERLAPPING SYNDROMES

A PBC/AIH overlap is the most frequently reported overlapping syndrome. In nearly all instances it would appear that PBC has been the primary diagnosis, the overlapping features being those of AIH. It may well be that, because the clinical symptomatology of AIH is so vague and non-specific, no overlapping clinical features have been described; rather the coexistent features have been biochemical, immunological and histological. When symptoms have been reported, all have had their symptoms attributed to PBC; i.e. fatigue and pruritus with or without additional non-hepatic complications such as the sicca syndrome. Both pruritus and sicca syndrome are extremely unusual in uncomplicated AIH.

Chazoullier et al.[7] reported in 1998 that 9.2% of their 130 patients given a primary diagnosis of PBC had features of AIH; however, rather than use the aforementioned AIH scoring system they used their own. Thus, definition of AIH in this study was defined as an ALT greater than $5 \times$ uln, a positive smooth muscle antibody and/or an IgG level of greater than 2-fold elevated, in addition to a liver biopsy showing evidence of piecemeal necrosis to a moderate or severe degree. However, Talwalker et al.[8], at the Mayo Clinic, did apply the 1999 AIH scoring system to 141 patients given a primary diagnosis of PBC, and found that, using this revised score, none of their patients had a score in the definite range but 19% scored within the 'probable' range. When Czaja[9] reviewed his patient population given a primary diagnosis of AIH or PBC he noted that 5% of AIH cases had features of PBC and 19% of PBC cases had features of AIH.

Lohse and colleagues[10] compared the liver histology of 20 individuals given a diagnosis of AIH with 20 thought to have PBC with a further 20 whom they described as having an overlap of PBC and AIH. Whereas all but four of the 20 individuals with AIH had absolutely no evidence of bile duct damage on liver histology, all of those in the overlap group, and all of the PBC patients, had overt bile duct disease on liver biopsy. As the common link between these diseases is that they are all probably mediated by autoimmune processes, it is to be expected that there may be certain class II HLA associations. Individuals with AIH are more likely to have DR3 and DR4 alleles, and Lohse et al.[10] reported that this was also the pattern in his PBC/AIH overlap patients, but Czaja and co-workers[9,11], in their description of variant syndromes of autoimmune liver disease, found no specific HLA association in individuals with an apparent PBC/AIH overlap!

This discussion concerning PBC/AIH overlap may have been clinically irrelevant if it were not for the paper by Corpechot et al.[12], who suggest that, for individuals with PBC, those who have histological evidence of piecemeal necrosis (a feature thought to be typical of AIH) have a worse outcome. However, this observation could not be confirmed by Joshi et al.[13], who were unable to show that patients with PBC with apparent AIH overlap had a survival any different over 7 years of follow-up from patients with PBC without AIH features. Thus it remains to be clarified whether patients with PBC with features of AIH do or do not need additional therapy with immunosuppressive agents, as was suggested by Chazoullier et al.[7].

Bile duct injury in individuals with otherwise clear-cut AIH

It has generally been thought that bile duct lesions on liver biopsy are confined to patients who have biliary disease. However, a recent review of 80 cases of otherwise clear-cut autoimmune hepatitis indicated that 24% had some evidence, albeit often mild, of cholangitis and/or bile duct loss[14]. Three of these cases of AIH with a destructive cholangitis had a 'definite' AIH score; another three had somewhat lower AIH scores. Four individuals had overt ductopenia, three of whom had a 'definite' AIH score, and 10 further patients with obvious AIH had a non-destructive cholangitis. These patients with AIH and bile duct lesions on biopsy rarely had IBD, and response to immunosuppressive therapy was similar whether or not duct lesions were present.

Two sequential autoimmune liver diseases (changing diagnosis)

Such cases are relatively rare, and hence can still be published as isolated case reports. Columbato et al.[15] described an individual who was initially diagnosed with PBC and who later changed to overt AIH. Whereas PBC changing to AIH is easy to validate as the clinical symptomatology – the liver biochemistry, the serology and the liver biopsy findings all could be seen to change dramatically – it is harder to prove in cases of AIH, who seem to have changed to PSC, that the PSC was not present at the time of the original diagnosis. However, Abdo et al.[16] have recently published six cases of clear-cut AIH all with a 'definite' AIH score, and none with any liver biopsy features of biliary tract disease who were subsequently shown to have the typical features on ERCP of PSC. Three of these six patients had previously been shown to have a normal ERCP. Although it is possible that all six did indeed have PSC at baseline, at present we have no better definitive test for PSC than the cholangiographic findings, liver biopsy being notoriously unhelpful in PSC[17]. All but two of these individuals were young – less than 25, again indicating that the overlap or crossover of AIH to PSC is something which is almost always limited to children and young adults.

OUTLIER SYNDROMES

The term outlier syndrome refers to cases of *presumed* autoimmune liver disease, presumed because some features are contradictory or missing: cases of apparent

PBC who test negative for AMA, cases of AIH who test positive for AMA and some patients who present with an active 'cryptogenic' hepatitis who have no detectable non-organ specific antibodies.

AMA-negative PBC

In 1965 mitochondrial antibodies were first reported to be a helpful serological marker of PBC[18]; this observation has held up since that time. The standard method of testing remains immunofluorescence, as this is simple, sensitive and inexpensive. However, now the specific antigens involved in this antibody response have been identified. This allows the development of much more specific tests using ELISA and immunoblotting techniques. In the study published by Michieletti et al.[19], patients were described who had the typical features of PBC, who had even been referred for entry into a therapeutic trial in PBC, but on testing by immunofluoresence their sera had no detectable AMA. Twenty such cases were described, and when their sera were retested by immunoblotting, 17 remained without detectable AMA, either to the common antigen, pyruvate dehydrogenase complex (PDC), or to 2-oxoglutarate dehydrogenase complex or to branched-chain 2-oxoacid dehydrogenase complex. There were no clinical features which distinguished AMA-negative from AMA-positive PBC, but biochemically there was a significant difference in the levels of AST and IgM, both being somewhat lower in the AMA-negative cases. Both Michieletti et al., and later Taylor et al.[20] noted that individuals with AMA-negative PBC usually had high-titre ANA. There have now been several reports of AMA-negative PBC with long-term follow-up, the largest coming from Italy, published by Invernizzi et al. in 1997[21]. In none of these reports could the pathologists distinguish AMA-negative from AMA-positive PBC. To date the only feature that distinguished AMA-positive and AMA-negative PBC is the HLA pattern. Whereas there is an increased prevalence of DR8 in AMA-positive PBC, this particular class II HLA was not observed in any AMA-negative cases[22]. Response to treatment with UDCA is exactly the same in AMA-positive and AMA-negative PBC[23].

AMA-positive AIH

Kenny et al.[24] reported that some patients with otherwise overt AIH had low-titre AMA. Subsequently it was identified that some of these individuals really had antimicrosomal and not antimitochondrial antibodies. However, there are isolated case reports of otherwise clear-cut AIH[25], who test positive for antimitochondrial antibodies. Long-term follow-up of these cases has not shown transition to PBC.

Cryptogenic chronic hepatitis

Czaja et al. have described 12 cases of 'cryptogenic' chronic hepatitis[26]. These patients presented similarly to classical AIH but tested negative for ANA; SMA and AMA and baseline IgG levels, although elevated, were lower than those observed in 94 cases of AIH. The response to corticosteroids in these 'cryptogenic' cases was excellent, and of the five cases who underwent rebiopsy on follow-up only one developed cirrhosis. However, these cases are rare; the more usual scenario is that cases of AIH may at presentation be seronegative but repeat serological testing a few weeks after the acute presentation may then reveal the presence of ANA and/or SMA and hypergammaglobulinaemia.

SUMMARY

Presumably there are only so many ways in which the liver can respond to immune attack, the damage affecting either hepatocytes or the biliary system or both. So with the likely diverse array of endogenous and exogenous antigenic stimulants, coupled with the profusion of genetic polymorphisms of all the many immune response elements, it is not surprising that the pattern of liver injury may sometimes cross the 'boundaries' that physicians have arbitrarily imposed. These overlaps and outliers are of great interest to the academic, as well as being clinically challenging. As no formal diagnosis can be made both the affected individual and the clinician remain frustrated. These curious syndromes are sufficiently rare for it to be impossible to precisely define (using evidence-based methods) what may be the best therapeutic approach in each case.

References

1. Gregorio GV, Portmann B, Karani J et al. Autoimmune hepatitis/sclerosing cholangitis overlap syndrome in childhood: a 16-year prospective study. Hepatology. 2001;33:544–53.
2. Alverez F, Berg PA, Bianchi FB et al. International autoimmune hepatitis group report: Review of criteria for diagnosis of autoimmune hepatitis. J Hepatol. 1999;31:929–38.
3. Wilshanski M, Chait P, Wade JA et al. Primary sclerosing cholangitis in 32 children: clinical, laboratory, and radiographic features with survival analysis. Hepatology. 1995;22:1415–22.
4. Boberg KM, Fausa O, Haaland T et al. Features of autoimmune hepatitis in primary sclerosing cholangitis: an evaluation of 114 primary sclerosing cholangitis patients according to a scoring system for the diagnosis of autoimmune hepatitis. Hepatology. 1996;23:1369–76.
5. Kaya M, Angulo P, Lindor KD. Overlap of autoimmune hepatitis and primary sclerosing cholangitis: an evaluation of a modified scoring system. J Hepatol. 2000;33:537–42.
6. van Buuren HR, van Hoogstraten HJF, Terkivatan T, Schalm SW, Vleggaar FP. High prevalence of autoimmune hepatitis among patients with primary sclerosing cholangitis. J Hepatol. 2000;33:543–8.
7. Chazouiller O, Wendum D, Serfaty L, Montembault S, Rosmorduc O, Poupon R. Primary biliary cirrhosis–autoimmune hepatitis overlap syndrome: clinical features and response to therapy. Hepatology. 1998;28:296–301.
8. Talwalker JA, Keach JC, Angulo P, Lindor K. Overlap hepatitis and primary biliary cirrhosis: an evaluation of a modified scoring system. Am J Gastroenterol. 2002;97:1191–7.
9. Czaja AJ. Frequency and nature of the variant syndromes of autoimmune liver disease. Hepatology. 1998;28:362.
10. Lohse AW, Meyer zum Buschenfelde KH, Franz B, Kanzler S, Gerken G, Dienes HP. Characterization of the overlap syndrome of primary biliary cirrhosis (PBC) and autoimmune hepatitis: evidence for it being a hepatic form of PBC in genetically susceptible individuals. Hepatology. 1999;29:1078–84.
11. Czaja AJ, Carpenter HA, Santrach PJ, Moore SB. Autoimmune cholangitis within the spectrum of autoimmune liver disease. Hepatology. 2000;31:1231–8.
12. Corpechot C, Carrat F, Poupon R, Poupon RE. Primary biliary cirrhosis: incidence and predictive factors of cirrhosis development in ursodiol-treated patients. Gastroenterology. 2002;122:652–8.
13. Joshi S, Cauch-Dudek K, Wanless IR, Heathcote EJ. Response to ursodeoxycholic acid in primary biliary cirrhosis patients with additional features of autoimmune hepatitis. Hepatology. 2002;35:409–13.
14. Czaja AJ, Carpenter HA. Autoimmune hepatitis with incidental histologic features of bile duct injury. Hepatology. 2001;34:659–65.

15. Columbato LA, Alvarez F, Cote J, Huet PM. Autoimmune cholangiopathy: the result of consecutive primary biliary cirrhosis and autoimmune hepatitis? Gastroenterology. 1994;107:1839–43.
16. Abdo AA, Bain VG, Kichian K, Lee SS. Evolution of autoimmune hepatitis to primary sclerosing cholangitis: a sequential syndrome. Hepatology. 2002;36:1393–9.
17. Burak KW, Angulo P, Lindor K. Is there a role for liver biopsy in primary sclerosing cholangitis? Am J Gastroenterol. 2003;98:1155–8.
18. Walker JG, Doniach D, Roitt IM, Sherlock S. Serological tests in diagnosis of primary biliary cirrhosis. Lancet. 1965:1:827–31.
19. Michieletti P, Wanless IR, Katz A et al. Antimitochondrial antibody negative primary biliary cirrhosis: a distinct syndrome of autoimmune cholangitis. Gut. 1994;35:260–5.
20. Taylor SL, Dean PJ, Riely CA. Primary autoimmune cholangitis. An alternative to antimitochondrial antibody-negative primary biliary cirrhosis. Am J Surg Pathol. 1994;18:91–9.
21. Invernizzi P, Crosigani A, Battezzati PM et al. Comparison of the clinical features and clinical course of antimitochondrial antibody-positive and -negative primary biliary cirrhosis. Hepatology. 1997;25:1090–5.
22. Stone J, Wade JA, Cauch-Dudek K, Ng C, Lindor KD, Heathcote EJ. Human leukocyte antigen class II associations in serum antimitochondrial antibodies (AMA)-positive and AMA negative primary biliary cirrhosis. J Hepatol. 2002;36:8–13.
23. Kim WR, Poterucha JJ, Jorgensen RA et al. Does antimitochondrial antibody status affect response to treatment in patients with primary biliary cirrhosis? Outcomes of ursodeoxycholic acid therapy and liver transplantation. Hepatology. 1997;26:22–6.
24. Kenny RP, Czaja AJ, Ludwig J et al. Frequency and significance of antimitochondrial antibodies in severe chronic active hepatitis. Dig Dis Sci. 1986;31:705–11.
25. Yanagchua T, Miyakawa H, Shibata M et al. Immunoreactivity to pyruvate dehydrogenase complex-E2 in well defined patients with autoimmune hepatitis. Hepatol Res. 2003;26:81–6.
26. Czaja AJ, Carpenter H, Santrach PJ, Moore B, Homberger HA. The nature and prognosis of severe cryptogenic chronic active hepatitis. Gastroenterology. 1993;104:1757–61.

13
The autoimmune hepatitis/ hepatitis C overlap syndrome: does it exist?

A. J. CZAJA

INTRODUCTION

Autoimmune hepatitis (AIH) is not a viral syndrome by international consensus[1,2]. The presence of viraemia, however, does not preclude the diagnosis[1,2], and 11% of North American white adults with classical AIH can have hepatitis C virus (HCV) RNA in serum[3]. These patients must be distinguished from individuals with chronic hepatitis C who have autoantibodies and/or concurrent immune diseases that resemble AIH[4–8]. Differentiation is important since interferon therapy can enhance the immune manifestations[9–14] and immunosuppressive treatment can increase the viral load[15].

The detection of viral markers in patients with AIH and the presence of immune features in patients with chronic hepatitis C have generated the hypothesis of an overlap syndrome[16–19]. This concept implies the existence of a discrete clinical entity in which typical features of a classical disorder are blended with findings associated commonly with another disease. The overlap syndrome is presumed to have a characteristic phenotype, independent existence, and disease-specific pathogenic mechanisms; as such it must be distinguished from variations of classical disease and from coincidental conditions that are unrelated[20,21].

The clinical boundaries which encompass the classical syndromes have not been rigorously defined, and the variations of a classical disorder that are still acceptable for a single diagnosis are imprecise[20]. Consequently, an overlap syndrome may be within the spectrum of classical disease and its legitimacy unacknowledged. Alternatively, two unrelated conditions may coexist, and the designation of overlap syndrome may be erroneously applied. International panels have codified the diagnoses of AIH[1] and chronic hepatitis C[22], and an overlap syndrome between the entities has not been promulgated. Whereas individuals with chronic hepatitis C and immune manifestations are designated as "chronic hepatitis C with autoimmune features"[22], patients with AIH and HCV infection remain unclassified[16]. Distinctions between the entities depend on the predominant (viral versus autoimmune) manifestations of each syndrome.

The goals of this review are to describe the immune features shared by patients with AIH and those with chronic hepatitis C, present the histological findings in patients with mixed autoimmune and viral features, explore common pathogenic risk factors, and develop a logical, albeit empiric, management algorithm. In this fashion the validity of AIH with true HCV infection as an independent clinical entity (overlap syndrome) or as a serendipitous event (coincidental concurrence) can be determined.

IMMUNE MANIFESTATIONS OF CHRONIC HEPATITIS C

Antinuclear antibodies (ANA) and/or smooth muscle antibodies (SMA) occur in 20–40% of patients with chronic hepatitis C[4–8,23–27]; antibodies to liver/kidney microsome type 1 (anti-LKM1) are detectable in 6% of adults and 10–33% of children with HCV infection[28–33]; immune diseases that are viral antigen-driven (cryoglobulinaemia, glomerulonephritis, and vasculitis) or autoantigen-driven (autoimmune thyroiditis, Sjögren's syndrome, Graves' disease, and lichen planus) can coexist with HCV infection[26,34–37]; and corticosteroids may be effective in some patients[21,33,38–42]. Autoantibodies, concurrent immune diseases, or both autoantibodies and concurrent immune diseases have been demonstrated in 52% of patients with chronic hepatitis C (Figure 1A). These findings underscore the immune nature of chronic hepatitis C, but they do not detract from the essential viral basis of the syndrome.

The immune manifestations of chronic hepatitis C are frequently non-specific background reactivities that reflect hepatic injury and inflammatory activity[4,5,8], immune responses based on molecular mimicry[28–32], and microvascular injury driven by viral antigen (immune complex deposition)[35,36] (Table 1). These immune features are mainly humoral events that reflect inflammatory reactions and/or viral proliferation, and they do not implicate a primary immunopathic mechanism for the liver disease[26].

Concurrent immune disorders, such as Sjögren's syndrome[34] and autoimmune thyroiditis[36,37], are cell-mediated immune diseases that are autoantigen-driven, and their occurrence in chronic hepatitis C does implicate immune mechanisms based on mistaken self-identity (Table 1). Host rather than viral factors may facilitate their expression, and an immune phenotype characterized by female gender and the presence of HLA-DR3 or DR4 may identify these individuals[24,25,43,44]. The role of the virus in the expression of these diseases is uncertain, but the clonal expansion of promiscuous cytotoxic T cells stimulated by HCV and directed to diverse targets by molecular mimicry may result in their production[45,46]. The frequency of cell-mediated, autoantigen-driven diseases associated with chronic hepatitis C is similar to that of the humoral, viral antigen-driven disorders (Figure 2).

CHOLESTATIC LIVER DISEASES

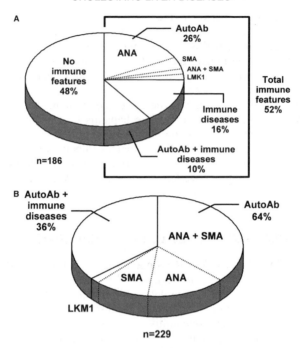

Figure 1 **A**: Frequency of immune manifestations in chronic hepatitis C. Autoantibodies (AutoAb) are the most common immune features, especially antinuclear antibodies (ANA). Smooth muscle antibodies (SMA) occur less commonly, and antibodies to liver/kidney microsome type 1 (LKM1) and concurrent SMA and ANA are rare in white North American patients. Immune diseases may be present in isolation (16%) or in combination with autoantibodies (10%). Original data. **B**: Frequency of immune manifestations in autoimmune hepatitis. Autoantibodies are the principal immune findings, and in contrast with chronic hepatitis C, concurrent SMA and ANA are common. Antibodies to LKM1 occur in only 4% of adult white North American patients. Original data

Table 1 Type and nature of principal immune manifestations

Liver disease	Principal immune manifestations	Putative mechanism
Chronic hepatitis C	Cryoglobulinaemia	Immune complex deposition
	Glomerulonephritis	Immune complex deposition
	Vasculitis	Immune complex deposition
	Smooth muscle antibodies	Bystander reactivity
	Antinuclear antibodies	Bystander reactivity
	Anti-liver/kidney microsome 1	Molecular mimicry
	Porphyria cutanea tarda	Viral-driven metabolic effect
	Autoimmune thyroiditis	Autoantigen-driven
	Graves' disease	Autoantigen-driven
	Sjögren's syndrome	Autoantigen-driven
	Lichen planus	Autoantigen-driven
Autoimmune hepatitis	Autoimmune thyroiditis	Autoantigen-driven
	Graves' disease	Autoantigen-driven
	Ulcerative colitis	Autoantigen-driven
	Rheumatoid arthritis	Autoantigen-driven

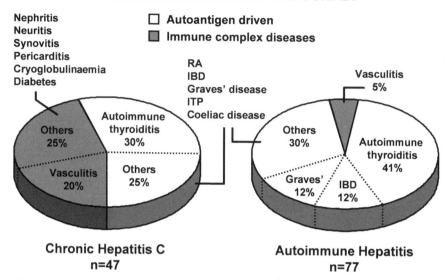

Figure 2 Nature of immune diseases associated with chronic hepatitis C and classical autoimmune hepatitis. Autoantigen-driven immune diseases reflective of cell-mediated immune responses are more common in classical autoimmune hepatitis than in chronic hepatitis C. Conversely, immune complex diseases reflective of humoral immune responses are more common in chronic hepatitis C than in classical autoimmune hepatitis. Immune complex diseases may be viral antigen-driven. Autoimmune thyroiditis is the most common autoantigen-driven disease in both autoimmune hepatitis and chronic hepatitis C. Other cell-mediated immune diseases, including rheumatoid arthritis (RA), idiopathic thrombocytopenic purpura (ITP), and inflammatory bowel disease (IBD) occur sporadically in both conditions. Original data

IMMUNE MANIFESTATIONS OF AIH

ANA, SMA, and anti-LKM1 are the hallmarks of AIH[1,2], and they are present in 95% of patients with the diagnosis[47]. Concurrent immune diseases are found in 36% of patients with AIH and, in contrast to chronic hepatitis C, SMA and ANA are commonly expressed together (Figure 1B). Furthermore, the nature of the immune diseases in classical AIH typically reflects cell-mediated, autoantigen-driven rather than humoral, viral antigen-driven immune responses[26] (Table 1 and Figure 2). Autoimmune thyroiditis, Graves' disease, and inflammatory bowel disease are the most common concomitant immune disorders in AIH, whereas vasculitis, glomerulonephritis, and symptomatic cryoglobulinaemia are rare[23,48] (Figure 2). The clinical and laboratory manifestations of humoral (autoantibody production) and cellular (autoantigen-driven) immune responses permeate the syndrome of AIH, and they support the concept of a primary immunopathic disorder[23,49].

CLINICAL AND SEROLOGICAL DISTINCTIONS

The nature and degree of the associated immune manifestations distinguish AIH with background HCV infection from chronic hepatitis C with autoimmune features. Concurrent immune diseases that reflect a cell-mediated response against autoantigens typify an autoimmune process, and they occur more commonly in AIH than in chronic hepatitis C[23] (Figure 2). They are also more likely to have clinical consequences if exacerbated during antiviral therapy than the manifestations of a humoral immune response[9–11,13,14,50–52].

Autoantibodies are common in both classical AIH and chronic hepatitis C, but their expression in AIH is stronger than in chronic hepatitis C[23] (Figure 3). In contrast to AIH, serum titres of ANA and/or SMA in chronic hepatitis C are typically less than 1 : 80 and infrequently above 1 : 320. Whereas ANA and SMA commonly occur together in AIH (Figure 1B), they rarely do so in chronic hepatitis C (Figure 1A)[23,53]. Furthermore, patients with AIH have higher serum levels of aspartate aminotransferase (AST), γ-globulin and immunoglobulin G than patients with chronic hepatitis C (Figure 4)[23].

High serum titres (≥ 1 : 320), marked hypergammaglobulinaemia, or the presence of autoantigen-driven concurrent immune diseases indicate an autoimmune predominant syndrome, and they justify liver biopsy evaluation to further define the nature of the process[54–58]. In chronic hepatitis C the presence of autoantibodies has been associated with increased inflammatory activity[8,59,60], and this observation has supported the likelihood that their production is secondary to tissue injury. In AIH, autoantibody production does not closely correlate with disease severity, and their production may reflect an underlying immune-mediated pathogenic process[49,61].

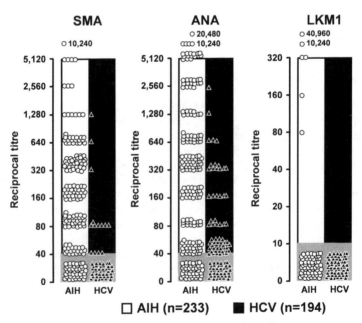

Figure 3 Reciprocal serum titres of smooth muscle antibodies (SMA), antinuclear antibodies (ANA), and antibodies to liver/kidney microsome type 1 (LKM1) in autoimmune hepatitis (AIH) and chronic hepatitis C (HCV). Serum titres of SMA and ANA are rarely ≥1 : 320 in chronic hepatitis C, and LKM1 are rare in North American patients with chronic hepatitis C. Original data

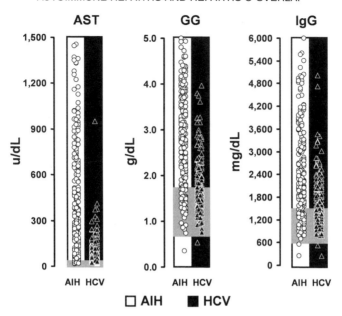

Figure 4 Serum levels of aspartate aminotransferase (AST), gamma-globulin (GG), and immunoglobulin G (IgG) in autoimmune hepatitis (AIH) and chronic hepatitis C (HCV). Serum AST, GG, and IgG levels are commonly higher in AIH than in chronic hepatitis C. Original data

HISTOLOGICAL DISTINCTIONS

Liver tissue examination is essential to determine the autoimmune or viral nature of a syndrome with mixed clinical and laboratory features[54–58]. Patients with classical AIH more commonly have severe interface hepatitis (23% versus 0%, $p = 0.02$), moderate to severe portal plasma cell infiltration (66% versus 21%, $p = 0.005$), and panacinar hepatitis (47% versus 16%, $p = 0.04$) than patients with typical chronic hepatitis C[56] (Table 2). In contrast, patients with typical chronic hepatitis C have a higher frequency of portal lymphoid aggregates (76% versus 42%, $p = 0.02$) and steatosis (52% versus 16%, $p = 0.006$) than patients with classical AIH[55] (Table 2).

The histological features of moderate–severe interface hepatitis, portal plasma cell infiltration, and panacinar hepatitis constitute a pattern (autoimmune pattern) that typifies AIH, whereas the histological features of portal lymphoid aggregation and steatosis constitute a pattern (viral pattern) that typifies chronic hepatitis C. The histological diagnoses based on these patterns have high specificity (81% and 91%) and predictability (62% and 82%) for AIH and chronic hepatitis C, respectively, but low sensitivity (40% and 57%) for each clinical diagnosis[56].

Patients with typical histological patterns of AIH or chronic hepatitis C have compelling evidence by which to define the predominant nature of their syndrome[54–58]. The histological changes are presumed to be more reflective of the true basis of the disease than the clinical trappings, and the histological findings override the clinical manifestations in establishing the diagnosis. When patients with chronic hepatitis C are separated by their predominant histological pattern, those individuals with interface hepatitis in the absence of portal lymphoid aggregates and steatosis (autoimmune pattern) have a different clinical phenotype than those who have portal lymphoid aggregates and steatosis (viral pattern)[57].

Patients with HCV infection and a pure autoimmune histological pattern (interface hepatitis, portal plasma cells, and panacinar hepatitis) have higher serum levels of γ-globulin and immunoglobulin G, greater frequency of autoantibodies, higher histological scores of inflammatory activity, and more frequent occurrence of cirrhosis than patients with HCV and a pure viral histological pattern (portal lymphoid aggregates and steatosis)[57] (Table 3). Patients with HCV infection and an autoimmune histological pattern that is pure or intermixed with background viral features have greater frequencies of high titre (titres $\geq 1:320$) SMA (13% versus 0%, $p = 0.05$) and HLA-DR3 (48% versus 15%, $p = 0.01$) than patients with a pure viral histological pattern[57]. Whilst these changes

Table 2 Histological distinctions between chronic hepatitis C and autoimmune hepatitis (percentages)

Histological features	Autoimmune hepatitis	Chronic hepatitis C
Interface hepatitis (severe)	23[c]	0[c]
Portal plasma cells (moderate)	66[a]	21[a]
Panacinar hepatitis	47[e]	16[e]
Portal lymphoid aggregates	42[d]	76[d]
Steatosis	16[b]	52[b]
Destructive cholangitis	5	5
Ductopenia	7	5

Significantly different from each other at level of [a]$p = 0.005$, [b]$p = 0.006$, [c,d]$p = 0.02$, and [e]$p = 0.04$. Adapted from ref. 56.

Table 3 Distinctions in chronic hepatitis C based on predominant histological pattern

Feature	Autoimmune histological pattern	Viral histological pattern
Gamma-globulin (nl 0.7–1.6 g/dl)	2.6 ± 0.3[a]	1.6 ± 0.1[a]
Immunoglobulin G (nl 700–1500 mg/dl)	2452 ± 363[c]	1414 ± 149[c]
SMA $\geq 1:320$	23%	0%
ANA $\geq 1:40$	62%	36%
Concurrent immune disease	23%	9%
HLA-DR3	54%	18%
A1-B8-DR3	36%	9%
Cirrhosis	46%[d]	0%[d]
Knodell score	12.1 ± 1.2[b]	7.1 ± 1.4[b]

Significantly different from each other at level of [a]$p = 0.005$, [b]$p = 0.01$, and [c,d]$p = 0.02$. Adapted from ref. 57.

may simply reflect differences in disease severity among patients with chronic hepatitis C[8,60], they might also connote different pathogenic pathways (auto-immune versus viral mechanisms)[45,46,49,62]. The association of HLA-DR3 with the autoimmune histological pattern suggests that autoimmune pathways modulate the disease in these individuals[57].

Only 40% of patients with chronic hepatitis C have histological changes that are classifiable as autoimmune (22%) and viral (18%) patterns[57]. Seventeen per cent have mixed (autoimmune and viral) histological patterns with interface hepatitis and portal lymphoid aggregates and/or steatosis, and 43% have non-discriminative patterns. Similarly, only 40% of individuals with classical AIH have histological changes of moderate–severe interface hepatitis, portal plasma cell infiltration, and panacinar hepatitis that confidently support the clinical diagnosis[56]. Consequently, less than half of the patients with mixed clinical and laboratory features have histological changes that compel a diagnosis. These individuals may be further categorized by the scoring system of the International Autoimmune Hepatitis Group (IAHG)[1].

DIAGNOSTIC SCORING SYSTEM

The scoring system of the IAHG was developed to quantify the strength of the diagnosis of AIH and to prevent isolated, weak, or inconsistent findings from discounting the disease[1]. The sensitivity of the scoring system for AIH ranges from 97% to 100%[63–66], and its specificity for excluding AIH in patients with chronic hepatitis C ranges from 66% to 92%[67,68]. The scoring system can classify patients as probable or definite AIH prior to corticosteroid therapy despite active viraemia if other autoimmune features are sufficiently numerous and/or strong. The scoring system provides a template that ensures the uniform assessment of all pertinent features of AIH, and in patients with mixed findings it can determine if AIH is the predominant syndrome. Since it has not been derived by direct comparisons between patients with AIH and those with chronic hepatitis C, the scoring system is not a discriminative index but rather a useful clinical tool in supporting clinical judgement[69].

TRANSITIONS BETWEEN AIH- AND VIRAL-PREDOMINANT SYNDROMES

The principal manifestations of a mixed syndrome can vary during the course of illness and treatment, and reclassification of the disease may be necessary[10,39,70,71]. Autoantibodies can develop *de novo* in individuals with classical chronic hepatitis C who are treated with interferon[72–74]. Concurrent autoimmune diseases, such as lichen planus[50,51] and ulcerative colitis[52], can be exacerbated during antiviral therapy, and the clinical findings and histological pattern can transform from a viral phenotype to an autoimmune phenotype (Figure 5A) or revert to a viral phenotype (Figure 5B) depending on the nature of the treatment that is applied (antiviral versus immunosuppressive therapy). Transitions, if they occur, usually do so after institution of a therapeutic regimen that favours emergence of the recessive component.

A

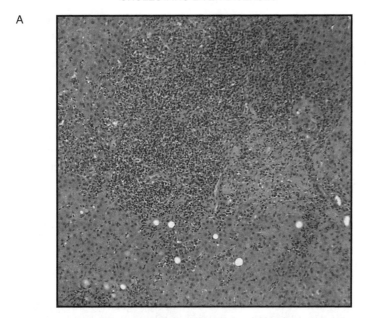

B

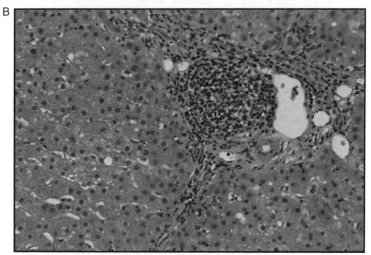

Figure 5 **A**: Emergence of autoimmune histological pattern in a patient with chronic hepatitis C who has been treated with interferon. The portal tract is expanded by a mononuclear infiltrate which contains plasma cells. Interface hepatitis is present in the absence of portal lymphoid aggregates and marked steatosis. Panacinar hepatitis is also present. The histological changes have been accompanied by clinical and laboratory deteriorations. (Haematoxylin and eosin; original magnification ×100.) **B**: Emergence of a viral histological pattern in the same patient with chronic hepatitis C after treatment with corticosteroids. The portal inflammation has decreased, and the interface hepatitis and panacinar hepatitis have disappeared. Portal lymphoid aggregates are now evident, and mild steatosis is present. The histological findings now more closely resemble a viral- rather than autoimmune-predominant process. The histological improvement has been mirrored by a clinical and laboratory improvement (Haematoxylin and eosin; original magnification ×200.)

140

PATHOGENIC MECHANISMS

The pathogenic mechanisms of an overlap syndrome between AIH and chronic hepatitis C require a molecular mimicry between self and viral antigens that produces coexistent autoimmune and viral features of comparable clinical significance[45,46]. AIH triggered by HCV infection persists after viral clearance and not in conjunction with it[75]. Homologies have been described between the HCV genome and an antigenic target of AIH (CYP2D6), but only non-pathogenic crossreacting antibodies have been characterized[76–79]. An Italian study demonstrated a high frequency of genotype 2a in patients with chronic hepatitis C and mixed cryoglobulinaemia, especially those with autoantibodies[80], and these findings suggested that certain HCV genomes had a greater immune stimulatory effect than others, possibly because of crossreacting epitopes. Genotype-related immune reactivities, however, were mainly humoral responses to viral antigen, not immunocyte-mediated responses against self-antigens, and the findings have been unconfirmed by French[81] and North American[82] studies.

Descriptions of cellular crossreactivities between autoantigens and HCV antigens have not been forthcoming[83], and a shared genetic predisposition for an overlap syndrome has not been found[24,43,84,85]. Furthermore, the clinical descriptions of the mixed AIH/HCV syndromes have not indicated a confusing hybrid condition. The patients with predominant features of AIH typically have background viraemia as their only viral manifestation[3], and patients with predominant features of HCV typically have low titre autoantibodies or associated immune complex diseases as their only immune manifestations[23,86,87].

Viraemia without clinical expression is insufficient to constitute an overlap syndrome, as are weak immune reactivities within a viral syndrome. Hypotheses based on crossreacting humoral and cellular mechanisms of immune reactivity, even if validated in overlap syndromes, are unnecessary to explain the coincidental, background autoimmune and viral features that typify patients with mixed AIH/HCV features[23,86,87].

EMPIRICAL MANAGEMENT ALGORITHM

The treatment of patients with mixed features of AIH and chronic hepatitis C should be appropriate for the predominant disease (Figure 6). A true overlap syndrome implies that autoimmune and viral features are blended in a distinctive clinical entity with shared pathogenic mechanisms. The clinical disorders with mixed features of AIH and HCV infection are not blended in this fashion, and typically the autoimmune or viral character of the condition is evident. It is this aspect that should be treated with the prescribed regimen, and the manifestations of another condition should be regarded as coincidental background findings. Criteria for instituting therapy are the same for each classical syndrome, and some patients with mixed features may not warrant treatment.

Patients with AIH and HCV viraemia are candidates for conventional corticosteroid therapy if they satisfy international clinical and/or scoring criteria for AIH (Figure 6). These patients usually have high titres of SMA and/or ANA

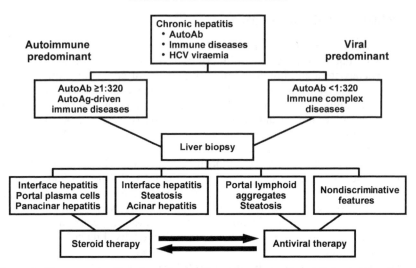

Figure 6 Treatment algorithm for patients with autoimmune and viral features. Therapies are empirical, but appropriate for the predominant character of the disease as defined by clinical, laboratory, and histological findings. Patients should have autoantibodies (AutoAb) and active hepatitis C virus (HCV) infection. Changes in the predominant character of the disease during one type of therapy justify substitution of another type of therapy more appropriate to the current manifestations. Criteria for instituting therapy are the same for each classical syndrome, and some patients with mixed features may not warrant treatment

(titres $\geq 1:320$), hypergammaglobulinaemia, and liver tissue examinations that show moderate to severe interface hepatitis with or without portal plasma cells or panacinar hepatitis[23,24,57]. Titres of anti-LKM1 do not differentiate autoimmune and viral syndromes, and the presence of anti-LKM1 in any titre requires a constellation of other clinical, laboratory, and histological findings before its proper interpretation[12,28–31,88].

Patients with a typical viral syndrome and low titre autoantibodies and histological features, including at least portal lymphoid aggregates and steatosis, are candidates for conventional antiviral treatment, especially if they have viral antigen-driven, immune complex disease[23,56,57,86,87] (Figure 6). Concurrent autoimmune diseases, such as autoimmune thyroiditis, lichen planus or ulcerative colitis, do not alter the diagnosis or treatment strategy. Multiple case reports have indicated that antiviral treatment can intensify autoantibody expression, exacerbate concurrent immune diseases, and decompensate the liver disease[9–14,50–52]. These consequences, however, have been rare in large experiences from Italy[86,89] and the United States[87], and they do not compel another therapeutic approach. Patients with immune features who are receiving interferon therapy, however, should be monitored closely for exacerbations that might justify discontinuation of the drug or its replacement with corticosteroids[10,11,71].

Combinations of immunosuppressive and antiviral drugs should be avoided since they counteract each other, and they are not justified by the clinical syndrome. Immunosuppressive and antiviral drugs can be administered in sequence as the predominant character of the syndrome changes[42,71] (Figures 5A and 5B).

142

An autoimmune liver disease can evolve from a viral liver disease undergoing interferon therapy, and it can respond to immunosuppressive drugs that replace the antiviral agents[10,11,71]. Similarly, a viral-predominant liver disease can emerge from an autoimmune liver disease treated with corticosteroids, and it can respond to antiviral drugs after discontinuation of the corticosteroids[42]. Responses to treatments in sequence must be measured by indices that reflect reductions in inflammatory activity rather than frequencies of sustained remission after drug withdrawal or virological clearance.

SUMMARY

Patients with AIH can have concurrent HCV infection, and patients with chronic hepatitis C can have autoantibodies and/or associated immunological diseases. These mixed syndromes are reflective of either coincidental viraemia (AIH and HCV infection) or background non-specific immune responses (chronic hepatitis C and autoimmune features). They are not distinct clinical entities that are independent of AIH or chronic hepatitis C, and they do not have responses to therapy that are different from the classical disease with which they are associated. Treatment is directed against the principal component of the syndrome with recognition that corticosteroids can increase viral load and interferon can exacerbate immune manifestations. Transition in the nature of the disease during one therapy may warrant implementation of the other therapy.

References

1. Alvarez F, Berg PA, Bianchi FB et al. International Autoimmune Hepatitis Group report: Review of criteria for diagnosis of autoimmune hepatitis. J Hepatol. 1999;31:929–38.
2. Czaja AJ, Freese DK. Diagnosis and treatment of autoimmune hepatitis. Hepatology. 2002;36:479–97.
3. Czaja AJ, Magrin S, Fabiano C et al. Hepatitis C virus infection as a determinant of behavior in type 1 autoimmune hepatitis. Dig Dis Sci. 1995;40:33–40.
4. Abuaf N, Lunel F, Giral P et al. Non-organ specific autoantibodies associated with chronic C virus hepatitis. J Hepatol. 1993;18:359–64.
5. Fried MW, Draguesku JO, Shindo M et al. Clinical and serological differentiation of autoimmune and hepatitis C virus-related chronic hepatitis. Dig Dis Sci. 1993;38:631–6.
6. Heintges T, Niederau C. Differentiation between autoimmune hepatitis and hepatitis C virus related liver disease. Z Gastroenterol. 1993;31:285–8.
7. Pawlotsky J-M, Deforges L, Bretagne S et al. Hepatitis C virus can mimic type 1 (antinuclear antibody positive) autoimmune chronic active hepatitis. Gut. 1993;34:S66–8.
8. Cassani F, Cataleta M, Valentini P et al. Serum autoantibodies in chronic hepatitis C: comparison with autoimmune hepatitis and impact on the disease profile. Hepatology. 1997;26:561–6.
9. Vento S, DiPerri G, Garofano T et al. Hazards of interferon therapy for HBV-seronegative chronic hepatitis. Lancet. 1989;2:926.
10. Shindo M, Di Bisceglie AM, Hoofnagle JH. Acute exacerbation of liver disease during interferon alfa therapy for chronic hepatitis C. Gastroenterology. 1992;102:1406–8.
11. Papo T, Marcellin P, Bernuau J, Durand F, Poynard T, Benhamou J-P. Autoimmune chronic hepatitis exacerbated by alpha-interferon. Ann Intern Med. 1992;116:51–3.
12. Vento S, Cainelli F, Conchia E, Ferraro T. Steroid and interferon therapy in liver/kidney microsomal antibody-positive patients with chronic hepatitis C. J Hepatol. 1997;26:955–6.
13. Lunel F, Cacoub P. Treatment of autoimmune and extrahepatic manifestations of hepatitis C virus infection. J Hepatol. 1999;31:210–16.

14. Lunel F, Cacoub P. Treatment of autoimmune and extra-hepatic manifestations of HCV infection. Ann Med Intern. 2000;151:58–64.
15. Magrin S, Craxi A, Fabiano C et al. Hepatitis C virus replication in 'autoimmune' chronic hepatitis. J Hepatol. 1991;13:364–7.
16. Czaja AJ. Chronic active hepatitis: the challenge for a new nomenclature. Ann Intern Med. 1993;119:510–17.
17. Czaja AJ. The variant forms of autoimmune hepatitis. Ann Intern Med. 1996;125:588–98.
18. Czaja AJ. Overlap of chronic viral hepatitis and autoimmune hepatitis. In: Willson RA, editor. Viral Hepatitis: Diagnosis, Treatment, Prevention. New York: Marcel Dekker, 1997:371–99.
19. Ben-Ari Z, Czaja AJ. Autoimmune hepatitis and its variant syndromes. Gut. 2001;49:589–94.
20. Heathcote J. Variant syndromes of autoimmune hepatitis. Clin Liver Dis. 2002;6:669–84.
21. Lohse AW, Gerken G, Meyer zum Buschenfelde K-H. Autoimmune hepatitis and hepatitis C virus infection. Curr Stud Hematol Blood Transfus. 1998;62:152–60.
22. Desmet VJ, Gerber M, Hoofnagle JH, Manns M, Scheuer PJ. Classification of chronic hepatitis: diagnosis, grading and staging. Hepatology. 1994;19:1513–20.
23. Czaja AJ, Carpenter HA, Santrach PJ, Moore SB, Taswell HF, Homburger HA. Evidence against hepatitis viruses as important causes of severe autoimmune hepatitis in the United States. J Hepatol. 1993;18:342–52.
24. Czaja AJ, Carpenter HA, Santrach PJ, Moore SB. Immunologic features and HLA associations in chronic viral hepatitis. Gastroenterology. 1995;108:157–64.
25. Czaja AJ, Carpenter HA, Santrach PJ, Moore SB. Genetic predispositions for immunological features in chronic liver diseases other than autoimmune hepatitis. J Hepatol. 1996;24:52–9.
26. Czaja AJ. Extrahepatic immunologic features of chronic viral hepatitis. Dig Dis. 1997;15:125–44.
27. Zauli D, Cassani F, Bianchi FB. Auto-antibodies in hepatitis C. Biomed Pharmocother. 1999;53:234–41.
28. Todros L, Touscoz G, D'Urso N et al. Hepatitis C virus-related chronic liver disease with autoantibodies to liver-kidney microsomes (LKM). Clinical characterization from idiopathic LKM-positive disorders. J Hepatol. 1991;13:128–31.
29. Lunel F, Abuaf N, Frangeul L et al. Liver/kidney microsome antibody type 1 and hepatitis C virus infection. Hepatology. 1992;16:630–6.
30. Lunel F, Abuaf N, Frangeul L et al. Liver/kidney microsome antibody type 1 and hepatitis C virus infection. Hepatology. 1992;16:630–6.
31. Giostra F, Manzin A, Lenzi M et al. Low hepatitis C viremia in patients with anti-liver/kidney microsomal antibody type 1 positive chronic hepatitis. J Hepatol. 1996;25:433–8.
32. Vergani D. NOSA in HCV infection: markers or makers of disease? Gut. 1999;45:328–9.
33. Bortolotti F, Muratori L, Jara P et al. Hepatitis C virus infection associated with liver–kidney microsomal antibody type 1 (LKM1) autoantibodies in children. J Pediatr. 2003;142: 185–90.
34. Haddad J, Deny P, Munz-Gotheil C et al. Lymphocytic sialadenitis of Sjögren's syndrome associated with chronic hepatitis C virus liver disease. Lancet. 1992;339:321–3.
35. Lunel F, Musset L, Cacoub P et al. Cryoglobulinemia in chronic liver diseases: role of hepatitis C virus and liver damage. Gastroenterology. 1994;106:1291–300.
36. Pawlotsky J-M, Yahia MB, Andre C et al. Immunological disorders in C virus chronic active hepatitis: a prospective case–control study. Hepatology. 1994;19:841–8.
37. Marcellin P, Pouteau M, Benhamou J-P. Hepatitis C virus infection, alpha interferon therapy and thyroid dysfunction. J Hepatol. 1995;22:364–9.
38. Fong T-L, Valinluck B, Govindarajan S, Charboneau F, Adkins RH, Redeker AG. Short-term prednisone therapy affects aminotransferase activity and hepatitis C virus RNA levels in chronic hepatitis C. Gastroenterology. 1994;107:196–9.
39. Bellary S, Schiano T, Hartman G, Black M. Chronic hepatitis with combined features of autoimmune chronic hepatitis and chronic hepatitis C: favorable response to prednisone and azathioprine. Ann Intern Med. 1995;123:32–4.
40. Tran A, Benzaken S, Yang G et al. Chronic hepatitis C and autoimmunity: good response to immunosuppressive therapy. Dig Dis Sci. 1997;42:778–80.
41. Yoshikawa M, Toyohara M, Yamane Y et al. Disappearance of serum HCV-RNA after short-term prednisolone therapy in a patient with chronic hepatitis C associated with autoimmune hepatitis-like serological manifestations. J Gastroenterol. 1999;34:269–74.

42. Schiano TD, Te HS, Thomas RM, Hussain H, Bond K, Black M. Results of steroid-based therapy for the hepatitis C–autoimmune overlap syndrome. Am J Gastroenterol. 2001;96: 2984–91.
43. Czaja AJ, Carpenter HA, Santrach PJ, Moore SB. Significance of human leukocyte antigens DR3 and DR4 in chronic viral hepatitis. Dig Dis Sci. 1995;40:2098–106.
44. Czaja AJ, Dos Santos RM, Porto A, Santrach PJ, Moore SB. Immune phenotype of chronic liver disease. Dig Dis Sci. 1998;43:2149–55.
45. Vergani D, Choudhuri K, Bogdanos DP, Mieli-Vergani G. Pathogenesis of autoimmune hepatitis. Clin Liver Dis. 2002;6:727–37.
46. Vogel A, Manns MP, Strassburg CP. Autoimmunity and viruses. Clin Liver Dis. 2002;6: 739–53.
47. Baeres M, Herkel J, Czaja AJ et al. Establishment of standardized SLA/LP immunoassays: specificity for autoimmune hepatitis, worldwide occurrence, and clinical characteristics. Gut. 2002;51:259–64.
48. Czaja AJ, Carpenter HA, Santrach PJ, Moore SB. Genetic predispositions for the immunological features of chronic active hepatitis. Hepatology. 1993;18:816–22.
49. Czaja AJ. Understanding the pathogenesis of autoimmune hepatitis. Am J Gastroenterol. 2001;96:1224–31.
50. Dupin N, Chosidow O, Frances C et al. Lichen planus after alpha-interferon therapy for chronic hepatitis C. Eur J Dermatol. 1994;4:535–6.
51. Protzer U, Ochsendorf FR, Leopolder-Ochsendorf A, Holtermuller KH. Exacerbation of lichen planus during interferon alfa-2a therapy for chronic active hepatitis C. Gastroenterology. 1993;104:903–5.
52. Mitoro A, Yoshikawa M, Yamamoto K et al. Exacerbation of ulcerative colitis during alpha-interferon therapy for chronic hepatitis C. Intern Med. 1993;32:327–31.
53. Cassani F, Muratori L, Manotti P et al. Serum autoantibodies and the diagnosis of type-1 autoimmune hepatitis in Italy: a reappraisal in the light of hepatitis C virus infection. Gut. 1992;33:1260–3.
54. Scheuer PJ, Ashrafzadeh P, Sherlock S, Brown D, Dusheiko GM. The pathology of hepatitis C. Hepatology. 1992;15:567–71.
55. Bach N, Thung SN, Schaffner F. The histological features of chronic hepatitis C and autoimmune chronic hepatitis: a comparative analysis. Hepatology. 1992;15:572–7.
56. Czaja AJ, Carpenter HA. Sensitivity, specificity and predictability of biopsy interpretations in chronic hepatitis. Gastroenterology. 1993;105:1824–32.
57. Czaja AJ, Carpenter HA. Histological findings in chronic hepatitis C with autoimmune features. Hepatology. 1997;26:459–66.
58. Hano H, Takasaki S, Nakayama J. Autoimmune forms of chronic hepatitis associated with hepatitis C virus (HCV) infection with and without HCV-RNA: histological differences from pure autoimmune hepatitis and chronic hepatitis C. Pathol Int. 2000;50:106–12.
59. Abuaf N, Lunel F, Giral P et al. Non-organ specific autoantibodies associated with chronic hepatitis C viral hepatitis. J Hepatol. 1993;18:359–64.
60. Lenzi M, Bellentani S, Saccoccio G et al. Prevalence of non-organ specific autoantibodies and chronic liver disease in the general population: a nested case-control study of the Dionysos cohort. Gut. 1999;45:435–41.
61. Czaja AJ. Behavior and significance of autoantibodies in type 1 autoimmune hepatitis. J Hepatol. 1999;30:394–401.
62. Gonzalez-Peralta RP, Davis GL, Lau JYN. Pathogenetic mechanisms of hepatocellular damage in chronic hepatitis C virus infection. J Hepatol. 1994;21:255–9.
63. Bianchi FB, Cassani F, Lenzi M et al. Impact of International Autoimmune Hepatitis Group scoring system in definition of autoimmune hepatitis. An Italian experience. Dig Dis Sci. 1996;41:166–71.
64. Czaja AJ, Carpenter HA. Validation of a scoring system for the diagnosis of autoimmune hepatitis. Dig Dis Sci. 1996;41:305–14.
65. Boberg KM, Fausa O, Haaland T et al. Features of autoimmune hepatitis in primary sclerosing cholangitis: an evaluation of 114 primary sclerosing cholangitis patients according to a scoring system for the diagnosis of autoimmune hepatitis. Hepatology. 1996;23:1369–76.
66. Omagari K, Masuda J, Kato Y et al. Re-analysis of clinical features of 89 patients with autoimmune hepatitis using the revised scoring system proposed by the International Autoimmune Hepatitis Group. Intern Med. 2000;39:1008–12.

67. Toda G, Zeniya M, Watanabe F et al. Present status of autoimmune hepatitis in Japan – correlating the characteristics with international criteria in an area with a high rate of HCV infection. J Hepatol. 1997;26:1207–12.

68. Dickson RC, Gaffey MJ, Ishitani MB, Roarty TP, Driscoll CJ, Caldwell SH. The international autoimmune hepatitis score in chronic hepatitis C. J Viral Hepat. 1997;4:121–8.

69. Talwalkar JA, Keach JC, Angulo P, Lindor KD. Overlap of autoimmune hepatitis and primary biliary cirrhosis: an evaluation of a modified scoring system. Am J Gastroenterol. 2002;97: 1191–7.

70. Silva MO, Reddy KR, Jeffers LJ, Hill M, Schiff ER. Interferon-induced chronic active hepatitis? Gastroenterology. 1991;101:840–2.

71. Garcia-Bury L, Garcia-Monzon C, Rodriguez S et al. Latent autoimmune hepatitis triggered during interferon therapy in patients with chronic hepatitis C. Gastroenterology. 1995;108:1770–7.

72. Noda K, Enomoto N, Arai K et al. Induction of antinuclear antibody after interferon therapy in patients with type-C chronic hepatitis: its relation to the efficacy of therapy. Scand J Gastroenterol. 1996;31:716–22.

73. Bayraktar Y, Bayraktar M, Gurakar A, Hassanein TI, Van Thiel DH. A comparison of the prevalence of autoantibodies in individuals with chronic hepatitis C and those with autoimmune hepatitis: the role of interferon in the development of autoimmune diseases. Hepato-Gastroenterology. 1997;44:417–25.

74. Dumoulin FL, Leifeld L, Sauerbruch T, Spengler U. Autoimmunity induced by interferon-α therapy for chronic viral hepatitis. Biomed Pharmacother. 1999;53:242–54.

75. Vento S, Cainelli F, Renzini C, Concia E. Autoimmune hepatitis type 2 induced by HCV and persisting after viral clearance. Lancet. 1997;350:1298–9.

76. Manns MP, Griffin KJ, Sullivan KF, Johnson EF. LKM-1 autoantibodies recognize a short linear sequence in P450IID6, a cytochrome P-450 monooxygenase. J Clin Invest. 1991;88:1370–8.

77. Yamamoto AM, Cresteil D, Homberg JC, Alvarez F. Characterization of the anti-liver–kidney microsome antibody (anti-LKM1) from hepatitis C virus-positive and -negative sera. Gastroenterology. 1993;104:1762–67.

78. Klein R, Zanger UM, Berg T, Hopf U, Berg PA. Overlapping but distinct specificities of anti-liver–kidney microsome antibodies in autoimmune hepatitis II and hepatitis C revealed by recombinant native CYP2D6 and novel peptide groups. Clin Exp Immunol. 1999;118:290–7.

79. Mackie FD, Peakman M, Yun M et al. Primary and secondary liver/kidney microsomal antibody response following infection with hepatitis C virus. Gastroenterology. 1994;106:1672–5.

80. Zignego AL, Ferri C, Giannini C et al. Hepatitis C virus genotype analysis in patients with type II mixed cryoglobulinemia. Ann Intern Med. 1996;124:31–4.

81. Pawlotsky J-M, Roudot-Thoraval F, Simmonds P et al. Extrahepatic immunologic manifestations in chronic hepatitis C and hepatitis C serotypes. Ann Intern Med. 1995;122:169–73.

82. Zein NN, Persing DH, Czaja AJ. Viral genotypes as determinants of autoimmune expression in chronic hepatitis C. Mayo Clin Proc. 1999;74:454–60.

83. Koskinas J, McFarlane BM, Nouria-Aria K et al. Cellular and humoral immune reactions against autoantigens and hepatitis C viral antigens in chronic hepatitis C. Gastroenterology. 1994;107: 1436–42.

84. Czaja AJ, Santrach PJ, Moore SB. Shared genetic risk factors in autoimmune liver disease. Dig Dis Sci. 2001;46:140–7.

85. Czaja AJ, Carpenter HA, Santrach PJ, Moore SB. DR human leukocyte antigens and disease severity in chronic hepatitis C. J Hepatol. 1996;24:666–73.

86. Saracco G, Touscoz A, Durazzo M et al. Antibodies and response to alpha-interferon in patients with chronic viral hepatitis. J Hepatol. 1990;11:339–43.

87. Clifford BD, Donahue D, Smith L et al. High prevalence of serological markers of autoimmunity in patients with chronic hepatitis C. Hepatology. 1995;21:613–19.

88. Muratori L, Lenzi M, Cataleta M et al. Interferon therapy in liver/kidney microsomal antibody type 1-positive patients with chronic hepatitis C. J Hepatol. 1994;21:199–203.

89. Fattovich G, Giustina G, Favarato S, Ruol A. A survey of adverse events in 11,241 patients with chronic viral hepatitis treated with alfa interferon. J Hepatol. 1996;24:38–47.

14
Histopathology of overlap syndromes in the liver

H. P. DIENES and A. W. LOHSE

INTRODUCTION

The term 'overlap syndrome' of autoimmune liver diseases has been challenged ever since its introduction in the literature, and is probably the most overused and abused term currently in use in hepatology[1]. However, this term applies mainly to groups of patients with autoimmune liver diseases that do not completely fit into the categories of autoimmune hepatitis, primary biliary cirrhosis or primary sclerosing cholangitis (AIH, PBC or PSC) regarding clinical symptoms[2], serology, biochemistry and histopathology. Diagnostic criteria of the autoimmune liver diseases (AIH[3], PBC[4], PSC[5]) are not well defined and there are no unique pathognomonic features or tests that allow precise diagnostic designation. In order to classify patients who have symptoms or data on the serological histological and biochemical level exceeding one disease entity the term 'overlap syndrome' has been coined[6]; synonyms include variants of PBC, PSC with features of AIH[7].

This chapter will try to provide histopathological data of patients who suffer from two autoimmune liver diseases displaying overlap syndromes, or who have one disease with additional histological features of another syndrome.

Overlap syndromes of autoimmune liver diseases have been the subject of many publications, with AIH and PBC being the most frequent players[8–11] and AIH and PSC being only secondary. The overlap syndrome of PBC and PSC seems to be unique, with only one report covering this issue[12].

Before outlining the histopathology of the overlap syndromes the individual disease entities constituting the syndrome will be described in detail.

DIAGNOSIS OF AIH

In clinical practice the diagnosis of AIH is clear-cut in female patients with the spectrum of autoantibodies, such as ANA, SLA, γGT, AP elevation, transaminase elevation and genetic background of HLA. However, there are no specific autoantibodies that are key diagnostic components, and about 10–20% of patients lack all autoantibodies[13,14]. In order to establish the diagnosis with more reliability a scoring system has been suggested by the International Autoimmune Hepatitis Group that has been widely accepted[15]. The issues of the scoring system include gender, autoantibodies, genetic background and histological features with characteristics such as interface hepatitis, lymphoplasmocytic infiltrate and rosetting of liver cells. The lesions are by no means pathognomonic. The exclusion of biliary changes, however, is questionable for two reasons: (a) in about 20% of liver biopsies from patients with AIH bile duct lesions may occur to some degree[16], and (b) the occurrence of overlap syndrome with PBC does not exclude the existence of AIH.

There are few descriptions of the histopathology of AIH, perhaps due to lack of security of the diagnosis. Two publications[17,18] have tried to define histological features in AIH after detection and identification of the hepatitis C virus (HCV) (at that time the non-A–non-B agent) at the end of the 1980s. Due to the fact that AIH could now be better differentiated from non-A–non-B hepatitis by virological and serological tests, histologic features could be attributed to AIH with greater certainty. Both studies found severe interface hepatitis (Figure 1) in about 80%. In the periportal area parenchymal collapse was found in 50% and

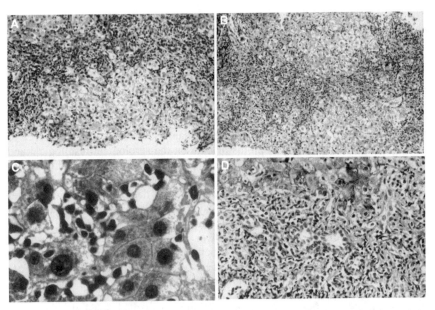

Figure 1 Autoimmune hepatitis with severe activity. **A**: Portal and periportal activity of the necroinflammatory lesion is evident with severe interface hepatitis (original magnification ×120; HE). **B**: Autoimmune hepatitis with bridging hepatic necrosis and rosetting of liver cells (original magnification ×120; HE). **C**: Liver damage is linked to the presence of lymphocytes frequently presenting as emperipolesis (original magnification ×630; HE). **D**: Bile duct lesions in autoimmune hepatitis with lymphocytes infiltrating the bile duct epithelia but without destruction (original magnification ×240; HE)

Table 1   Histopathology of AIH (from ref. 19)

Interface hepatitis
Lymphocytic/lymphoplasmocytic infiltrates
Emperipolesis
BHN
Hepatocellular polymorphism: ballooning,
  acidophilic shrinkage, apoptosis
Hepatic rosette formation
Lymphocytic cholangitis

Table 2   Percentage bile duct lesions in
AIH; 84 patients (from ref. 16)

Destructive cholangitis	7
Non-destructive cholangitis	11
Bile duct loss	4

67% respectively. There was severe lobular inflammation. Rosetting of hepatocytes occurred in about 62%. Plasma cells made up about 16% of the inflammatory infiltrate. Both studies agreed that there are characteristic but by no means pathognomonic features of the disease.

A more extensive review on the histopathology of AIH (Table 1) has been presented by Czaja and Carpenter[19] in the textbook by McSween et al. Besides the above-mentioned features interface hepatitis, emperipolesis of lymphocytes and hepatocellular polymorphism are extensively described. The involvement of bile ducts in AIH (Figure 1D) is included in the review. In a recent publication the authors investigated bile duct lesions in AIH (Table 2) in more detail, including 84 patients in the study[16]. They found destructive cholangitis in about 7%, lymphocytic non-destructive cholangitis in about 11% and bile duct loss in 4% of patients. The destruction of bile ducts in AIH, however, was not accompanied by granuloma formation with lymphoepithelial lesions. In this investigation bile duct loss is reported; however, it did not result in overt ductopenia, i.e. loss of bile ducts in more than 50% of the portal tracts. Summarizing the involvement of bile ducts in AIH, destructive cholangitis may occur, but without granulomatous destruction of bile ducts and with no overt ductopenia. There may be some ductular reaction in AIH with increasing number of ductules; however, when staining for cytokeratin 7 and 19 the liver cells do not display ductular metaplasia, in contrast to PBC (H. Dienes, unpublished observation).

DIAGNOSIS OF PBC

The diagnosis of PBC is based on three parameters[4] (Table 3): (a) elevation of cholestatic liver tests, (b) AMA2 greater than 1 : 40 and (c) histopathology that is diagnostic or should be compatible with the diagnosis (Figure 2). Histological lesions that are pathognomonic for PBC may be seen in liver biopsies in about 30% of cases. The purpose of taking a biopsy in PBC is therefore mainly to exclude other diseases that may have cholestatic liver enzyme elevation, such as steatohepatitis.

Table 3 Diagnosis of PBC (from ref. 4)

Elevation of cholestatic liver tests
AMA2 greater than 1 : 40
Histopathology, compatible or diagnostic

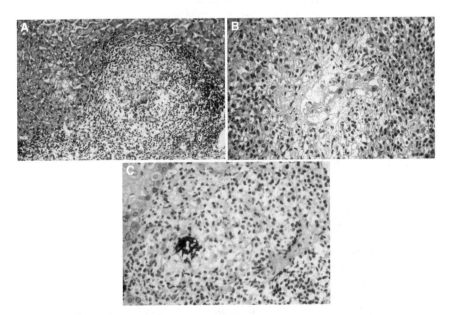

Figure 2 **A**: PBC stage 1, ductular lesion; the portal tract is enlarged and rounded with a bile duct in the centre of a granuloma undergoing destruction. **B**: Higher magnification displays the loss of basement membrane and bile duct epithelia undergoing apoptosis. **C**: Immunohistology for cytokeratin 7 to appreciate the lymphoepithelial lesion of the bile duct. Hepatocytes of the limiting plate are stained as well as sign for cholestasis (original magnification ×240; antibody against cytokeratin 7; counterstain with Mayer's Hämalaun)

Bile duct destruction in PBC is pathognomonic at the histological level[20], including disruption of the basement membrane and necrosis or apoptosis of bile duct epithelia. Invasion of bile duct epithelia by lymphocytic infiltrates can be better appreciated when staining for cytokeratin 7, and this so-called lymphoepithelial lesion is very characteristic of PBC. Staining for cytokeratin 7 may also reveal hepatocellular cholestasis by staining periportal hepatocytes as an indicator for ductular metaplasia (Figure 2C). Ductular metaplasia is an important feature of differential diagnosis to AIH when affection of bile ducts may occur in AIH. On the other hand, bridging hepatic necrosis and lobular inflammation may occur in PBC, as Portmann et al.[21] had shown, especially in stage 2 of PBC.

Exact and definite diagnosis of PBC should therefore include serology with presence of AMA, cholestatic liver tests and histopathology, either diagnostic or at least compatible with the diagnosis.

DIAGNOSIS OF AIH/PBC OVERLAP SYNDROME

The diagnosis of an overlap syndrome should be made only when both disease entities, AIH and PBC, present simultaneously[8]. For AIH the scoring should be greater than 15 points, meaning definite AIH. PBC should present with AMA2 greater than 1 : 40, cholestatic liver test elevation and corresponding liver pathology. The main features of AIH and PBC should be present in the liver tissue at the time of biopsy (Table 4). The frequency of AIH/PBC overlap syndromes is given in the literature in a range from 4.8% of PBC and up to 20% of AIH[8,9] (Table 5).

Histopathology is characterized by histological features of PBC[20] in the portal tracts, which means granulomatous destruction of bile ducts with disruption of basement membranes (Figure 3). There is necrosis of bile duct epithelia with lymphoepithelial lesions. There is a broad spill-over of lymphocytes and plasma cells onto the periportal hepatocytes by destroying the limiting plate. In the lobule there is conspicuous emperipolesis and much continuous necroinflammatory activity from periportal area to central zone. When grading interface hepatitis, lobular spotty necrosis and infiltration and bile duct lesions on an arbitrary scale from 1 to 8, we found (in comparing three groups of patients[8] with autoimmune hepatitis, PBC and overlap syndrome), that patients with overlap syndrome equalled the scoring of interface hepatitis and spotty necrosis with AIH and bile duct lesions with PBC. Concluding from this study we could show that, on the histopathology level, patients with overlap syndrome present the salient and pathognomonic features of both diseases in the same biopsy (Tables 6 and 7).

The association of AIH and PBC based on the unifying concept of autoimmune liver diseases[22] can also be demonstrated by reports in the literature on the development of AIH in liver grafts after liver transplantation for end-stage PBC[23]. We have observed another patient in reversed circumstances (unpublished observation): a 63-year-old female received a new liver because of end-stage PBC with decompensated cirrhosis. At that time autoimmune antibodies were positive with ANA at a titre of 1 : 128 and SMA 1 : 40. Three years after transplantation the patient developed a period of cholestatic enzyme elevation, moderate transaminase elevation and positivity of AMA2 at a titre of 1 : 80 that had been negative at the point of transplantation. Histopathology in the liver biopsy taken 3 years

Table 4   Diagnosis of AIH/PBC/OLS (from refs 1, 8 and 9)

AIH: scores greater than 15
PBC: (definite) AMA2 greater than 1 : 40, cholestatic
 liver tests, histopathology
Histopathology of AIH and PBC in the same biopsy

Table 5   Frequency of AIH/PBC overlap syndrome

Czaja and Carpenter 1998[19]: 8% AIH + PBC
Chazouillières et al. 1998[9]: 9.2% of PBC
Lohse et al. 1999[8]: 20% of AIH
Joshi et al. 2002[1]: 4.8% of PBC

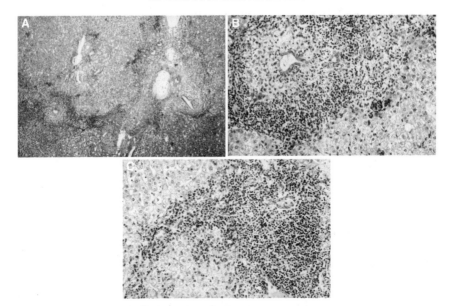

Figure 3 Female patient with AIH/PBC overlap syndrome. **A**: Even at low magnification portal tracts with biliary lesions and bridging hepatic necrosis between portal tracts are evident (original magnification ×80; HE). **B**: Same patient with higher magnification of portal tract showing bile duct destruction within a granuloma and above that interface hepatitis around the portal tract (original magnification ×160; HE). **C**: Same biopsy with abundant lymphoplasmocytic infiltrate in portal tract and spilling over into the parenchyma accompanying a bridging hepatic necrosis (original magnification ×160; HE)

Table 6 Histological features of PBC/AIH overlap syndrome

PBC	AIH
Lymphoepithelial lesions of bile duct epithelia	Severe interface hepatitis
Epithelial granulomas	Rosetting of liver cells
Disruption of basement membrane	Conspicuous emperipolesis
Dense portal lymphocytic infiltrates	Continuous necroinflammatory activity

Table 7 Assessment of necroinflammatory lesions of bile ducts and liver lobules ($n = 30$/cohort)

	AIH	Overlap	PBC
Interface hepatitis	6.5	6.3	2.4
Spotty necrosis, inflammation	5.8	5.5	0.9
Bile duct lesions	0.3	3.4	3.9

Scoring is adapted to the suggestion of Bianchi et al.[37] regarding HAI, and Ishak et al.[38] on a scale from 0 to 9.

after transplantation showed chronic destructive non-suppurating cholangitis corresponding to PBC stage 2.

DIAGNOSIS OF PSC

The diagnosis of PSC should include[24] cholestatic biochemistry, histopathology compatible or diagnostic for PSC including lesions of fibrous obliterative cholangitis, distinctive cholangiography, and association with idiopathic bowel disease (Table 8).

When present the histological features of PSC are quite characteristic[20], including sclerosing spanding of portal tracts with a periductual fibrous cuff around bile ducts (Figure 4). There is characteristic hyaline thickening of basement

Table 8 Diagnosis of PSC (from ref. 24)

Cholestatic biochemistry
Histopathology of fibrous obliterative
cholangitis
Distinctive cholangiography
Association with idiopathic bowel disease

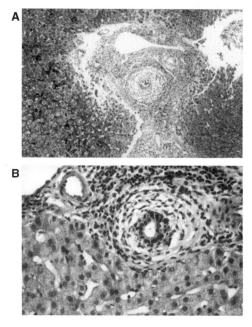

Figure 4 A 35-year-old male patient with PSC. **A**: The portal tract is enlarged with a bile duct in the centre surrounded by onion-skin-like fibrous tissue. Inflammation is only moderate (original magnification ×120; Masson's trichrome). **B**: Higher magnification of a small bile duct displaying typical features of PSC with a fibrous cuff, scanty lymphocytes and atrophic biliary epithelia (original magnification ×360; PASD)

membrane obvious in PASD staining, and atrophy or destruction of bile ducts. Bile duct epithelia are then shrunken with nuclear pyknosis and condensation of the cytoplasm of the epithelia. In later stages bile ducts are disappearing, and are substituted by a fibrous scar that has been named the tombstone of bile duct. The inflammatory reaction during PSC is variable. Especially in the early stages the inflammatory infiltrates may be quite vivid, with lymphohistiocytic infiltrates in portal tracts and spilling over to the parenchyma. There are no obvious apoptotic bodies of bile duct epithelia or lymphoepithelial lesions. Disruption of basement membrane or piecemeal necroses are generally absent.

By histopathology there is no difference between common PSC and so-called small-duct PSC.

OVERLAP SYNDROME OF AIH AND PSC

The AIH/PSC overlap syndrome in adults seems to be less frequent than the PBC/AIH overlap. Figures show between 1.4% and 8% of patients with PSC[25–28] or 6.5% of patients with AIH[29] (Table 9). With regard to PBC/AIH overlap syndrome the diagnosis of AIH/PSC overlap syndrome should be established on the simultaneous or consecutive criteria of cholangiographic lesions, cholestatic parameters and an IAIHG score corresponding to definite AIH.

The histopathology[30] of AIH/PSC overlap syndrome displays portal and periportal lymphocytic infiltration with disruption of the limiting plate. Piecemeal necrosis or interface hepatitis is present, and lymphocytic infiltrates dominate in the lobule with a periportal to central gradient. Bile ducts are infiltrated by lymphocytes and show periductal fibrosis to a varying degree (Figure 5). Basement membrane is conspicuous with hyaline thickening in the PASD stain. In the lobule spotty necrosis of hepatocytes is visible, and bridging hepatic necrosis between portal tracts and central veins may be detected. In the PSC/AIH overlap syndrome histopathology shows a more florid bile duct lesion, and the features of PSC may be obscured. However, not all of the bile ducts are affected at the same time, and when carefully screening the biopsy there may be one bile duct displaying the typical lesion of PSC.

Whereas in PBC/AIH overlap syndrome both disease entities occur simultaneously, in the overlap syndrome of AIH/PSC there may be a consecutive sequence of events (Table 10). There are nine reports of this overlap syndrome in the literature[26–34] and about five report a simultaneous occurrence of both diseases[31–34]. However, there may also be a first manifestation of AIH followed by PSC, as has been demonstrated by Abdo et al.[29] and by Lüth et al.[29,34]. The other way around, with PSC starting, is still less frequent, and only two patients are mentioned in the literature who first developed PSC[25,34] and then showed AIH after treatment of the first disease.

Table 9 Frequency of AIH/PSC overlap syndrome

Kaya et al. 2000[26]: 1.4% of patients with PSC
van Buuren et al. 2000[27]: 8% of patients with PSC
Abdo et al. 2002[29]: 6.5% of patients with AIH

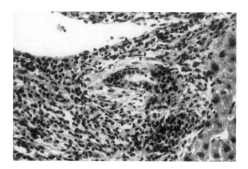

Figure 5 Liver biopsy from a patient with AIH/PSC overlap simultaneously; there is intense lymphocytic infiltration of the portal tract with interface hepatitis and features of PSC with fibrous cuff around a bile duct with inflammatory changes (original magnification ×480; HE)

Table 10 AIH/PSC: sequence of events

	No. of patients	References
AIH/PSC	2	Minuk et al. 1988[31]
	1	Rabinovitz et al. 1992[32]
	5	Lüth et al. 2003[34]
	1	Lawrence et al. 1994[33]
	3	Gohlke et al. 1996[30]
AIH→PSC	10	Lüth et al. 2003[34]
	6	Abdo et al. 2003[29]
PSC→AIH	1	McNair et al. 1998[25]
	1	Lüth et al. 2003[34]

AIH/PSC OVERLAP SYNDROME IN CHILDREN

In children PSC and the overlap with AIH seems to be different from that in adults[35,36]; it is more frequent and displays more features of autoimmune hepatitis. Because of its own clinical symptoms and onset of disease it has been termed 'autoimmune sclerosing cholangitis', based on a larger study by Gregorio et al.[35]. Histopathology is similar to that of simultaneous AIH and PSC (Figure 6).

In a large study the authors could demonstrate that, in liver biopsies from children with autoimmune sclerosing cholangitis, features of sclerosing cholangitis were prominent, besides the histopathology of AIH. The lobular activity was conspicuous and periportal hepatitis, inflammatory and sclerosing lesions of bile ducts were present. The most salient features were portal tract inflammation, septal and bridging fibrosis, copper-binding protein was positive and sclerosing and inflammatory cholangitis were either acute or chronic. The majority of patients showed the manifestations of both disease entities simultaneously at a high degree; so by histopathology there seems to be no difference from the overlap syndrome of PSC and AIH in adults; however, responsiveness to immunosuppressive therapy was

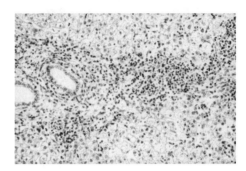

Figure 6 Liver biopsy from a 15-year-old girl with autoimmune sclerosing cholangitis. The enlarged portal tract contains two bile ducts with circumferential loose connective tissue and moderate lymphocytic infiltrates spilling over to the lobule (original magnification ×280; HE)

more favourable, and the results of the follow-up showed a better prognosis regarding histopathology, cholangiography and inflammatory lesions.

SUMMARY

The diagnosis of an overlap syndrome, either of AIH and PBC or AIH and PSC, should be presumed only when both disease entities meet all criteria. The theory is that it is a manifestation of two disease entities, and not a gradual transformation from one disease into the other. Histopathology should help to establish the diagnosis which is not possible in all cases, however, on a single biopsy. A biopsy should be able to exclude other diseases. Only the ensemble of patient's history, clinics, serology and histology provides the basis for correct diagnosis and treatment that is different in overlap syndromes and a common disease without overlap.

References

1. Heathcote EJ. Overlap of autoimmune hepatitis and primary biliary cirrhosis: an evaluation of a modified scoring system. Am J Gastroenterol. 2002;97:1090–1.
2. Woodward J, Neuberger J. Autoimmune overlap syndromes. Hepatology. 2001;33:994–1002.
3. McFarlane IG. The relationship between autoimmune markers and different clinical syndromes in autoimmune hepatitis. Gut. 1998;42:599–602.
4. James OFW. Definition and epidemiology of primary biliary cirrhosis. In: Neuberger J, editor. Primary Biliary Cirrhosis. Eastbourne: West End Studios, 2000:53–9.
5. Wiesner RH, LaRusso NF, Ludwig J, Dickson ER. Comparison of the clinicopathological features of primary sclerosing cholangitis and primary biliary cirrhosis. Gastroenterology. 1985; 88:108–14.
6. Geubel AP, Baggenstoss AH, Summerskill WHJ. Responses to treatment can differentiate chronic active liver disease with cholangitic features from the primary biliary cirrhosis syndrome. Gastroenterology. 1976;71:444–9.
7. Czaja AJ. Frequency and nature of the variant syndromes of autoimmune liver diseases. Hepatology. 1998;28:360–5.
8. Lohse AW, zum Büschenfelde K-HM, Franz B, Kanzler S, Gerken G, Dienes H-P. Characterization of the overlap syndrome of primary biliary cirrhosis (PBC) and autoimmune hepatitis:

evidence for its being a hepatitic form of PBC in genetically susceptible individuals. Hepatology. 1999;29:1078–84.

9. Chazouillieres O, Wendum D, Serfaty L, Montembault S, Rosmorduc O, Poupon R. Primary biliary cirrhosis–autoimmune hepatitis overlap syndrome: clinical features and response to therapy. Hepatology. 1998;28:296–301.

10. Wurbs D, Klein R, Terracciano L-M, Berg PA, Bianchi L. A 28-year old woman with a combined hepatitic/cholestatic syndrome. Hepatology. 1995;22:1598–605.

11. Horsmans Y, Piet A, Brenard R, Rahier J, Geubel AP. Autoimmune chronic active hepatitis responsive to immunosuppressive therapy evolving into a typical primary biliary cirrhosis syndrome: a case report. J Hepatol. 1994;21:194–8.

12. Rubel LR, Seeff LB, Patel V. Primary biliary cirrhosis–primary sclerosing cholangitis overlap syndrome. Arch Pathol Lab Med. 1984;108:360–1.

13. McFarlane IG. Clinical spectrum and heterogeneity of autoimmune hepatitis. In: zum Büschenfelde K-HM, Hoofnagel JH, Manns M, editors. Falk Symposium 70: Immunology and Liver. London: Kluwer, 1993:179–92.

14. Lohse AW, Gerken G, Mohr H et al. Relation between autoimmune liver diseases and viral hepatitis: clinical and serological characteristics in 859 patients. Z Gastroenterol. 1995;33: 527–33.

15. Alvarez F, Berg PA, Bianchi FB et al. International Autoimmune Hepatitis Group report: review of criteria for diagnosis of autoimmune hepatitis. J Hepatol. 1999;31:929–38.

16. Czaja AJ, Carpenter HA. Autoimmune hepatitis with incidental histologic features of bile duct injury. Hepatology. 2001;34:659–65.

17. Dienes H-P, Popper H, Manns M, Baumann W, Thoenes W, Meyer zum Büschenfelde KH. Histologic features in autoimmune hepatitis. Z Gastroenterol. 1989;27:325–30.

18. Bach N, Thung SN, Schaffner F. The histological features of chronic hepatitis C and autoimmune chronic hepatitis: a comparative analysis. Hepatology. 1992;15:572–7.

19. Czaja AJ, Carpenter HA. Autoimmune hepatitis. In: MacSween RNM, Burt AD, Portmann BC, Ishak KG, Scheuer MD, Anthony PP, editors. Pathology of the Liver. London: Churchill Livingstone, 2002:415–34.

20. Portmann BC, Nakanuma Y. Diseases of the bile ducts. In: MacSween RNM, Burt AD, Portmann BC, Ishak KG, Scheuer MD, Anthony PP, editors. Pathology of the Liver. London: Churchill Livingstone, 2002:435–506.

21. Portmann BC, Popper H, Neuberger J, Williams R. Sequential and diagnostic features in primary biliary cirrhosis based on serial histologic study in 209 patients. Gastroenterology. 1985;88: 1777–90.

22. Doniach D, Walker JG. A unified concept of autoimmune hepatitis. Lancet. 1969;1:813–15.

23. Jones DE, James OF, Portmann B, Burt AD, Williams R, Hudson M. Development of autoimmune hepatitis following liver transplantation for primary biliary cirrhosis. Hepatology. 1999;30:53–7.

24. Chapman RW, Arborgh BMA, Rhodes JM, Summerfield JA, Dick R, Scheuer PJ. Primary sclerosing cholangitis: a review of its clinical features, cholangiography and hepatic histology. Gut. 1980;21:870–7.

25. McNair ANB, Moloney M, Portmann BC, Williams R, McFarlane IG. Autoimmune hepatitis overlapping with primary sclerosing cholangitis in five cases. Am J Gastroenterol. 1998;93: 777–84.

26. Kaya M, Angulo P, Lindor K. Overlap of autoimmune hepatitis and primary sclerosing cholangitis: an evaluation of a modified scoring system. J Hepatol. 2000;33:537–42.

27. vanBuuren HR, van Hoogstraten HJF, Terkivatan T, Schalm S, Vleggaar FP. High prevalence of autoimmune hepatitis among patients with primary sclerosing cholangitis. J Hepatol. 2000;33:543–8.

28. Chazouillieres O. Diagnosis of primary sclerosing cholangitis–autoimmune hepatitis overlap syndrome: to score or not to score? J Hepatol. 2000;33:661–3.

29. Abdo A, Bain VG, Kichian K, Lee SS. Evolution of autoimmune hepatitis to primary sclerosing cholangitis: a sequential syndrome. Hepatology. 2002;36:1393–9.

30. Gohlke F, Lohse AW, Dienes HP et al. Evidence for an overlap syndrome of autoimmune hepatitis and primary sclerosing cholangitis. J Hepatol. 1996;24:699–705.

31. Minuk G, Sutherland LR, Pappas C. Autoimmune chronic active hepatitis (lupoid hepatitis) and primary sclerosing cholangitis in two young adult females. Can J Gastroenterol. 1988; 2:22–7.

32. Rabinowitz M, Demetris AJ, Bou-Abboud CF, Van Thiel D. Simultaneous occurrence of primary sclerosing cholangitis and autoimmune chronic active hepatitis in a patient with ulcerative colitis. Dig Dis Sci. 1992;37:1606–11.
33. Lawrence SP, Sherman KE, Lawson JM, Goodman ZD. A 39 year old man with chronic hepatitis. Semin Liver Dis. 1994;14:97–105.
34. Lüth S, Kanzler S, Vieth A, Dienes HP, Galle PR, Lohse AW. Clinical characteristics and longterm prognosis of autoimmune hepatitis/primary sclerosis overlap syndrome. Hepatology. 2003;4(Suppl.1):490A.
35. Gregorio GV, Portmann B, Karani J et al. Autoimmune hepatitis/sclerosing cholangitis overlap syndrome in childhood: a 16-year prospective study. Hepatology. 2001;33:544–53.
36. Roberts EA. Primary sclerosing cholangitis in children. J Gastroenterol Hepatol. 1999;14:588–93.
37. Bianchi L, Gudat F. Chronic hepatitis. In: MacSween RNM, Anthony PP, Scheuer MD, Burt AD, Portmann BC, Ishak KG, editors. Pathology of the Liver. London: Churchill Livingstone, 1994:349–6.
38. Ishak K, Baptista A, Bianchi L et al. Histologic grading and staging of chronic hepatitis. J Hepatol. 1995;22:696–9.

Section V
Treatment of primary biliary cirrhosis

15
Mechanisms of action of ursodeoxycholic acid in cholestasis

U. BEUERS, C. RUST, T. PUSL, G. DENK and
G. PAUMGARTNER

INTRODUCTION

Ursodeoxycholic acid (UDCA: $3\alpha,7\beta$-dihydroxy-5β-cholanoic acid) is a dihydroxy bile acid which is used for the treatment of chronic cholestatic liver diseases such as primary biliary cirrhosis (PBC) or primary sclerosing cholangitis (PSC)[1-5]. UDCA is a physiological constituent of human bile, albeit in low amounts of 1–3% of total bile acids. In the Western literature the beneficial effects of UDCA on serum liver tests in cholestatic disorders were first reported less than 20 years ago[6-8], but effects of UDCA treatment in liver disease were published earlier in Japan. In Chinese traditional medicine UDCA was used as a remedy for liver diseases in the form of dried black bear's bile[9], in which UDCA constitutes the predominant bile acid (about 50–60% of total bile acids).

PHARMACOKINETICS AND METABOLISM OF UDCA

After oral administration, UDCA is solubilized in mixed micelles of endogenous bile acids in the proximal jejunum. UDCA is absorbed by passive non-ionic diffusion, mainly in the small intestine. Its absorption rate is affected by the availability of endogenous bile acids in the intestinal lumen, which is high during meals and low under cholestatic conditions[10]. After uptake into the liver, UDCA is mostly conjugated with glycine or, to a lesser degree, taurine and UDCA conjugates are secreted into bile. UDCA conjugates are reabsorbed mainly from the distal ileum via an active Na^+-dependent transport mechanism undergoing an effective enterohepatic circulation. Non-absorbed UDCA and UDCA conjugates enter the colon and, after bacterial deamidation of conjugates, are mostly converted to lithocholic acid by bacterial enzymes and eliminated via the faeces. Only small amounts of the poorly soluble lithocholic acid are reabsorbed via the colonic mucosa, sulphated in the liver, secreted into bile and excreted via the faeces.

SITES AND MECHANISMS OF ACTION OF UDCA IN CHOLESTASIS

Cholangiocytes

Protection of injured cholangiocytes against toxic effects of hydrophobic bile acids

In chronic cholestatic liver diseases such as PBC and PSC, biliary epithelia are the primary target of an immune-mediated attack. Although the exact molecular mechanisms underlying the immunological damage of biliary epithelia are incompletely understood in these disorders, bile, with its high millimolar concentration of hydrophobic bile acids, has been assumed to aggravate cholangiocellular damage due to its extracellular cytotoxic potential[11–13]. UDCA has been shown to counteract membrane-damaging effects of hydrophobic bile acids *in vitro*, presumably by effects on the formation and structure of simple and mixed micelles rather than by direct membrane interactions[14].

UDCA treatment at therapeutic doses of 13–15 mg/kg per day results in a relative enrichment of UDCA to about 40–50% of total biliary bile acids, and renders the bile acid composition of bile less hydrophobic. UDCA may decrease the degree of cholangiocellular injury, portal inflammation and ductular proliferation in the Mdr2-knockout mouse[15], an experimental model of cholestasis which shares morphological features with PSC[16]. Similarly, the (peri)portal inflammatory reaction is less severe in patients with PBC and PSC under UDCA treatment as compared to those treated with placebo[17–20]. UDCA may protect cholangiocytes not only by rendering bile less toxic to the cholangiocytes; it may also impair apical uptake of hydrophobic bile acids via an apical Na^+-dependent bile acid transporter (ASBT) in cholangiocytes under cholestatic conditions and decrease the intracellular concentration of hydrophobic bile acids, thereby reducing intracellular toxicity[21]. This might explain why UDCA feeding prevented ductular proliferation in bile duct-ligated rats[21]. The effects of UDCA conjugates in cholangiocytes are apparently mediated by Ca^{2+}- and protein kinase Cα (PKCα)-dependent mechanisms which have been implicated in stimulation of biliary secretion in cholestatic hepatocytes[22–25] as outlined below.

Stimulation of cholangiocyte HCO_3^- secretion

Cholangiocytes secrete a HCO_3^--rich fluid which represents about 25% of daily bile formation in humans. In cystic fibrosis, Cl^--dependent HCO_3^- secretion is impaired due to a mutation of the *CFTR* gene which encodes for a Ca^{2+}-independent Cl^- channel. UDCA is known to stimulate HCO_3^- secretion in rats and in humans. It has been speculated that UDCA may stimulate cholangiocyte HCO_3^- secretion by Ca^{2+}-dependent mechanisms via activation of a Ca^{2+}-dependent Cl^- channel and concomitant stimulation of Cl^-/HCO_3^- exchange via the anion exchanger 2 (AE2). UDCA conjugates increase cytosolic free calcium $[Ca^{2+}]_i$ in cholangiocytes and induce membrane binding of Ca^{2+}-dependent

PKCα[21], mechanisms similar to those observed in hepatocytes[22,23,26–28]. In addition, UDCA conjugates might also increase $[Ca^{2+}]_i$ in cholangiocytes indirectly by stimulation of hepatocellular ATP secretion into bile, which then may induce Ca^{2+}-dependent Cl^- secretion via apical P2Y ATP receptors[29–31].

AE2 expression and HCO_3^- secretion are impaired in patients with PBC and are up-regulated after treatment with UDCA[32,33]. Thus, stimulation of cholangiocellular HCO_3^- secretion may contribute to the anticholestatic effect of UDCA in those biliary diseases in which HCO_3^- secretion is impaired.

Hepatocytes

Stimulation of hepatobiliary secretion

Cholestatic disorders are characterized by an impairment of hepatobiliary secretion. Bile acids and other potentially toxic cholephiles accumulate in the hepatocyte and may lead to hepatocyte injury, apoptosis and necrosis. UDCA stimulates biliary secretion of bile acids and other organic anions (e.g. bilirubin glucuronides, glutathione conjugates) in experimental cholestasis, and counteracts cholestasis induced by hydrophobic bile acids in rat liver[24,34–36]. In patients with PBC and PSC, UDCA stimulates biliary secretion of bile acids[37] and decreases elevated serum levels of the hydrophobic bile acid, chenodeoxycholic acid[38] and of bilirubin[17,19,39,40]. Thus, UDCA may exert beneficial effects in cholestatic liver disease by stimulating the elimination of toxic compounds from the hepatocytes.

The secretory capacity of the hepatocytes is determined by the number and activity of carrier proteins in the canalicular membrane. Carrier expression is regulated at a transcriptional and post-transcriptional level. It has recently been shown that UDCA stimulates the expression of transporter proteins for biliary secretion in the liver[32,41] and the targeting and insertion of transporter molecules into the canalicular membrane[24,42,43]. While effects of UDCA on mRNA and protein levels of transporters may be important for long-term regulation, the effects on the insertion of transporters (targeting) into the canalicular membrane and on the activity of transporters may regulate short-term secretion. By up-regulation of synthesis, apical insertion, and activation of the bile salt export pump (BSEP), the conjugate export pump (MRP2) and the anion exchanger 2 (AE2), UDCA might enhance bile salt-dependent and bile salt-independent bile flow.

Transcriptional regulation of synthesis of transporter proteins

The transcriptional regulation of canalicular transporter proteins by UDCA and cholic acid (CA) has recently been studied in mice fed a UDCA or CA supplemented diet[41]. Both UDCA and CA up-regulated hepatocellular Bsep mRNA and Mrp2 mRNA. Since this effect was not specific for UDCA, its role for the anticholestatic action of UDCA remains unclear.

Post-transcriptional regulation of targeting and membrane insertion of carriers

Vesicle-mediated targeting of proteins to the canalicular membrane is impaired in cholestasis[44]. Experimental evidence suggests that the taurine conjugate of

UDCA (TUDCA), by activating a complex network of signals, stimulates hepatobiliary vesicular exocytosis and insertion of carrier proteins into the apical membrane of the hepatocyte[22–24,42,43,45–47]. In cholestatic rat liver, TUDCA significantly enhances the density of the conjugate export pump, Mrp2, and the bile salt export pump, Bsep, in canalicular membranes of the hepatocyte and thereby stimulates biliary secretion of potentially toxic compounds[24,43].

Cytosolic free calcium $[Ca^{2+}]_i$ and Ca^{2+} influx seem to be critical for TUDCA-induced exocytosis in the model of the perfused rat liver[22]. TUDCA, but not the trihydroxy bile acid taurocholic acid (TCA), induces a sustained elevation of $[Ca^{2+}]_i$ and stimulates Ca^{2+} influx in isolated hepatocytes[22,26,27]. TUDCA also selectively induces translocation of the Ca^{2+}-sensitive α-isoform of PKC, a key mediator of regulated exocytosis, to hepatocellular membranes and activates membrane-bound PKC[23,28]. Inhibition of PKCα by the PKC inhibitor bisindolylmaleimide-I markedly impairs TUDCA-induced secretion of the model Mrp2 substrate dinitrophenyl-S-glutathione (GS-DNP) in experimental cholestasis[24] and antagonizes taurolithocholic acid (TLCA)-induced impairment in rat hepatocyte couplets by Ca^{2+}- and PKC-dependent mechanisms[25], supporting the concept that TUDCA exerts anticholestatic effects, at least in part, by Ca^{2+}- and PKCα-dependent mechanisms[5,22].

Interestingly, the cholestatic bile acid TLCA has been shown to selectively translocate the novel and Ca^{2+}-independent ε-isoform of PKC to canalicular membranes[48] and to exert cholestatic effects including retrieval of apical transporters Mrp2 and Bsep from the canalicular membrane by phosphatidylinositol-3 kinase (PI3K)- and putatively PKCε-dependent mechanisms[49]. Thus, it is attractive to speculate that cholestatic (e.g. TLCA) and anticholestatic (e.g. TUDCA) bile acids, by differential modulation of PKC isoforms[24,49], affect transporter density and activity in the canalicular membrane in an opposite fashion.

TUDCA may stimulate canalicular bile acid secretion independent of PKC via alternative signalling pathways in normal rat liver[42,46]. TUDCA has recently been shown to interact with membrane integrins and, thereby, to activate a dual signalling cascade including the small GTP-binding protein Ras and the mitogen-activated protein kinases (MAPK), extracellular signal-regulated kinase (Erk)-1 and Erk-2 on the one hand and the Ras/Raf-independent p38[MAPK] on the other hand. Both mechanisms lead to stimulation of bile acid secretion in the normal perfused rat liver[42,46] accompanied by enhanced insertion of Bsep into the canalicular membrane[42].

In summary, UDCA conjugates may improve the impaired secretory capacity of the cholestatic liver by modulating complex intracellular signalling cascades including calcium, PKCα and different MAP kinases.

Activation/inactivation of transporter proteins

Phosphorylation/dephosphorylation of transporter proteins at their site of action has been regarded as another possible mechanism by which UDCA modulates apical secretion in hepatocytes. The mouse Bsep is phosphorylated by PKCα in insect cells overexpressing PKCα after transfection[50]. Whether this finding *in vitro* is related to an increased transport capacity of the bile salt export pump *in vivo* remains to be shown.

In conclusion, UDCA modulates hepatobiliary secretion by transcriptional and post-transcriptional mechanisms in experimental models *in vivo* and *in vitro*. Thus, up-regulation of synthesis, apical targeting and insertion and activation of key canalicular transporters such as BSEP, MRP2 and AE2 may represent key mechanisms to explain the anticholestatic action of UDCA in patients with cholestatic liver disease.

Inhibition of apoptosis

Accumulation of hydrophobic bile acids in cholestatic hepatocytes may lead to apoptosis and necrosis of cells, subsequent inflammatory changes and liver fibrosis. The mechanisms of bile acid-induced apoptosis are increasingly being understood. Glycochenodeoxycholic acid (GCDCA) or glycodeoxycholic acid (GDCA) induce apoptosis by ligand-independent activation of the Fas death receptor[51] possibly involving PKC- and c-Jun N-terminal kinase-dependent transient heterodimerization of the Fas death receptor and epidermal growth factor receptor (EGFR) as shown for the hydrophobic bile acid taurolithocholic acid sulphate[52]. Subsequent steps include activation of caspase 8 and Bid which chaperones Bax to the mitochondrial membrane inducing mitochondrial membrane permeability transition (MMPT). A sudden increase in permeability of the inner mitochondrial membrane to ions is followed by mitochondrial swelling, release of cytochrome-c to the cytosol, interaction of cytochrome-c with the apoptotic protease-activating factor 1 (APAF-1), activation of caspase 9 and apoptotic cell death[2].

Antiapoptotic effects of UDCA *in vitro* and *in vivo* in the rat[53,54] and in human hepatocytes[55] were associated with a reduction of the MMPT and mitochondrial cytochrome-c release[2,54]. UDCA diminishes Fas ligand-induced apoptosis in mouse hepatocytes, possibly via direct effects on the mitochondrial membrane[56] and protects rat hepatocytes against bile acid-induced apoptosis by preventing bile acid-induced, c-Jun N-terminal kinase-dependent Fas trafficking to the plasma membrane[57]. UDCA also inhibits apoptosis by activation of the epidermal growth factor receptor (EGFR). EGFR stimulates mitogen-activated protein kinases (MAPK) which induce a survival signal and inhibit bile acid-induced apoptosis[58]. Blockage of this MAPK survival pathway, however, renders UDCA toxic[58]. It remains to be noted that the role of antiapoptotic mechanisms for the beneficial effects of UDCA in cholestatic liver disease remains unclear at present.

Stimulation of detoxification of hydrophobic bile acids

Preliminary evidence suggests that UDCA stimulates drug and steroid metabolism[59,60]. UDCA, TUDCA and taurohyodeoxycholic acid induce cytochrome P450 (CYP) in mouse liver[59,60]. CYP3A-linked enzyme activities such as testosterone 6β-hydroxylase were increased by UDCA and decreased by DCA[60]. CYP3A is of major importance for drug metabolism and is involved in the metabolism of more than 50% of all drugs currently available, as well as a number of hydrophobic bile acids[61]. The expression of CYP enzymes is regulated by the pregnane X receptor/steroid and xenobiotic receptor (PXR/SXR). UDCA was reported to activate PXR/SXR in primary human hepatocytes and to induce CYP3A4[62]. In patients with gallstones, UDCA stimulates CYP3A4-dependent formation of 4β-hydroxycholesterol[63]. Whether UDCA exerts this effect directly by binding to PXR/SXR or by its metabolite lithocholic acid (LCA), a potent ligand of PXR/SXR, is unclear. Thus, it could be speculated that UDCA-induced metabolism of toxic hydrophobic bile acids to hydrophilic, less toxic compounds is a hepatoprotective mechanism.

Ileocytes

Competitive inhibition/down-regulation of ileal bile acid carriers

Ileal uptake of conjugated bile acids via the apical sodium-dependent bile acid transporter, ASBT, may be affected by UDCA treatment. In healthy individuals the retention of [^{75}Se]homotaurocholic acid (SeHCAT), a TCA analogue, was diminished during administration of UDCA[64]. In patients with ileoanal pouch, the loss of primary bile acids (CDCA, CA) was markedly increased when UDCA was administered[65]. SeHCAT retention in patients with PBC was reported to be increased when compared to healthy controls. In these patients UDCA administration led to a decrease of SeHCAT retention in parallel to improvement of cholestasis comparable to SeHCAT retention of controls[66]. However, pool sizes of major hydrophobic bile acids, CDCA and DCA, were not reduced in cholestatic patients during UDCA treatment when markers of cholestasis improved[67,68]. Thus, it remains unclear whether UDCA-induced changes of bile acid uptake by ileocytes have an impact on the anticholestatic action of UDCA.

OTHER SITES

A number of other potential sites of action of UDCA in chronic cholestatic liver diseases have been discussed. It should be considered, however, that actions of UDCA in cell types which do not express bile acid carriers appear unlikely at therapeutic low micromolar levels in humans. *In-vitro* studies suggested direct immunomodulating effects of UDCA on cytokine secretion of peripheral monocytes. The physiological relevance of these studies, however, has been questioned due to methodological concerns[69]. Modulation of cell-mediated immunity by UDCA, such as reversal of aberrant expression of HLA class I molecules on hepatocytes[19,70], has been observed, but appears to be secondary to the anticholestatic effect of UDCA.

CONCLUSION

Several sites and mechanisms of action of UDCA have been proposed based on experimental and clinical observations. Their relative contribution to the anticholestatic action of UDCA remains unclear, and may depend on the type of the cholestatic injury. In early-stage PBC the protection of injured cholangiocytes against toxic effects of bile acids may prevail over other mechanisms, whereas stimulation of hepatobiliary secretion may be most relevant in more advanced cholestasis. In drug-induced cholestasis with impaired function of apical hepatocellular transporters, stimulation of apical transporter insertion and hepatobiliary secretion may be essential. In cystic fibrosis, stimulation of cholangiocellular Ca^{2+}-dependent Cl^-/HCO_3^- secretion may be of major value. Finally, in case of bile acid retention in hepatocytes, inhibition of bile acid-induced hepatocyte apoptosis may become important. Thus, different sites and mechanisms of action may contribute to the anticholestatic action of UDCA under diverse cholestatic conditions.

References

1. Paumgartner G, Beuers U. Ursodeoxycholic acid in cholestatic liver disease: mechanisms of action and therapeutic use revisited. Hepatology. 2002;36:525–31.
2. Lazaridis KN, Gores GJ, Lindor KD. Ursodeoxycholic acid 'mechanisms of action and clinical use in hepatobiliary disorders'. J Hepatol. 2001;35:134–46.
3. Poupon R, Chazouilleres O, Poupon RE. Chronic cholestatic diseases. J Hepatol. 2000;32:129–40.
4. Trauner M, Graziadei IW. Review article: mechanisms of action and therapeutic applications of ursodeoxycholic acid in chronic liver diseases. Aliment Pharmacol Ther. 1999;13:979–96.
5. Beuers U, Boyer JL, Paumgartner G. Ursodeoxycholic acid in cholestasis: potential mechanisms of action and therapeutic applications. Hepatology. 1998;28:1449–53.
6. Leuschner U, Leuschner M, Sieratzki J, Kurtz W, Hubner K. Gallstone dissolution with ursodeoxycholic acid in patients with chronic active hepatitis and two years follow-up. A pilot study. Dig Dis Sci. 1985;30:642–9.
7. Poupon R, Chretien Y, Poupon RE, Ballet F, Calmus Y, Darnis F. Is ursodeoxycholic acid an effective treatment for primary biliary cirrhosis? Lancet. 1987;1:834–6.
8. Leuschner U, Fischer H, Kurtz W et al. Ursodeoxycholic acid in primary biliary cirrhosis: results of a controlled double-blind trial. Gastroenterology. 1989;97:1268–74.
9. Hagey LR, Crombie DL, Espinosa E, Carey MC, Igimi H, Hofmann AF. Ursodeoxycholic acid in the Ursidae: biliary bile acids of bears, pandas, and related carnivores. J Lipid Res. 1993; 34:1911–17.
10. Hofmann AF. Pharmacology of ursodeoxycholic acid, an enterohepatic drug. Scand J Gastroenterol Suppl. 1994;204:1–15.
11. Hofmann AF. Bile acids: the good, the bad, and the ugly. News Physiol Sci. 1999;14:24–9.
12. Guldutuna S, Zimmer G, Imhof M, Bhatti S, You T, Leuschner U. Molecular aspects of membrane stabilization by ursodeoxycholate. Gastroenterology. 1993;104:1736–44.
13. Heuman DM, Pandak WM, Hylemon PB, Vlahcevic ZR. Conjugates of ursodeoxycholate protect against cytotoxicity of more hydrophobic bile salts: in vitro studies in rat hepatocytes and human erythrocytes. Hepatology. 1991;14:920–6.
14. Heuman DM, Bajaj RS, Lin Q. Adsorption of mixtures of bile salt taurine conjugates to lecithincholesterol membranes: implications for bile salt toxicity and cytoprotection. J Lipid Res. 1996;37:562–73.
15. Van Nieuwkerk CM, Elferink RP, Groen AK et al. Effects of ursodeoxycholate and cholate feeding on liver disease in FVB mice with a disrupted mdr2 P-glycoprotein gene. Gastroenterology. 1996;111:165–71.
16. Fickert P, Trauner M, Fuchsbichler A, Stumptner C, Zatloukal K, Denk H. Cytokeratins as targets for bile acid-induced toxicity. Am J Pathol. 2002;160:491–9.
17. Poupon RE, Balkau B, Eschwege E, Poupon R. A multicenter, controlled trial of ursodiol for the treatment of primary biliary cirrhosis. UDCA–PBC Study Group. N Engl J Med. 1991;324:1548–54.
18. Pares A, Caballeria L, Rodes J et al. Long-term effects of ursodeoxycholic acid in primary biliary cirrhosis: results of a double-blind controlled multicentric trial. UDCA-Cooperative Group from the Spanish Association for the Study of the Liver. J Hepatol. 2000;32:561–6.
19. Beuers U, Spengler U, Kruis W et al. Ursodeoxycholic acid for treatment of primary sclerosing cholangitis: a placebo-controlled trial. Hepatology. 1992;16:707–14.
20. Stiehl A. Ursodeoxycholic acid therapy in treatment of primary sclerosing cholangitis. Scand J Gastroenterol Suppl. 1994;204:59–61.

21. Alpini G, Baiocchi L, Glaser S et al. Ursodeoxycholate and tauroursodeoxycholate inhibit cholangiocyte growth and secretion of BDL rats through activation of PKC alpha. Hepatology. 2002;35:1041–52.
22. Beuers U, Nathanson MH, Isales CM, Boyer JL. Tauroursodeoxycholic acid stimulates hepatocellular exocytosis and mobilizes extracellular Ca^{++} mechanisms defective in cholestasis. J Clin Invest. 1993;92:2984–93.
23. Beuers U, Throckmorton DC, Anderson MS et al. Tauroursodeoxycholic acid activates protein kinase C in isolated rat hepatocytes. Gastroenterology. 1996;110:1553–63.
24. Beuers U, Bilzer M, Chittattu A et al. Tauroursodeoxycholic acid inserts the apical conjugate export pump, Mrp2, into canalicular membranes and stimulates organic anion secretion by protein kinase C-dependent mechanisms in cholestatic rat liver. Hepatology. 2001;33:1206–16.
25. Milkiewicz P, Roma MG, Elias E, Coleman R. Hepatoprotection with tauroursodeoxycholate and beta muricholate against taurolithocholate induced cholestasis: involvement of signal transduction pathways. Gut. 2002;51:113–19.
26. Beuers U, Nathanson MH, Boyer JL. Effects of tauroursodeoxycholic acid on cytosolic Ca2+ signals in isolated rat hepatocytes. Gastroenterology. 1993;104:604–12.
27. Bouscarel B, Fromm H, Nussbaum R. Ursodeoxycholate mobilizes intracellular Ca2+ and activates phosphorylase a in isolated hepatocytes. Am J Physiol. 1993;264:G243–51.
28. Stravitz RT, Rao YP, Vlahcevic ZR, Gurley EC, Jarvis WD, Hylemon PB. Hepatocellular protein kinase C activation by bile acids: implications for regulation of cholesterol 7 alpha-hydroxylase. Am J Physiol. 1996;271:G293–303.
29. Nathanson MH, Burgstahler AD, Masyuk A, Larusso NF. Stimulation of ATP secretion in the liver by therapeutic bile acids. Biochem J. 2001;358:1–5.
30. Roman RM, Feranchak AP, Salter KD, Wang Y, Fitz JG. Endogenous ATP release regulates Cl⁻ secretion in cultured human and rat biliary epithelial cells. Am J Physiol. 1999;276:G1391–400.
31. Dranoff JA, Masyuk AI, Kruglov EA, LaRusso NF, Nathanson MH. Polarized expression and function of P2Y ATP receptors in rat bile duct epithelia. Am J Physiol Gastrointest Liver Physiol. 2001;281:G1059–67.
32. Medina JF, Martinez A, Vazquez JJ, Prieto J. Decreased anion exchanger 2 immunoreactivity in the liver of patients with primary biliary cirrhosis. Hepatology. 1997;25:12–17.
33. Prieto J, Garcia N, Marti-Climent JM, Penuelas I, Richter JA, Medina JF. Assessment of biliary bicarbonate secretion in humans by positron emission tomography. Gastroenterology. 1999;117:167–72.
34. Kitani K, Ohta M, Kanai S. Tauroursodeoxycholate prevents biliary protein excretion induced by other bile salts in the rat. Am J Physiol. 1985;248:G407–17.
35. Scholmerich J, Baumgartner U, Miyai K, Gerok W. Tauroursodeoxycholate prevents taurolithocholate-induced cholestasis and toxicity in rat liver. J Hepatol. 1990;10:280–3.
36. Heuman DM, Mills AS, McCall J, Hylemon PB, Pandak WM, Vlahcevic ZR. Conjugates of ursodeoxycholate protect against cholestasis and hepatocellular necrosis caused by more hydrophobic bile salts. In vivo studies in the rat. Gastroenterology. 1991;100:203–11.
37. Jazrawi RP, de Caestecker JS, Goggin PM, Britten AJ, Joseph AE, Maxwell JD, Northfield TC. Kinetics of hepatic bile acid handling in cholestatic liver disease: effect of ursodeoxycholic acid. Gastroenterology. 1994;106:134–42.
38. Poupon RE, Chretien Y, Poupon R, Paumgartner G. Serum bile acids in primary biliary cirrhosis: effect of ursodeoxycholic acid therapy. Hepatology. 1993;17:599–604.
39. Heathcote EJ, Cauch-Dudek K, Walker V et al. The Canadian Multicenter Double-blind Randomized Controlled Trial of ursodeoxycholic acid in primary biliary cirrhosis. Hepatology. 1994;19:1149–56.
40. Lindor KD. Ursodiol for primary sclerosing cholangitis. Mayo Primary Sclerosing Cholangitis–Ursodeoxycholic Acid Study Group. N Engl J Med. 1997;336:691–5.
41. Fickert P, Zollner G, Fuchsbichler A et al. Effects of ursodeoxycholic and cholic acid feeding on hepatocellular transporter expression in mouse liver. Gastroenterology. 2001;121:170–83.
42. Kurz AK, Graf D, Schmitt M, Vom Dahl S, Haussinger D. Tauroursodesoxycholate-induced choleresis involves p38(MAPK) activation and translocation of the bile salt export pump in rats. Gastroenterology. 2001;121:407–19.
43. Dombrowski F, Stieger B, Beuers U. Tauroursodeoxycholic acid inserts the bile salt export pump into canalicular membranes in cholestatic rat liver. Hepatology. 2003;38:688A.
44. Larkin JM, Palade GE. Transcytotic vesicular carriers for polymeric IgA receptors accumulate in rat hepatocytes after bile duct ligation. J Cell Sci. 1991;98:205–16.

45. Haussinger D, Saha N, Hallbrucker C, Lang F, Gerok W. Involvement of microtubules in the swelling-induced stimulation of transcellular taurocholate transport in perfused rat liver. Biochem J. 1993;291:355–60.

46. Schliess F, Kurz AK, vom Dahl S, Haussinger D. Mitogen-activated protein kinases mediate the stimulation of bile acid secretion by tauroursodeoxycholate in rat liver. Gastroenterology. 1997;113:1306–14.

47. Kurz AK, Block C, Graf D, Dahl SV, Schliess F, Haussinger D. Phosphoinositide 3-kinase-dependent Ras activation by tauroursodesoxycholate in rat liver. Biochem J. 2000;350:207–13.

48. Beuers U, Probst I, Soroka C, Boyer JL, Kullak-Ublick GA, Paumgartner G. Modulation of protein kinase C by taurolithocholic acid in isolated rat hepatocytes. Hepatology. 1999;29:477–82.

49. Beuers U, Denk GU, Soroka CJ et al. Taurolithocholic acid exerts cholestatic effects via phosphatidylinositol 3-kinase-dependent mechanisms in perfused rat livers and rat hepatocyte couplets. J Biol Chem. 2003;278:17810–18.

50. Noe J, Hagenbuch B, Meier PJ, St-Pierre MV. Characterization of the mouse bile salt export pump overexpressed in the baculovirus system. Hepatology. 2001;33:1223–31.

51. Faubion W, Guicciardi M, Miyoshi H et al. Toxic bile salts induce rodent hepatocyte apoptosis via direct activation of Fas. J Clin Invest. 1999;103:137–45.

52. Reinehr R, Graf D, Haussinger D. Bile salt-induced hepatocyte apoptosis involves epidermal growth factor receptor-dependent CD95 tyrosine phosphorylation. Gastroenterology. 2003;125:839–53.

53. Benz C, Angermuller S, Tox U et al. Effect of tauroursodeoxycholic acid on bile-acid-induced apoptosis and cytolysis in rat hepatocytes. J Hepatol. 1998;28:99–106.

54. Rodrigues C, Fan G, Wong P, Kren B, Steer C. Ursodeoxycholic acid may inhibit deoxycholic acid-induced apoptosis by modulating mitochondrial transmembrane potential and reactive oxygen species production. Mol Med. 1998;4:165–78.

55. Benz C, Angermuller S, Otto G, Sauer P, Stremmel W, Stiehl A. Effect of tauroursodeoxycholic acid on bile acid-induced apoptosis in primary human hepatocytes. Eur J Clin Invest. 2000;30:203–9.

56. Azzaroli F, Mehal W, Soroka CJ et al. Ursodeoxycholic acid diminishes Fas-ligand-induced apoptosis in mouse hepatocytes. Hepatology. 2002;36:49–54.

57. Graf D, Kurz AK, Fischer R, Reinehr R, Haussinger D. Taurolithocholic acid-3 sulfate induces CD95 trafficking and apoptosis in a c-Jun N-terminal kinase-dependent manner. Gastroenterology. 2002;122:1411–27.

58. Qiao L, Yacoub A, Studer E et al. Inhibition of the MAPK and PI3K pathways enhances UDCA-induced apoptosis in primary rodent hepatocytes. Hepatology. 2002;35:779–89.

59. Paolini M, Pozzetti L, Piazza F, Cantelli-Forti G, Roda A. Bile acid structure and selective modulation of murine hepatic cytochrome P450-linked enzymes. Hepatology. 1999;30:730–9.

60. Paolini M, Pozzetti L, Montagnani M et al. Ursodeoxycholic acid (UDCA) prevents DCA effects on male mouse liver via up-regulation of CYP [correction of CXP] and preservation of BSEP activities. Hepatology. 2002;36:305–14.

61. Thummel KE, Wilkinson GR. In vitro and in vivo drug interactions involving human CYP3A. Annu Rev Pharmacol Toxicol. 1998;38:389–430.

62. Schuetz EG, Strom S, Yasuda K et al. Disrupted bile acid homeostasis reveals an unexpected interaction among nuclear hormone receptors, transporters, and cytochrome P450. J Biol Chem. 2001;276:39411–18.

63. Bodin K, Bretillon L, Aden Y et al. Antiepileptic drugs increase plasma levels of 4beta-hydroxy-cholesterol in humans: evidence for involvement of cytochrome p450 3A4. J Biol Chem. 2001;276:38685–9.

64. Marteau P, Chazouilleres O, Myara A, Jian R, Rambaud JC, Poupon R. Effect of chronic administration of ursodeoxycholic acid on the ileal absorption of endogenous bile acids in man. Hepatology. 1990;12:1206–8.

65. Stiehl A, Raedsch R, Rudolph G. Acute effects of ursodeoxycholic and chenodeoxycholic acid on the small intestinal absorption of bile acids. Gastroenterology. 1990;98:424–8.

66. Lanzini A, De Tavonatti MG, Panarotto B et al. Intestinal absorption of the bile acid analogue 75Se-homocholic acid-taurine is increased in primary biliary cirrhosis, and reverts to normal during ursodeoxycholic acid administration. Gut. 2003;52:1371–5.

67. Beuers U, Spengler U, Zwiebel FM, Pauletzki J, Fischer S, Paumgartner G. Effect of ursodeoxycholic acid on the kinetics of the major hydrophobic bile acids in health and in chronic cholestatic liver disease. Hepatology. 1992;15:603–8.

68. Rudolph G, Endele R, Senn M, Stiehl A. Effect of ursodeoxycholic acid on the kinetics of cholic acid and chenodeoxycholic acid in patients with primary sclerosing cholangitis. Hepatology. 1993;17:1028–32.
69. Bergamini A, Dini L, Baiocchi L et al. Bile acids with differing hydrophilic-hydrophobic properties do not influence cytokine production by human monocytes and murine Kupffer cells. Hepatology. 1997;25:927–33.
70. Calmus Y, Gane P, Rouger P, Poupon R. Hepatic expression of class I and class II major histocompatibility complex molecules in primary biliary cirrhosis: effect of ursodeoxycholic acid. Hepatology. 1990;11:12–15.

16
Primary biliary cirrhosis: long-term therapy with ursodeoxycholic acid

R. POUPON, C. CORPECHOT, F. CARRAT and R. E. POUPON

INTRODUCTION

Primary biliary cirrhosis (PBC) is a chronic cholestatic liver disease of unknown cause, most often diagnosed in middle-aged women. Morphologically, PBC is characterized by portal inflammation and necrosis of biliary cells in the small and medium-sized bile ducts. These lesions result in the focal destruction of the interlobular and septal bile ducts, with progressive cholestasis. As in other forms of chronic obstructive cholestasis, lobular lesions and cirrhosis can occur. Although PBC is generally a progressive disease, the rate of progression varies greatly from one patient to another. The terminal phase is characterized by hyperbilirubinaemia (>100 µmol/L), a major decrease in the number of intrahepatic bile ducts, and extensive fibrosis or cirrhosis.

During the past three decades our understanding of the natural history and pathogenesis has considerably progressed. It is now well established that orthotopic liver transplantation (OLT) is the treatment of choice for patients entering the terminal phase of the disease.

A variety of therapeutic agents have been proposed for treatment of patients with PBC. However, when tested in clinical trials, most have been found ineffective or too toxic to be widely used. In contrast, there is evidence from large well-designed therapeutic trials and long-term observational studies that long-term administration of ursodeoxycholic acid (UDCA) is safe and prolongs survival free of OLT. UDCA has also been combined with other drugs, in particular corticosteroids, colchicine, and methotrexate, in an attempt to enhance favourable effects on the outcome of patients with PBC, or provide beneficial effects in the subset of patients who have suboptimal response to UDCA therapy alone. In this chapter we describe briefly the natural history and prognosis of PBC, and review the data showing that UDCA improves the natural history of PBC.

NATURAL HISTORY AND PROGNOSIS

Most of the patients in whom PBC was diagnosed when asymptomatic will develop symptoms in the following years. In a 40-month period, 10–30% of asymptomatic patients become symptomatic. The mean duration of the asymptomatic phase is extremely variable but is of the order of 6 years. The 5-year survival rate of asymptomatic patients is about 90%. After 5 years of progression the proportion of survivors is significantly lower than in a paired control population. The duration of the symptomatic phase varies greatly, but can last for 10 years. The mean 5-year survival rate among symptomatic patients is 50%, with a range of 30–70%. The terminal phase of the disease is defined when serum bilirubin level is higher than 100 μmol/L, with or without signs of portal hypertension (gastrointestinal bleeding, ascitis or encephalopathy)[1].

In 1979 Shapiro and co-workers[2] showed the importance of serum bilirubin as a factor prognostic for survival in PBC. They noted that, after a relatively stable phase, serum bilirubin increased sharply in the months preceding death. In patients with serum bilirubin levels above 34 μmol/L (2 mg/dl), the mean survival was 4 years; in those with values above 102 μmol/L (60 mg/dl) 2 years, and in those with values above 170 μmol/L (10 mg/dl) 1.4 years. The extraordinary importance of bilirubin for short-term and long-term survival was confirmed in all later studies. The other parameters more constantly found to be the best predictors of death were age, serum albumin level, prothrombin time, and the presence of cirrhosis on histopathological examination. Several prognostic models have been proposed to improve the prognostic value of serum bilirubin. Because these models are complex, or are not highly superior to serum bilirubin alone, they are not widely used.

It is important to emphasize that the prognostic value of serum bilirubin level for survival free of OLT is similar in UDCA-treated patients as in non-treated patients. The European multicentre study[3], initially aimed at evaluating the efficacy of azathioprine in PBC, supplied the most precise and complete data on the natural history of the disease. The Popper and Schaffner classification was used for histological staging, and disease progression was assessed in 236 patients[4]. At enrollment 14% were in histological stage I, 40% in stage II, 19% in stage III, and 27% in stage IV. During a 4-year period 30% and 28% of the patients developed hepatomegaly and splenomegaly. Cirrhosis, diagnosed histologically, developed in about half the patients. Ascites and gastrointestinal bleeding occurred in a quarter of the patients. Similarly, 25–35% of the patients developed major laboratory test abnormalities (serum bilirubin >105 μmol in one-quarter of cases, serum albumin <29 g/L in 35%). Overall, during a 4-year period, it seems reasonable to expect that one-quarter to one-third of patients will reach the terminal phase of the disease and may qualify for OLT.

In sum, PBC progresses through three irreversible states: (a) cirrhosis; (b) a terminal phase defined when serum bilirubin reaches 100 μmol/L (with or without gastrointestinal bleeding, ascites, or encephalopathy); and (c) death unless OLT is performed.

The long-term natural course of this rare disease (10–15 years since diagnosis) explains the lack of power and weaknesses of the majority of past clinical trials in terms of assessment of survival. It has been estimated, by calculating the predictive survival of patients using a prognostic model for PBC, that death or OLT are unrealistic end-points to estimate the efficacy of a drug unless a sufficient number of patients with sufficient severity of the disease are assessed during a sufficient follow-up period[5]. For these reasons, and because most of the UDCA clinical trials were not designed to test the efficacy of the drug on survival, a combined analysis of individual data of three major trials was performed[6]. Only this study had the power to detect an effect on survival without OLT.

THE MULTISTATE MODELLING APPROACH

Long-term observational studies and/or a multistate modelling approach can overcome these difficulties. We[7,8] and others[9] used these approaches to determine the impact of UDCA therapy as well as the impact of clinical, biochemical, and histological parameters on the natural history of PBC. Indeed, PBC can be viewed as a multistate progressive disease with four successive histological stages, a terminal phase defined by a serum bilirubin higher than 105 μmol/L with or without ascites, and bleeding and eventually death or OLT.

When a disease with a long natural course progresses through well-defined stages, a peculiar statistical approach, named 'continuous time Markov or multistate modelling' may be applied. With this method the transition rates between stages and the potential effect of a treatment may be determined. The transition probabilities are computed for the observed follow-up, the accuracy of the model is validated by comparing the number of predicted transitions with those observed, and lastly, the predictions are extended beyond the observed follow-up.

UDCA AS THE FIRST-LINE THERAPY OF PBC

The increasing use of UDCA as the first-line therapy is based on a body of evidence showing that this bile acid slows the progression of the disease towards the irreversible terminal phase.

This chapter will not address the issue of the combination therapies aimed at managing patients with PBC resistant to UDCA therapy, and will focus on long-term observational studies.

Optimal dose of UDCA

Among all the published clinical trials only three used the initially proposed dose, i.e. 13–15 mg/kg per day. Two clinical trials were conducted to address the issue of the optimal daily dose[10,11]. These two studies show that doses ranging from 13 to 20 mg/kg per day afford the optimal enrichment in biliary UDCA, as well as the most significant changes of liver tests. Doses equal to 10 mg/kg per day or less should be considered as suboptimal for treating PBC.

However, it should be emphasized that the dose regimen must be adapted to the patient status. In particular, in patients having pruritus, hyperbilirubinaemia, severe ductopenia or cirrhosis, we recommend: (a) starting with a low dose, i.e. 200 mg/day, to avoid side-effects; and (b) checking serum bile acid and bilirubin levels every month. The optimal daily dose may be reached only 6–8 months after the onset of treatment. Ideally, serum UDCA and endogenous bile acid levels should be assessed to determine the optimal dose, which in fact may vary from one patient to another because of differences in absorption, metabolism of bile acids and liver metabolic activity.

Ten-year survival in UDCA-treated patients with PBC

UDCA treatment has been shown to increase survival free of OLT in patients with PBC at 4 years[12]. Whether this beneficial effect was maintained over the long term remained to be established. In a large cohort of UDCA-treated PBC patients followed for up to 10 years we aimed to determine the outcome of these patients using two endpoints: (a) survival free of OLT, and (b) survival[13].

The cohort comprised 225 patients with PBC treated with UDCA (13–15 mg/kg per day) followed for up to 10 years from the beginning of treatment until time of last follow-up, OLT or death. Because of the absence of a control group, survival free of OLT was compared with survival predicted by the Mayo model (first 7 years), and estimation of the observed survival with survival of a standardized control cohort of the French population.

Observed survival free of OLT of treated patients was significantly higher ($p < 0.04$) than survival predicted by the Mayo model. Observed survival was significantly lower ($p < 0.01$) than survival predicted from the French population. Observed survival of non-cirrhotic patients was not different ($p > 0.9$) from that of the French control population, but that of cirrhotic patients was significantly lower ($p < 0.0001$). Twenty-two patients died; 13 from hepatic causes and four after OLT.

Observed survival free of OLT of treated patients was higher than that predicted by the Mayo model. Survival of treated patients was slightly lower than that of an age- and sex-matched general population. Most of the patients died from hepatic causes. In addition, prognostic factors of survival were defined. The risk to receive OLT or to die was much higher in patients with high serum bilirubin levels (>1.6 mg/dl (27 μmol/L)) or presence of cirrhosis at the outset of treatment.

This would suggest that treating patients at early stages might prevent progression to cirrhosis, and underlines the need for adjuvant therapies in patients who do not respond to UDCA. Similar results have been reported elsewhere[14].

UDCA therapy decreases fibrosis progression

The benefit from UDCA therapy on the progression of PBC from its early stage towards extensive fibrosis and cirrhosis has not been clearly shown. The aim of our study was to assess the effect of UDCA therapy on liver fibrosis progression in PBC[7]. A Markov model was used to analyse the progression rates between early and late histological stages in 103 patients with PBC enrolled in a randomized, double-blind, placebo-controlled trial of UDCA. Early stage was defined by the presence of portal and periportal lesions without extensive fibrosis, whereas late stage was defined by the presence of numerous septa, bridging fibrosis, or cirrhosis. A total of 162 pairs of liver biopsy specimens were studied. The model accurately described the observed data. UDCA therapy was associated with a 5-fold lower progression rate from early-stage disease to extensive fibrosis or cirrhosis (7% per year under UDCA vs 34% per year under placebo, $p < 0.002$), but was not associated with a significant difference in regression rates (3% per year under both UDCA and placebo). At 4 years the probability of UDCA-treated patients to remain in early-stage disease is 76% (95% confidence interval 58–88%), as compared with 29% (15–52%) in placebo-treated patients. Thus, UDCA therapy significantly delays the progression of liver fibrosis in PBC. Markov modelling should prove useful in assessing the efficacy of future medical treatments in clinical trials involving histological endpoints.

We also aimed to evaluate the effect of UDCA treatment on histological progression in PBC[12]. Using combined individual histological findings from four clinical trials we selected the patients in whom paired liver-biopsy specimens were available with a time interval of about 36 months between biopsies. A total of 367 patients was selected (UDCA: 200 vs placebo: 167). Overall, there was no significant difference in the progression of the histological stage between the two groups. By contrast, in the subgroup of patients with initial stages I–II ($n = 177$) there was a significant decrease in the histological stage progression in the UDCA group relative to the placebo group ($p < 0.03$). Overall, there was a significant delay in the progression of periportal necroinflammatory lesions ($p = 0.03$), and an improvement in the degree of ductular proliferation ($p = 0.02$) in the UDCA group compared with the placebo group. There was no significant difference in the progression of other specific lesions.

In conclusion, a 2-year UDCA treatment reduces periportal necroinflammation and improves ductular proliferation and, when initiated at the earlier stages I–II of the disease, also delays the progression of histological stage. These data support the early initiation of the drug to prevent these histological features of PBC.

Incidence and predictive factors for development of cirrhosis in UDCA-treated patients

UDCA slows the progression of PBC. However, some UDCA-treated patients escape and progress towards cirrhosis and end-stage disease. This study aimed to assess the incidence of cirrhosis in UDCA-treated patients with PBC and to determine the predictive factors of cirrhosis development under this treatment[8].

A Markov model was used to describe the progression towards cirrhosis in 183 UDCA-treated patients with PBC. A total of 254 pairs of liver biopsy specimens collected during 655 patient-years were studied.

The incidence of cirrhosis after 5 years of UDCA treatment was 4%, 12%, and 59% among patients followed up from stages I, II, and III, respectively. At 10 years the incidence was 17%, 27%, and 76%, respectively. The median time for developing cirrhosis from stages I, II, and III was 25 years, 20 years, and 4 years, respectively. The independent predictive factors of cirrhosis development were serum bilirubin greater than 17 μmol/L, serum albumin less than 38 g/L, and moderate to severe lymphocytic piecemeal necrosis (Figure 1).

This study provides new data concerning the time-course of PBC under UDCA, and constitutes a rationale for the design and evaluation of clinical trials aimed to assess the efficacy of drugs associated with UDCA.

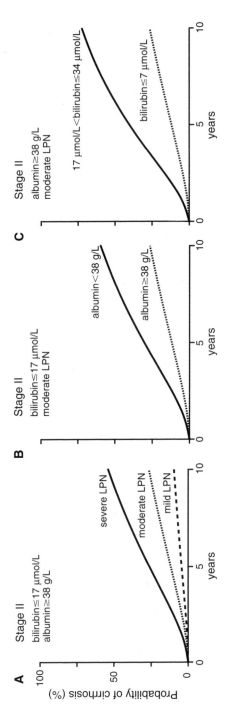

Figure 1 Incidence of cirrhosis in UDCA-treated patients with PBC as a function of three independent predictive variables: bilirubinaemia, albuminaemia, and severity of lymphocytic piecemeal necrosis (LPN). **A**: Predictive significance of LPN intensity in stage II patients with normal bilirubin and albumin levels; $p = 0.003$, Wald test. **B**: Predictive significance of serum albumin levels in stage II patients with moderate LPN and normal bilirubin level; $p = 0.011$, Wald test. **C**: Predictive significance of serum bilirubin levels in stage II patients with moderate LPN and normal albumin level; $p < 0.001$, Wald test

LONG-TERM SURVIVAL IN UDCA-TREATED PATIENTS

To assess the long-term survival (i.e. 10–20 years) in UDCA-treated patients we designed a Markov model with OLT or death as endpoints. The accuracy of the model was validated in 262 patients with a median follow-up of 10 years (1–22 years). A total of 874 observations collected during 2019 patient-years of follow-up was the data set for the analysis.

The proportion of patients treated from early histological stages (stage I or II according to Ludwig et al.[15]) remaining free of late histological stages, OLT or death was 59% and 40% at 10 and 20 years, respectively. In contrast the proportion of patients treated from early histological stages who have progressed towards OLT or death was 6% and 22% at 10 and 20 years, respectively; i.e. far less than that expected from available data from the natural history (see above).

Overall survival and survival without treatment failure were significantly longer than the 7-year survival free of OLT predicted by the updated Mayo model (RR 4.22, 95% CI 2.0–8.07, $p < 0.0001$; and RR 2.11, 95% CI 1.23–3.63, $p < 0.01$, respectively). In addition, survival of the patients was similar to that of an age- and sex-matched French population ($p = 0.3$).

CONCLUSION

UDCA as the first-line therapy of PBC prolongs survival of patients with PBC, especially when introduced at the early stages of the disease. We believe that results drawn from long-term observational studies will end the controversy regarding UDCA efficacy raised by meta-analysis of short-term clinical trials.

References

1. Poupon R, Poupon RE. Primary biliary cirrhosis. In: Zakim D, Boyer TD, editors. Hepatology. A Textbook of Liver Disease, 3rd edn. Philadelphia: W.B. Saunders, 1996:1329–65.
2. Shapiro JM, Smith H, Schaffner F. Serum bilirubin: a prognostic factor in primary biliary cirrhosis. Gut. 1979;20:137–40.
3. Christensen E, Crowe JP, Doniach D et al. Clinical pattern and course of disease in primary biliary cirrhosis based on an analysis of 236 patients. Gastroenterology. 1980;78:236–46.
4. Popper H, Schaffner F. Non-suppurative destructive chronic cholangitis and chronic hepatitis. In: Popper H, Schaffner F, editors. Progress in Liver Diseases. New York: Grune & Stratton, 1970:336–54.
5. Carithers RL. Primary biliary cirrhosis: specific treatment. In: Jenny HE, editor. Clinical Liver Disease, Vol. 7. Philadephia: W.B. Saunders, 2003:923–39.
6. Poupon RE, Lindor KD, Cauch-Dudek K, Dickson ER, Poupon R, Heathcote EJ. Combined analysis of randomized controlled trials of ursodeoxycholic acid in primary biliary cirrhosis. Gastroenterology. 1997;113:884–90.
7. Corpechot C, Carrat F, Bonnand A-M, Poupon RE, Poupon R. The effect of ursodeoxycholic acid therapy on liver fibrosis progression in primary biliary cirrhosis. Hepatology. 2000; 32:1196–99.
8. Corpechot C, Carrat F, Poupon R, Poupon RE. Primary biliary cirrhosis: incidence and predictive factors of cirrhosis development in ursodiol-treated patients. Gastroenterology. 2002;122:652–8.
9. Locke III GR, Therneau TM, Ludwig J, Dickson ER, Lindor KD. Time course of histological progression in primary biliary cirrhosis. Hepatology. 1996;23:52–6.
10. van Hoogstraten HJF, de Smet MBM, Renooij W et al. A randomized trial in primary biliary cirrhosis comparing ursodeoxycholic acid in daily doses of either 10/mg/kg or 20 mg/kg. Aliment Pharmacol Ther. 1998;12:965–71.

11. Angulo P, Dickson ER, Therneau TM et al. Comparison of three doses of ursodeoxycholic acid in the treatment of primary biliary cirrhosis: a randomized trial. J Hepatol. 1999;30:830–5.
12. Poupon RE, Lindor KD, Parès A, Chazouilleres O, Poupon R, Heathcote EJ. Combined analysis of the effect of treatment with ursodeoxycholic acid on histologic progression in primary biliary cirrhosis. J Hepatol. 2003;39:12–16.
13. Poupon RE, Bonnand A-M, Chrétien Y, Poupon R and the UDCA-PBC Study Group. Ten-year survival in ursodeoxycholic acid-treated patients with primary biliary cirrhosis. Hepatology. 1999;29:1668–71.
14. Lindor KD, Therneau TM, Jorgensen R, Malinchoc M, Dickson ER. Effects of ursodeoxycholic acid on survival in patients with primary biliary cirrhosis. Gastroenterology. 1996;110:1515–18.
15. Ludwig J, Dickson ER, MacDonald GSA. Staging of chronic nonsuppurative destructive cholangitis (syndrome of primary biliary cirrhosis). Virchows Arch Pathol Anat. 1978;379:103–12.

17
Combination therapy of primary biliary cirrhosis and overlap syndromes

U. LEUSCHNER

COMBINATION THERAPY IN PATIENTS WITH PRIMARY BILIARY CIRRHOSIS

Since 1985 ursodeoxycholic acid (UDCA) is the treatment of choice for patients with primary biliary cirrhosis (PBC) and primary sclerosing cholangitis (PSC). UDCA improves laboratory data, delays the development of fibrosis and consequently the development of oesophageal varices, and prolongs the interval free of liver transplantation. In patients with initially lower cholestasis indicating parameters (alkaline phosphatase below 240 U/L and gamma-glutamyl transpeptidase below 27 U/L), UDCA normalizes liver biochemistry within 2–3 years, but in 70% of patients with higher pretreatment data a plateau above the upper limit of normal develops[1]. Except in a few Japanese studies, UDCA is unable to eradicate antimitochondrial antibodies. UDCA monotherapy is unable to cure the disease.

UDCA improves cholestasis, reduces inflammation and has immunomodulatory properties; but UDCA is not an immunosuppressant. The rationale for combining UDCA with immunosuppressants is as follows: PBC is an autoimmune disease (as well as a cholestatic disease) which presents with characteristic autoantibodies, an augmentation of immunoglobulins, immunocompetent cells in liver infiltrates, concomitant autoimmune diseases and overlaps with autoimmune hepatitis.

In a prospective, controlled 3-year study from 1992 it has been shown[2] that prednisone alone obviously has no influence on PBC; but in this study a decrease of all immunoglobulins and of antimitochondrial antibodies was observed, whereas liver histology deteriorated in the placebo group. Although there were no statistically significant differences between the two groups, this study showed that the immunosuppressant prednisolone obviously has some beneficial effects.

In 1994 a group from the Netherlands[3] showed that the therapeutic effect of UDCA was increased by adding prednisone, and normalization of AST and AP was achieved as early as within 3 months (Figure 1).

Based on these data in 1996 we treated 15 patients with UDCA and placebo and 15 with UDCA and prednisolone, 10 mg/day for 9 months[4]. A statistically significant decrease of GLDH, ALT, AST, γ-GT and IgM ($p < 0.001$) was observed in both groups compared to the pretreatment data, revealing no difference between the two treatment groups; however, concerning IgG, IgA and liver histology ($p < 0.003$), UDCA plus prednisolone was superior to UDCA plus placebo (Table 1).

The data from this prospective placebo-controlled trial corroborated the results of the above-mentioned studies from the UK and the Netherlands: immunosuppressants obviously influence liver histology, immunoglobulins and AMA; UDCA, on the other hand, improves AP and γ-GT.

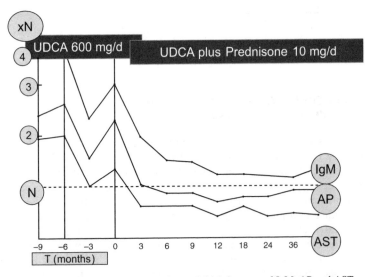

Figure 1 Effect of UDCA monotherapy: after an initial decrease of IgM, AP and AST a plateau had developed. After addition of prednisone the combination therapy of UDCA and prednisone induced further improvement and normalization of liver values (from ref. 3)

Table 1 UDCA plus placebo vs. UDCA plus prednisolone in primary biliary cirrhosis: results of a prospective double blind trial (from ref. 4)

Patient number: 30, stages I–III
Treatment time: 9 months

Group A: $n = 15$; 5 patients stage III: UDCA 13 mg/kg per day plus placebo
Group B: $n = 15$; 1 patient stage III: UDCA 13 mg/kg per day plus prednisolone 10 mg/day

In both groups ALT, AST, γ-GT, GLDH and IgM decreased significantly ($p < 0.001$) vs therapy onset. In group B IgG and IgA improved to a significantly greater extent than in group A, and liver histology also improved ($p < 0.003$).

As shown in 1998, not only does the combination of UDCA with one other immunosuppressant seem to be superior to UDCA monotherapy, but also triple therapy with UDCA, prednisone and azathioprine[5]. In this 1-year study prednisone was tapered off from 30 mg/day to 10 mg/day; however, this study and our own study with UDCA plus prednisolone revealed side-effects in about 30% of the patients. Although these side-effects in these short-term studies were of minor degree, long-term treatment with glucocorticoids could increase pre-existing osteoporosis.

Therefore, in 1997 we started a randomized, prospective, double-blind trial in which we compared UDCA (10–15 mg/kg per day) plus 3×3 mg budesonide (group A) versus UDCA plus placebo (group B)[6]. Budesonide is a topical glucocorticoid with high relative receptor-binding affinity, compared to conventional glucocorticoids, and a low systemic bioavailability of 15%. Therefore, we expected fewer side-effects and good treatment response. Our study was performed in 39 patients for 2 years. In the UDCA plus placebo group the well-known effects of UDCA were observed: AP, γ-GT, IgM and transaminases decreased significantly compared to the pretreatment data, and there was no change of antimitochondrial antibodies or of liver histology. These data improved to a greater extent in the UDCA plus budesonide group and the difference between the two study arms was statistically significant after only 6 months (Table 2). As in our study with UDCA plus prednisone, there was a marked improvement of liver histology after the end of the study. The point score of liver histology has improved by 30.3%, without change in the UDCA plus placebo group. When we analysed inflammation, bile duct injury and the amount of connective tissue separately, we found an improvement mainly of inflammation and fibrosis, while there was an increase of florid bile duct lesions (Table 3) in both groups. These findings were corroborated by a second evaluation of an earlier study with UDCA monotherapy from the United States[7] in which the prevalence of bile duct lesions dropped from 37.7% to 18.2% in the UDCA-treated group, and from 38.3% to 21.7% in the placebo group.

A study from the Mayo Clinic with budesonide and UDCA showed different results[8]. Only AP improved for a short period, but there were no further positive reactions and some patients complained of side-effects. However, the Mayo Clinic study and our study cannot be compared because of major differences: the Mayo Clinic study was an uncontrolled, open study over the short period of 1 year. The patient number was half of that of our study, they were not naive patients and many of them had late-stage disease. When we stopped UDCA/budesonide therapy in group A of our study, the liver enzymes increased again, but did not

Table 2 UDCA plus budesonide vs UDCA plus placebo in primary biliary cirrhosis: results of a randomized double blind trial (from ref. 6)

Patient number: 39, stages I–III
Treatment time: 24 months

Group A: $n = 20$; 10 patients stage III: UDCA 10–15 mg/kg per day plus budesonide 3×3 mg/day
Group B: $n = 19$; 8 patients stage III: UDCA plus placebo

In group A AP, GLDH, IgM and IgG improved to a greater extent than in group B
($p < 0.05$–0.001). Serum cortisol in group A did not drop below the lower reference line; ACTH-stimulated cortisol secretion was not suppressed by budesonide.

Table 3 Influence of UDCA plus budesonide and UDCA plus placebo on liver histology: results of a randomized double-blind trial (from ref. 6)

	Group A (UDCA 10–15 g/kg per day + budesonide 3 × 3 mg/day)	Group B (UDCA placebo)
Inflammation	−25.0	+3.2 ($p < 0.01$)
Fibrosis	−57.1	+16.0 ($p < 0.001$)
Bile duct lesions	+12.5	+16.0 (n.s.)
Total score	−30.3	+3.5 ($p < 0.001$)

Liver biopsies: before, after 12 months, after end of study.
Point score: 0 (not present) to 4 (severe alterations).
Deterioration (+) and improvement (−) of the point score are given in percentages.

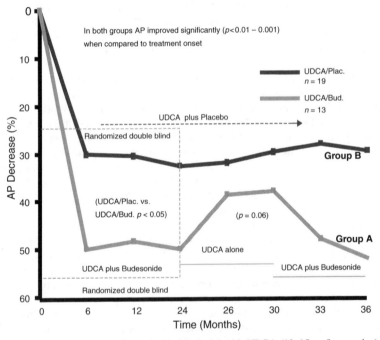

Figure 2 After a 2-year randomized, double-blind trial with UDCA (10–15 mg/kg per day) plus budesonide (3 × 3 mg/day), treatment with budesonide was stopped (group A lower line). AP (γ-GT, AST and ALT not shown) increased again (ns) and improved after combination therapy with UDCA and budesonide was resumed

reach the levels of UDCA monotherapy (Figure 2). When UDCA/budesonide therapy was resumed, data improved for a second time. These observations show that budesonide provides an additional beneficial effect.

The observation that immunosuppressants and anti-inflammatory compounds in combination with UDCA might be beneficial could also be shown in a study in which UDCA was combined with the old-fashioned NSAID sulindac[9]. Animal experiments proved that sulindac, in addition to its anti-inflammatory and immunosuppressant properties, stimulates choleresis 2–3-fold, and that one could expect that UDCA (a hypercholeretic bile acid) plus sulindac could be superior to UDCA monotherapy in cholestatic and autoimmune liver diseases. Therefore, in 11 patients who were under UDCA for a period of 7 years, and had developed a plateau above the upper limit of normal, sulindac was added in a dose of 100, 200 and 300 mg/day, while 12 patients remained on UDCA alone. In all patients treated with UDCA and sulindac for 2 more years there was a significant improvement of liver biochemistry ($p < 0.001$) while there was no change in the UDCA group.

In conclusion, there are at least six controlled studies showing that immuno-suppressive compounds added to UDCA are obviously superior to UDCA monotherapy. Therefore, future studies should concentrate on the following questions: which patients with PBC may profit from combination therapy; which is the most suitable immunosuppressant for combination therapy; are there major side-effects during long-term treatment with UDCA plus an immunosuppressant; and could more modern immunosuppressants, e.g. the topical steroid budesonide (which has a 25-fold higher relative receptor-binding affinity than conventional glucocorticoids and with 15% systemic bioavailability a lower spill-over into the systemic circulation), cyclosporin A or mycophenolate mofetil, both successfully used following liver transplatation, be better than UDCA monotherapy?

In 1987 Landon et al. observed, in a female patient with stage III PSC, a marked improvement of liver biochemistry when she became pregnant[10]. During the past few years we have gathered data from female patients with PBC and PSC who were treated with UDCA and became pregnant during therapy. Again, in all patients, AP, γ-GT, AST, ALT and IgM significantly improved. At delivery there was a steep increase of laboratory data, but within a couple of weeks they returned to the pre-pregnancy levels (Figure 3).

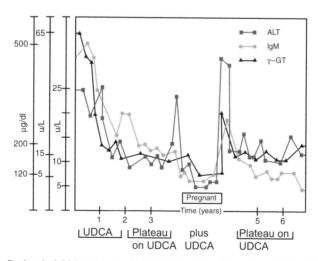

Figure 3 During the initial treatment with UDCA (10–15 mg/kg per day) AP (not shown), ALT, IgM and γ-GT decreased significantly. When the patient became pregnant the values even normalized. At delivery a flare-up was observed, but within 2–3 months all values returned to the prepregnancy levels

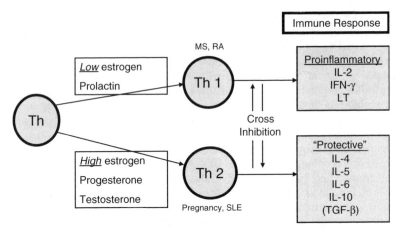

Figure 4 Pregnancy and high oestrogen concentrations stimulate the expression of Th2-mediated and more protective cytokines. Low oestrogen concentrations stimulate the expression of proinflammatory cytokines, similar to multiple sclerosis (MS) and rheumatoid arthritis (RA) (from ref. 11)

Explaining this phenomenon is difficult. Obviously the fetoplacental unit redirects maternal immunity from Th1 to Th2, that is a status of strong temporary immunosuppression. The cause of this redirection of maternal immunity to Th2 may be the higher oestrogen and progesterone concentrations in the maternal circulation (Figure 4). As has been shown previously, high oestrogen concentrations stimulate the expression of more protective cytokines such as IL-4, -5, -6, -10 and TGF-β[11]. This in our opinion highly interesting observation raises the question as to whether, for the treatment of primary biliary liver disease, the combination of UDCA with oestrogens with or without progesterone could cure the disease. Unlike as in studies with UDCA plus conventional glucocorticoids the combination of UDCA plus pregnancy not only improved but even normalized laboratory data. Further, these observations again raise the questions of why PBC is a predominantly female disease, whether the combination of UDCA and hormones could prevent the development or improve coexisting osteoporosis, and whether PBC is a Th1- or Th2-mediated disorder.

Other UDCA combination therapies for patients with PBC were performed with azathioprine, methotrexate[12–14], colchicine[15–17], silymarin and bezafibrate[18]. The data from these studies are contradictory; at the most the combination of UDCA and colchicine in a dosage of 1 mg/day could have some positive effects in selected patients.

COMBINATION THERAPY OF PBC OVERLAP SYNDROMES

At present there is no unequivocal definition of the overlap syndrome between PBC and autoimmune hepatitis (AIH). Variant I of the AIH/PBC overlap syndrome is also called autoimmune cholangitis (AIC) and is characterized by liver histology of PBC, cholestasis parameters and the absence of AMA (Figure 5).

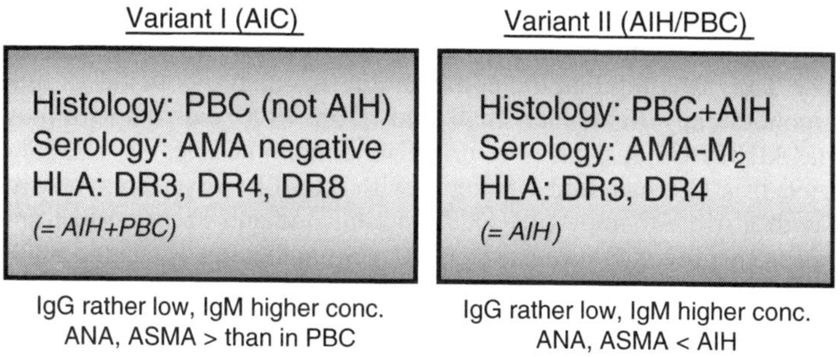

Variant I (AIC) Variant II (AIH/PBC)

Histology: PBC (not AIH) Serology: AMA negative HLA: DR3, DR4, DR8 *(= AIH+PBC)*	Histology: PBC+AIH Serology: AMA-M$_2$ HLA: DR3, DR4 *(= AIH)*

IgG rather low, IgM higher conc. IgG rather low, IgM higher conc.
ANA, ASMA > than in PBC ANA, ASMA < AIH

Figure 5 Whether variant I of the AIH/PBC overlap syndrome can be defined as overlap syndrome or is nothing else than an AMA-negative PBC is not known. At present there is no unequivocal definition of any overlap syndrome (AIC=autoimmune cholangitis)

Table 4 Treatment of the autoimmune hepatitis–primary biliary cirrhosis overlap syndrome (from ref. 19)

Definition of the OLS
AP > 2N, or γ-GT > 5N, ALT > 5N, AMA-positive, IgG > 2N or ASMA, bile duct lesions, piecemeal necrosis

130 consecutive patients with PBC: OLS 12 (9.2%); 10 female, 2 male

Treatment
 5 patients UDCA 13–15 mg/kg per day, 23 months: AP and γ-GT decreased =
 incomplete response
 6 patients corticosteroids 0.5 mg/kg per day, 4 months: AP, IgG and ALT decreased =
 incomplete response

Patients with persistent abnormal liver tests: *UDCA + corticosteroids*, 18 months: in all patients *further improvement* with near normalization. In two patients liver biopsy showed decrease of activity and stable fibrosis

---

Immunogenetically in some patients we find HLA-DR3, DR4 as in autoimmune hepatitis, and DR8 as in PBC. IgG is rather low; IgM is found in higher concentrations. The titres of ANA and ASMA are said to be higher than in patients with PBC. In these patients monotherapy with UDCA is sufficient and, therefore, will not be discussed further. In the second variant, histology is characterized by findings like those in PBC, but also like those in autoimmune hepatitis. This variant is AMA-positive; immunologically HLA-DR3 and DR4 are expressed as in autoimmune hepatitis.

There are only very few observational therapy studies with variant II of the AIH/PBC overlap syndrome with small patient numbers and short treatment times. In a French study from 1998 in 130 consecutive patients with PBC (Table 4), 12 patients (9.2%) had an overlap syndrome[19]. In this study the definition of the overlap syndrome was as follows: AP > 2N or γ-GT > 5N, ALT > 5N, AMA-positive, IgG > 2N or ASMA. Bile duct lesions and piecemeal necroses had to be present. Five out of the 12 patients were treated with UDCA and responded incompletely: AP and γ-GT decreased. The same happened to six patients who were treated with corticosteroids: AP, γ-GT and ALT improved. Subsequent treatment with the combination of UDCA plus corticoids further improved the laboratory data, showing that the combination treatment is obviously superior to UDCA monotherapy. In another small study from 1998, patients with the overlap syndrome AIH/PBC[20] responded to prednisone monotherapy.

In 1999, in a German study, patients with AIH/PBC overlap syndrome were treated with a triple therapy of UDCA, prednisone and azathioprine, and again combination therapy was superior to UDCA monotherapy[21].

SUMMARY

Although there is no general recommendation for the combination of UDCA with conventional or more modern immunosuppressants, all studies with combination therapy in some aspects were superior to UDCA monotherapy. Since UDCA, which remains the basic therapy of PBC, does not cure PBC, and since PBC is an autoimmune liver disease, it is necessary to investigate which patients will benefit from combination therapy and which anti-inflammatory or immunosuppressive compound could be the drug of choice. An interesting observation is made during pregnancy which, in addition to UDCA therapy, improved liver biochemistry of PBC and PSC. This raises the question of whether combination of UDCA with hormones could also be beneficial, at least for a limited period of treatment. For treatment of the AIH/PBC overlap syndrome the combination of UDCA plus prednisone is recommended. The experience with overlap syndromes is extremely small. Further investigations and study results are expected.

References

1. Leuschner M, Dietrich CF, You T et al. Characterization of patients with primary biliary cirrhosis responding to long term ursodeoxycholic acid treatment. Gut. 2000;46:121–6.
2. Mitchison HC, Palmer JM, Bassendine MF et al. A controlled trial of prednisolone treatment in primary biliary cirrhosis. Three-year results. J Hepatol. 1992;15:336–44.
3. Wolfhagen FHJ, van Buuren HR, Schalm SW. Combined treatment with ursodeoxycholic acid and prednisolone in primary biliary cirrhosis. Neth J Med. 1994;44:84–90.
4. Leuschner M, Güldütuna S, You T et al. Ursodeoxycholic acid and prednisolone versus ursodeoxycholic acid and placebo in the treatment of early stage of primary biliary cirrhosis. J Hepatol. 1996;25:49–57.
5. Wolfhagen FHJ, van Hoogstraten HJF, van Buuren HR et al. Triple therapy with ursodeoxycholic acid, prednisone and azathioprine in primary biliary cirrhosis: a 1-year randomized, placebo-controlled study. J Hepatol. 1998;29:736–42.
6. Leuschner M, Maier K-P, Schlichting J et al. Oral budesonide and ursodeoxycholic acid for treatment of primary biliary cirrhosis: Results of a prospective double-blind trial. Gastroenterology. 1999;117:918–25.
7. Combes B, Markin RS, Wheeler DE et al. The effect of ursodeoxycholic acid on the florid duct lesion of primary biliary cirrhosis. Hepatology. 1999;30:602–5.
8. Angulo P, Jorgensen RA, Keach JC et al. Oral budesonide in the treatment of patients with primary biliary cirrhosis with a suboptimal response to ursodeoxycholic acid. Hepatology. 2000;31:318–23.
9. Leuschner M, Holtmeier J, Ackermann H et al. The influence of sulindac on patients with primary biliary cirrhosis that responds incompletely to ursodeoxycholic acid: a pilot study. Eur J Gastroenterol Hepatol. 2002;14:1369–76.
10. Landon MB, Soloway RD, Freedman LJ et al. Primary sclerosing cholangitis and pregnancy. Obstet Gynecol. 1987;69:457–60.

11. Whitacre CC, Reingold SC, O'Looney PA et al. A gender gap in autoimmunity. Science. 1999;283:1277–8.
12. Buscher H-P, Zietschmann Y, Gerok W. Positive responses to methotrexate and ursodeoxycholic acid in patients with primary biliary cirrhosis responding insufficiently to ursodeoxycholic acid alone. J Hepatol. 1993;18:9–14.
13. Lindor KD, Dickson ER, Jorgensen RA et al. The combination of ursodeoxycholic acid and methotrexate for patients with primary biliary cirrhosis: The results of a pilot study. Hepatology. 1995;22:1158–62.
14. González-Koch A, Brahm J, Antezana C et al. The combination of ursodeoxycholic acid and methotrexate for primary biliary cirrhosis is not better than ursodeoxycholic acid alone. J Hepatol. 1997;27:143–9.
15. Shibata J, Fujiyama S, Honda Y et al. Combination therapy with ursodeoxycholic acid and colchicine for primary biliary cirrhosis. J Gastroenterol Hepatol. 1992;7:277–82.
16. Ikeda T, Tozuka S, Noguchi O et al. Effects of additional administration of colchicine in ursodeoxycholic acid-treated patients with primary biliary cirrhosis: a prospective randomized study. J Hepatol. 1996;24:88–94.
17. Poupon RE, Huet PM, Poupon R et al. A randomized trial comparing colchicine and ursodeoxycholic acid combination to ursodeoxycholic acid in primary biliary cirrhosis. Hepatology. 1996;24:1098–103.
18. Kanda T, Yokosuka O, Imazeki F et al. Bezafibrate treatment: a new medical approach for PBC patients? J Gastroenterol. 2003;38:573–8.
19. Chazouillères O, Wendum D, Serfaty L et al. Primary biliary cirrhosis–autoimmune hepatitis overlap syndrome: clinical features and response to therapy. Hepatology. 1998;28:296–301.
20. Czaja AJ. Frequency and nature of the variant syndromes of autoimmune liver disease. Hepatology. 1998;28:360–5.
21. Lohse AW, Meier zum Büschenfelde K-HM, Franz B et al. Characterization of the overlap syndrome of primary biliary cirrhosis (PBC) and autoimmune hepatitis: evidence for its being a hepatitic form of PBC in genetically susceptible individuals. Hepatology. 1999;29:1078–84.

18
Management of pruritus, fatigue and bone disease in patients with primary biliary cirrhosis

N. V. BERGASA

INTRODUCTION

Pruritus, fatigue and osteoporosis are complications of liver disease, including that secondary to primary biliary cirrhosis (PBC). These complications can have a marked negative impact on the quality of life of patients, and hence require specific addressing and treatment. In this chapter a general review on the treatment of these complications is provided.

PRURITUS IN PBC

A substantial number of patients with PBC have pruritus. The pruritus is believed to result from cholestasis, which is defined as impaired secretion of bile. The skin of patients with cholestasis and pruritus is devoid of primary pruritic skin lesions; however, excoriations and prurigo nodularis, consequences of scratching, abound. There are no universally satisfactory therapies to treat this form of pruritus.

The aetiology of the pruritus of cholestasis is unknown. It is believed that the pruritogen(s) is produced in the liver, excreted in bile, and that it accumulates in plasma as a result of cholestasis. The idea that pruritus arises from the stimulation of skin nerve fibres by retained 'pruritogen(s)' can be appealing but there are no data at present that prove that idea.

Over the past decade the hypothesis that the pruritus of cholestasis is mediated, at least in part, by endogenous opioids, has been advanced[1]. A central mechanism has been proposed[1]. In this context the increase in opioidergic neurotransmission by the central administration of drugs with agonist activity at opioid receptors, mostly the mu receptor, including morphine, is associated with pruritus[2-5]. This type of pruritus can be effectively treated with opiate antagonists[6]. This observation suggests that opiate-induced pruritus is mediated by an opioid receptor mechanism. There is evidence to suggest that, in cholestasis, the opioid neurotransmission is increased. This evidence can be summarized as follows: (1) patients with cholestasis can develop an opiate-withdrawal-like reaction when administered opiate antagonists[7-9], (2) plasma levels of endogenous opioids can be increased in cholestatic patients and in an animal model of cholestasis[7,10], (3) in the rat model of cholestasis secondary to bile duct resection there is a state of stereospecific naloxone-reversible antinociception (analgesia)[11], (4) there is down-regulation of opioid receptors in brain membranes of rats with cholestasis[12], and (5) the microinjection of plasma extracts from patients with cholestasis and pruritus into the medullary dorsal horn of monkeys is associated with naloxone-preventable scratching behaviour[13]. Accordingly, if the pharmacological increase in opioidergic tone can be associated with pruritus, increased opioidergic tone in cholestasis may also result in pruritus. The fact that the pruritus can be ameliorated by opiate antagonists supports the idea of opioid-mediated pruritus in cholestasis[7-9,14-18]. A central mechanism has been proposed, analogous to the mechanism by which central morphine causes pruritus. The neurophysiological changes that result in pruritus are unknown at present, but the medullary dorsal horn has been identified as a site in which opioid-mediated pruritus can be triggered[19,20].

The treatments for the pruritus of cholestasis can be classified according to the means by which the intervention is expected to exert its effect, as follows (Table 1).

Table 1 Selected treatments for the pruritus of cholestasis

Medication	Postulated antipruritic mechanism	Potential side-effects	Dose /mode of administration/frequency	Refs
Cholestyramine	Increased excretion of pruritogen(s)	Bloating, constipation, malabsorption of nutrients	4 g p.o. before and after breakfast; increase by 4 g at other mealtimes, not to exceed 16 g/day	*
Rifampicin	Unknown	Hepatotoxicity	150 mg p.o./b.i.d. if serum bilirubin > 3 mg/dl; 150 mg p.o./t.i.d. if serum bilirubin < 3	33
Naloxone	Decreased opioidergic tone	Opiate-withdrawal-like syndrome	0.2 μ/kg per minute i.v. continuous infusions preceded by 0.4 mg i.v. bolus	15
Naltrexone	Decreased opioidergic tone	Opiate-withdrawal-like syndrome, potential hepatotoxicity	25 mg p.o./b.i.d. on day 1 followed by 50 mg p.o. daily	17

* This regimen has not been tested in clinical trials but is based on the inference that the pruritogen(s) accumulates in the gallbladder during the overnight fast.

Treatments aimed at the removal of pruritogens from the circulation

The non-absorbable resins cholestyramine, colestipol and colesevalam fall into this category. There is a consensus that the administration of cholestyramine is associated with an improvement of the pruritus in a substantial number of patients. The improvement may be transient in many patients. The rationale for the use of these resins is to enhance the faecal excretion of the 'pruritogen(s)'. Interestingly, however, the administration of cholestyramine to human beings[21] and to laboratory animals[22] is associated with the release of cholecystokinin (CCK), an endogenous antiopiate[23]. Thus, the interesting possibility of an antipruritic effect of cholestyramine by an opiate-antagonist mechanism may be of relevance. Invasive procedures also aimed at the removal of circulating 'pruritogen(s)' include plasmapheresis[24] and recently extracorporeal albumin dialysis[25,26]. Surgical procedures have also been carried out to decrease the pruritus, including partial external diversion of bile[27] and partial ileal exclusion[28], which have been done in children. These procedures have not been submitted to controlled clinical trials. Their invasive nature requires a specific design; in addition, a placebo response has to be considered as contributing to the reported relief.

There is no evidence that histamine plays a role in the pruritus of cholestasis; however, antihistamines are commonly prescribed to treat this symptom. Antihistamines can be associated with reported improvement in some patients, which appears to be due to the sedating effect of this type of drug. Side-effects, including dry mouth, may worsen the symptoms of sicca syndrome in patients with PBC[29]. The use of antihistamines to treat this form of pruritus without a clear response to this type of drug does not seem justified.

Enzyme inducers

Rifampicin is an enzyme inducer, and it can alter the metabolism of bile acids[30]. Rifampicin is also associated with increased levels of serum bile acids in human beings[31]. In addition, it can precipitate an opiate-withdrawal reaction in methadone-maintained patients[32], without affecting the metabolism of the drug. Thus, an opiate antagonist effect of this drug has been considered, which may be relevant in the amelioration of the pruritus. Rifampicin is frequently used to treat the pruritus of cholestasis, based on controlled studies that applied subjective methodology[33–35].

Phenobarbital is also an enzyme inducer, with choleretic properties. It causes sedation, which may be a reason for the reported relief in the pruritus of cholestasis[36,37].

Opiate antagonists

The use of naloxone, an opiate antagonist, was reported to relieve the pruritus in a patient with PBC by Bernstein and Swift in 1979[38]. Several years later, in studies of plasma endogenous opioids and manifestation of liver disease, Thornton and Losowsky reported in their landmark publication that patients with cholestasis reported a decrease in their pruritus associated with the intake of nalmefene, another opiate antagonist[7]. These investigators proposed that the decrease in the pruritus might have been due to the blocking of the release of pruritogens by the drug[7]; however, they also reported that the administration of nalmefene was associated with a constellation of symptoms in all the patients, termed 'opiate withdrawal-like reaction', suggesting increased opioidergic tone in cholestasis. The development of an opiate-withdrawal-like reaction and the decrease in pruritus by an opiate antagonist inspired the hypothesis stating that, in cholestasis, the pruritus was mediated by increased central opioidergic neurotransmission[1]. The evidence connecting increased opioidergic tone with pruritus was reviewed above.

A major obstacle to progress in the field of pruritus had concerned methods of quantitation. Pruritus is a sensation; accordingly, it cannot be measured directly. In contrast, the behaviour that results from pruritus, scratching activity, can be measured, provided a suitable method is available. A scratching activity monitoring system (SAMS) was developed to record continuously scratching behaviour in human beings independent from gross body movements[39]. The anecdotal report of Bernstein and Swift, and the study of nalmefene that applied subjective methodology by Thornton and Losowsky, were followed by controlled clinical trials that applied behavioural methodology[8,9,14,15]. In these studies the administration of opiate antagonists was associated with a decrease in the perception of pruritus and in scratching activity[8,9,14,15]. Thus, objective data were provided for the first time supporting a role of a specific group of substances, endogenous opioids, as mediators of the pruritus of cholestasis. Opiate antagonists are currently used to treat the pruritus. A concern regarding their use is the precipitation of an opiate-withdrawal-like syndrome. The occurrence of this syndrome can be prevented by the introduction of opiate antagonists in low doses, as published[40,41].

Serotonin type 3 receptor antagonists

Anecdotal reports on the serotonin receptor type 3 antagonist, ondansetron, were published in the mid-1990s[42,43], followed by two controlled studies that applied subjective methodology in which ondansetron was associated with an amelioration of the pruritus[44,45]. In a study that applied quantitative methodology, however, ondansetron was not associated with decrease in scratching activity as compared to placebo[46].

Bright-light therapy reflected towards the eyes

In a placebo-controlled study of naloxone a 24-hour rhythm in scratching activity was detected in a group of patients[15]. This finding suggests that scratching activity may have circadian rhythmicity[15]. The most important regulator of circadian rhythms is light, via retinothalamic pathways[47]. To explore whether light altered scratching activity, the behaviour that results directly from pruritus, the effect of bright light therapy reflected towards the eyes was tested in a pilot study[47]. Light therapy administered in this fashion is the treatment of choice for seasonal affective disorders. Bright light therapy at doses of up to 60 minutes per day twice a day was associated with a decrease in scratching activity in the majority of patients, as well as with a decrease in the perception of pruritus[47]. In addition, the variability on scratching activity was significantly reduced in all the patients, suggesting the light therapy was associated with a decrease in the outbursts of pruritus[47]. If confirmed in properly controlled trials, bright light therapy may be a therapeutic alternative for the pruritus. A controlled study on this mode of treatment has not been conducted.

POTENTIAL NOVEL TREATMENTS

Anecdotal reports on the amelioration of the pruritus of cholestasis by sertraline[48], a serotonin re-uptake inhibitor, and by dronabinol[49], an agonist at the central cannabinoid receptor, have been published. Controlled studies on these drugs have not been performed. A study of the drug gabapentin, approved as an anticonvulsant for partial seizures in adults, is associated with increased threshold to experience nociception in animal models[50,51]. A behavioural study of this drug for the treatment of the pruritus of cholestasis is being completed at the time of this writing (NV Bergasa, unpublished).

FATIGUE IN PBC

The aetiology of fatigue in PBC is unknown. A central mechanism has been proposed[52]. It is a difficult symptom to study as only subjective methodology has been developed.

The hypothesis that increased serotonin neurotransmission[52,53] mediates fatigue in cholestasis was tested in a randomized double-blind placebo-controlled trial with a crossover design of the drug ondansetron in which 56 patients with PBC participated[54]. Ondansetron is a serotonin type 3 receptor antagonist. Ondansetron was reported to be associated with a decrease in the Fisk Fatigue Severity Score[54] (Table 2).

In evaluating patients with PBC who report fatigue, it is necessary to exclude the presence of conditions also associated with fatigue, including anaemia, depression and hypothyroidism, which should be treated specifically. Naps during the day are associated with improved energy levels in patients with PBC and fatigue anecdotally.

Table 2 Ondansetron for the treatment of fatigue in PBC

Intervention	Aim	Dose/mode of administration/frequency	Ref.
Ondansetron	To decrease serotoninergic tone	4 mg p.o./t.i.d.	54

BONE DISEASE IN PBC

Osteoporosis, as a specific complication of PBC, is being questioned in the emerging literature[55–57].

Sufficient calcium and vitamin D availability are necessary to prevent bone loss, generally speaking. The most important source of vitamin D in human beings is endogenous; thus, sufficient exposure to sunlight is necessary.

Etidronate, taken cyclically, was reported to be associated with reduced bone loss, as compared to sodium fluoride in patients with PBC in Spain[58]. In contrast, the use of this biphosphonate in a study of 2 years duration, conducted in Minnesota, did not report a higher effect of etidronate over placebo on bone loss in patients with PBC[59]. Recently, the results of a randomized study of 2 years duration, also from Spain, that compared the effect of alendronate to cyclical etidronate on bone mass in 32 patients with PBC and osteopenia was published. In that study both biphosphonates were associated with increased bone mineral density; the increase at the lumbar spine and proximal femur was greater in the group randomized to alendronate than in that of the group randomized to etidronate. New spinal fractures were not recorded in patients from any group, although peripheral fractures did occur in a total of three patients from both groups.

Table 3 Summary of selected publications on drug therapy in bone disease in PBC

Medication(s)	Dose/mode of administration/frequency	No. of Patients	Results	Refs
Etidronate[a] versus Fluoride[b]	[a]400 mg p.o./day × 14 days every 3 months [b]50 mg/day	16 subjects per group	[a]Increased mineral bone density at lumbar spine. No change in proximal femur[c]	58
Etidronate versus placebo	400 mg p.o./day × 14 days every 3 months	29 etidronate, 31 placebo	[d]No difference in bone density at lumbar spine or femur	59
Alendronate[e] versus etidronate	[e]10 mg p.o./day 400 mg/day × 14 days every 3 months	16 per group	[f]Increase in bone density at lumbar in both arms. Increase at lumbar spine and femur greater with alendronate than with etidronate	62

[c] Data from 13 patients in the etidronate group and 10 patients in the fluoride groups that completed 2 years of treatment.

[d] Sixty patients completed 1 year of treatment. Four patients in each group had fractures.

[f] Data from 13 patients per group at 2 years.

In a retrospective study the use of oestrogen was associated with a significant reduction in bone loss in a group of 46 postmenopausal patients with PBC as compared to an age-matched control group of patients with this liver disease who were not using oestrogens[60]. No side-effects associated with oestrogens were reported[60].

It has been recently recommended that, at the time of diagnosis of liver disease (e.g. PBC), patients undergo measurement of bone density with dual X-ray absorptiometry[61]. If the results do not suggest the presence of bone disease the incorporation of preventive measures, including weight-bearing exercise, is recommended. If the results of the study are consistent with the presence of osteopenia, bone measurements should be repeated in 2 years and preventive measures applied. If the diagnosis of osteoporosis is made, however, a systematic work-up to exclude other conditions that may lead to osteoporosis should be undertaken, and the use of biphosphonates considered. The referral of patients with PBC and osteopenia or osteoporosis to a bone specialist, however, is an open option in these recommendations. Referral to bone specialists seems prudent in the view of this writer, as the management of this complication requires specific expertise in many cases.

In summary, complications of PBC, including pruritus, fatigue and bone disease, can have a substantial negative impact in the lives of patients. It is necessary to establish if patients are suffering from these complications by history and by an appropriate work-up because specific therapy may be necessary and is available. Areas of uncertainty, however, are discerned more powerfully in clinical trials; thus patients' referral to studies is part of the management of patients with PBC.

References

1. Jones EA, Bergasa NV. The pruritus of cholestasis: from bile acids to opiate agonists. Hepatology. 1990;11:884–7.
2. Scott P, Fischer H. Spinal opiate analgesis and facial pruritus: a neural theory. Postgrad Med J. 1982;58:531–5.
3. Ballantyne JC, Loach AB, Carr DB. Itching after epidural and spinal opiates. Pain. 1988; 33:149–60.
4. Ballantyne JC, Loach AB, Carr DB. The incidence of pruritus after epidural morphine. Anaesthesia. 1989;44:863.
5. Abbound TK, Lee K, Zhu J et al. Prophylactic oral naltrexone with intrathecal morphine for cesarean section: effects on adverse reactions and analgesia. Anesth Analg. 1990;71:367–70.
6. Kjellberg F, Tramer MR. Pharmacological control of opioid-induced pruritus: a quantitative systematic review of randomized trials. Eur J Anaesthesiol. 2001;18:346–57.
7. Thornton JR, Losowsky MS. Opioid peptides and primary biliary cirrhosis. Br Med J. 1988; 297:1501–4.
8. Bergasa NV, Talbot TL, Schmitt JP et al. Open label trial of oral nalmefene therapy for the pruritus of cholestasis. Hepatology. 1998;27:679–84.
9. Bergasa NV, Alling DW, Talbot TL, Wells M, Jones EA. Oral nalmefene therapy reduces scratching activity due to the pruritus of cholestasis: a controlled study. J Am Acad Dermatol. 1999;41:431–4.
10. Swain MG, Rothman RB, Xu H, Vergalla J, Bergasa NV, Jones EA. Endogenous opioids accumulate in plasma in a rat model of acute cholestasis. Gastroenterology. 1992;103:630–5.
11. Bergasa NV, Alling DW, Vergalla J, Jones EA. Cholestasis in the male rat is associated with naloxone-reversible antinociception. J Hepatol. 1994;20:85–90.
12. Bergasa NV, Rothman RB, Vergalla J, Xu H, Swain MG, Jones EA. Down-regulation of delta opioid receptors in bile duct resected rats: further evidence for alteration in the opioid system in cholestasis. Gastroenterology. 1992;102:A946.

13. Bergasa NV, Thomas DA, Vergalla J, Turner ML, Jones EA. Plasma from patients with the pruritus of cholestasis induces opioid receptor-mediated scratching in monkeys. Life Sci. 1993; 53:1253–7.
14. Bergasa NV, Talbot TL, Alling DW et al. A controlled trial of naloxone infusions for the pruritus of chronic cholestasis. Gastroenterology. 1992;102:544–9.
15. Bergasa NV, Alling DW, Talbot TL et al. Naloxone ameliorates the pruritus of cholestasis: results of a double-blind randomized placebo-controlled trial. Ann Intern Med. 1995;123:161–7.
16. Carson KL, Tran TT, Cotton P, Sharara AI, Hunt CM. Pilot study of the use of naltrexone to treat the severe pruritus of cholestatic liver disease. Am J Gastroenterol. 1996;91:1022–3.
17. Wolfhagen FHJ, Sternieri E, Hop WCJ, Vitale G, Bertolotti M, van Buuren HR. Oral naltrexone treatment for cholestatic pruritus: a double-blind, placebo-controlled study. Gastroenterology. 1997;113:1264–9.
18. Terg R, Coronel E, Sorda J, Munoz AE, Findor J. Efficacy and safety of oral naltrexone treatment for pruritus of cholestasis, a crossover, double blind, placebo-controlled study. J Hepatol. 2002;37:717–22.
19. Thomas DA, Williams GM, Iwata K, Kenshalo DJ, Dubner R. Effects of central administration of opioids on facial scratching in monkeys. Brain Res. 1992;585:315–17.
20. Thomas DA, Hammond DL. Microinjection of morphine into the rat medullary dorsal horn produces a dose-dependent increase in facial scratching. Brain Res. 1995;695:267–70.
21. Koop I, Dorn S, Koop H et al. Dissociation of cholecystokinin and pancreaticobiliary response to intraduodenal bile acids and cholestyramine in humans. Dig Dis Sci. 1991;36:1625–32.
22. Kogire M, Gomez G, Uchida T, Ishizuka J, Greeley GH Jr, Thompson JC. Chronic effect of oral cholestyramine, a bile salt sequestrant, and exogenous cholecystokinin on insulin release in rats. Pancreas. 1992;7:15–20.
23. Wiertelak EP, Maier SF, Watkins LR. Cholecystokinin antianalgesia: safety cues abolished morphine analgesia. Science. 1992;256:830–3.
24. Ambinder EP, Cohen LB, Wolke AM et al. The clinical effectiveness and safety of chronic plasmapheresis in patients with primary biliary cirrhosis. J Clin Apheresis. 1985;2:219–23.
25. Doria C, Mandala L, Smith J et al. Effect of molecular adsorbent recirculating system in hepatitis C virus-related intractable pruritus. Liver Transplant. 2003;9:437–43.
26. Schachschal G, Morgera S, Kupferling S, Neumayer HH, Lochs H, Schmidt HH. Emerging indications for MARS dialysis. Liver. 2002;22(Suppl. 2):63–8.
27. Emerick KM, Whitington PF. Partial external biliary diversion for intractable pruritus and xanthomas in Alagille syndrome. Hepatology. 2002;35:1501–6.
28. Hollands CM, Rivera-Pedrogo FJ, Gonzalez-Vallina R, Loret-de-Mola O, Nahmad M, Burnweit CA. Ileal exclusion for Byler's disease: an alternative surgical approach with promising early results for pruritus. J Pediatr Surg. 1998;33:220–4.
29. Babe Jr KS, Serafin WE. Histamine, bradykinin, and their antagonists. In: Molinoff PB, Ruddon RW, editors. The Pharmacological Basis of Therapetics, 9th edn. New York: McGraw-Hill, 1996:581–600.
30. Wietholtz H, Marschall HU, Sjovall J, Matern S. Stimulation of bile acid 6 alpha-hydroxylation by rifampin. J Hepatol. 1996;24:713–18.
31. Galeazzi R. Rifampicin-induced elevation of serum bile acids in man. Dig Dis Sci. 1980; 25:108–12.
32. Kreek MJ, Garfield JW, Gutjahr CL, Giusti LM. Rifampicin-induced methadone withdrawal. N Engl J Med. 1976;294:1104–6.
33. Ghent CN, Carruthers SG. Treatment of pruritus in primary biliary cirrhosis with rifampicin. Results of a double-blind, crossover, randomized trial. Gastroenterology. 1988;94:488–93.
34. Bachs L, Parés A, Elena M, Piera C, Rodés J. Effects of long-term rifampicin administration in primary biliary cirrhosis. Gastroenterology. 1992;102:2077–80.
35. Bachs L, Parés A, Elena M, Piera C, Rodés J. Comparison of rifampicin with phenobarbitone for treatment of pruritus in biliary cirrhosis. Lancet. 1989;1:574–6.
36. Ghent CN, Bloomer JR, Hsia YE. Efficacy and safety of long-term phenobarbital therapy of familial cholestasis. J Pediatr. 1978;93:127–32.
37. Ghent CN, Bloomer JR, Hsia YE. Safety and efficacy of longterm treatment of familial intrahepatic cholestasis with phenobarbital. J Pediatr. 1978;93:127–32.
38. Bernstein JE, Swift R. Relief of intractable pruritus with naloxone. Arch Dermatol. 1979;115: 1366–7.

39. Talbot TL, Schmitt JM, Bergasa NV, Jones EA, Walker EC. Application of piezo film technology for the quantitative assessment of pruritus. Biomed Instrument Technol. 1991;25:400–3.
40. Jones EA, Dekker LR. Florid opioid withdrawal-like reaction precipitated by naltrexone in a patient with chronic cholestasis. Gastroenterology. 2000;118:431–2.
41. Jones EA, Neuberger J, Bergasa NV. Opiate antagonist therapy for the pruritus of cholestasis: the avoidance of opioid withdrawal-like reactions. Q J Med. 2002;95:547–52.
42. Raderer M, Muller C, Scheithauer W. Ondansetron for pruritus due to cholestasis. N Engl J Med. 1994;21:1540.
43. Schworer H, Ramadori G. Improvement of cholestatic pruritus by ondansetron. Lancet. 1993; 341:1277.
44. Muller C, Pongratz S, Pidlich J et al. Treatment of pruritus in chronic liver disease with the 5-hydroxytryptamine receptor type 3 antagonist ondansetron: a randomized, placebo-controlled, double-blind cross-over trial. Eur J Gastroenterol Hepatol. 1998;10:865–70.
45. Schworer H, Hartmann H, Ramadori G. Relief of cholestatic pruritus by a novel class of drugs: 5-hydroxytryptamine type 3 (5-HT3) receptor antagonists: effectiveness of ondansetron. Pain. 1995;61:33–7.
46. O'Donohue JW, Haigh C, Williams R. Ondansetron in the treatment of the pruritus of cholestasis: a randomised controlled trial. Gastroenterology. 1997;112:A1349.
47. Moore RY. Organization of the mammalian circadian system. In: Chadwick DJ, Ackrill K, editors. Circadian Clocks and their Readjustments. London: John Wiley, 1993:88–106.
48. Browning JD, Combes B, Mayo M. Sertraline: evidence for a role in the treatment of cholestatic pruritus T1105. Gastroenterology. 2002;123(Suppl. 1):66.
49. Neff GW, O'Brien CB, Reddy KR et al. Preliminary observation with dronabinol in patients with intractable pruritus secondary to cholestatic liver disease. Am J Gastroenterol. 2002;97: 2117–19.
50. Yoon MH, Yaksh TL. The effect of intrathecal gabapentin on pain behavior and hemodynamics on the formalin test in the rat. Anesth Analg. 1999;89:434–9.
51. Gustafsson H, Flood K, Berge OG, Brodin E, Olgart L, Stiller CO. Gabapentin reverses mechanical allodynia induced by sciatic nerve ischemia and formalin-induced nociception in mice. Exp Neurol. 2003;182:427–34.
52. Jones EA, Yurdaydin C. Is fatigue associated with cholestasis mediated by altered central neurotransmission? Hepatology. 1997;25:492–4.
53. Jones EA. Relief from profound fatigue associated with chronic liver disease by long-term ondansetron therapy. Lancet. 1999;354:397.
54. Theal J, Toosi MN, Girlan LM et al. Ondansetron ameliorated fatigue in patients with primary biliary cirrhosis (PBC). Hepatology. 2002;36:296A.
55. Le Gars L, Grandpierre C, Chazouilleres O et al. Bone loss in primary biliary cirrhosis: absence of association with severity of liver disease. Jt Bone Spine. 2002;69:195–200.
56. Newton J, Francis R, Prince M et al. Osteoporosis in primary biliary cirrhosis revisited. Gut. 2001;49:282–7.
57. Ormarsdottir S, Ljunggren O, Mallmin H et al. Longitudinal bone loss in postmenopausal women with primary biliary cirrhosis and well-preserved liver function. J Intern Med. 2002;252: 537–41.
58. Guanabens N, Pares A, Monegal A et al. Etidronate versus fluoride for treatment of osteopenia in primary biliary cirrhosis: preliminary results after 2 years. Gastroenterology. 1997;113:219–24.
59. Lindor KD, Jorgensen RA, Tiegs RD, Khosla S, Dickson ER. Etidronate for osteoporosis in primary biliary cirrhosis: a randomized trial. J Hepatol. 2000;33:878–82.
60. Menon KVN, Augulo P, Boe GM, Lindor KD. Safety and efficacy of estrogen therapy in preventing bone loss in primary biliary cirrhosis. Am J Gastroenterol. 2003;98:889–92.
61. Association AG. American Gastroenterological Association Medical Position Statement: Osteoporosis in Hepatic Disorders. Gastroenterology. 2003;125:937–40.
62. Guanabens N, Pares A, Ros I et al. Alendronate is more effective than etidronate for increasing bone mass in osteopenic patients with primary biliary cirrhosis. Am J Gastroenterol. 2003;98: 2268–74.

19
Liver transplantation, rejection and disease recurrence

S. BECKEBAUM, V. R. CICINNATI and C. E. BROELSCH

Primary biliary cirrhosis (PBC) is a chronic cholestatic liver disease leading to destruction of the small intrahepatic bile ducts with progressive ductopenia and potential development of liver failure. Therapy aims at preventing disease progression and treating complications such as fat-soluble vitamin deficiencies, pruritus, metabolic bone disease, and portal hypertension. Ursodeoxycholic acid (UDCA) is currently the only approved pharmacological therapy for PBC[1]. It has been shown to reduce bilirubin levels, and to delay the time point of liver transplantation (LT). However, UDCA can only slow disease progression. In PBC the severity of symptoms and the degree of liver damage do not always correlate well. Some patients with sufficient liver function can be severely affected by fatigue and pruritus.

Various studies have suggested that hepatocellular carcinoma (HCC) in cirrhotic PBC is a rare complication[2]. However, Jones et al. have recently found that HCC is a relatively common cause of death in male PBC patients with cirrhosis[3]. In their study the incidence of HCC was 20% in male patients with stage III or IV disease versus 4% in females. The data suggest careful screening for primary liver cancer and earlier rather than later transplantation in this patient group.

Many attempts have been undertaken to optimize the timing of liver transplantation for progressed chronic cholestatic liver disease. A number of investigators have developed prognostic indices using clinical and laboratory parameters for prediction of survival in PBC[4-6]. Independently of the prognostic model, serum bilirubin level is the most heavily weighted variable for prediction of survival. Several studies performed Cox multiple regression analyses, allowing multiple clinical variables to be analysed simultaneously. The Mayo Clinic Model has been accepted as an appropriate, well-validated tool for determination of a risk score[7]. This model considers prognostic variables such as serum levels of bilirubin and albumin, age, prothrombin time and the presence of peripheral oedema including response to diuretic therapy. It does not require invasive procedures such as liver biopsy and can be repeated over time. Based on the Mayo PBC

Survival Model the efficacy of liver transplantation has been assessed in 161 PBC patients undergoing LT at the University of Pittsburgh and at Baylor University in Dallas[8]. Results have shown that, 6 months after LT, the Kaplan–Meier survival probabilities in LT recipients were significantly higher than the Mayo Model estimated survival probabilities without LT ($p < 0.001$). Those patients having a risk score below 8.6 had a 4-month survival of 91% and those with a risk score of between 8.6 and 9.9 had a 4-month survival of 78%. In contrast, transplant recipients having a high risk score > 9.9 had a 4-month survival of only 57%. Analysis also revealed that, for each unit increase in risk score, the death rate increased by a factor of 1.6 during the first 90 days post-transplant. Further studies have clearly shown that patients with a high preoperative risk score accrued the highest hospital costs related to increased morbidity[9,10]. Based on these observations it has been suggested that optimal timing of LT in PBC patients may not only decrease mortality related to the transplant procedure but may also significantly decrease morbidity and the total charges. One disadvantage of the Original Mayo Model is the lack of time-dependency throughout the disease progression of PBC[10]. The Updated Mayo Model is a short-term survival model of patients with PBC, and has been developed for prediction of survival for 0–2 years.

Within the past two decades various attempts have been undertaken to develop survival models in PBC. Recently, a Japanese group found that hepatic receptor imaging with [99m]technetium galactosyl human serum albumin (GSA) is useful for the evaluation of hepatic functional reserve and for prognosis of PBC independently of blood tests that may be affected by treatment[11]. However, a longitudinal study with a larger number of patients is required to confirm these results.

The model for end-stage liver disease (MELD), originally developed to predict the survival of patients undergoing transjugular intrahepatic portosystemic shunt (TIPS), can also be applied to predict survival of patients with PBC. However, this model is not specific to PBC but validated for liver diseases in general. Bonsel et al. investigated the follow-up of 30 patients with PBC after LT between 1978 and 1989, and found a cumulative survival of only 65% after 1 year and of 60% after 5 years[12]. Survival after LT now shows a progressive improvement due to developments in surgical techniques and immunosuppressive therapy, and due to the trend that patients are being evaluated in earlier stages for LT. Thus, recent studies report survival rates at 1 year and 5 years of more than 80% and 70% respectively[13,14].

Rejection seems to occur more often in patients with autoimmune indications including PBC as compared to those transplanted for other diseases. Farges et al. found that the incidence of acute rejection (48% at 1 year) and chronic rejection (10% at 3 years) in PBC patients was significantly higher than that of patients transplanted for hepatitis B virus-related cirrhosis (21% at 1 year and 0% at 3 years, respectively). Furthermore the incidence of acute but not chronic rejection was significantly lower in alcoholic cirrhosis as compared to patients with cholestatic liver disease[15,16].

Quality of life before and after LT in patients with cholestatic liver disease has been evaluated in various studies. Gross et al. reported that distress from symptoms of liver disease was reduced after LT, as well as limitations to functioning in areas such as mobility, sex life, and social life[17]. However, life is not as 'normal' as in the general population, and limitations in physical activity contribute to the situation in which only a small percentage of post-transplant patients are working full- or part-time.

The incidence of PBC recurrence in liver allografts has been discussed controversially[13,18,19]. Data regarding the frequency of disease recurrence vary widely throughout the literature; however, most investigators report recurrence rates of between 8% and 20% at 5 years after transplantation[20,21]. Diagnosis of PBC in the transplanted liver is often more challenging than diagnosis in the native liver[20]. Immunoglobulin M (IgM) and antimitochondrial antibodies (AMA) often persist after LT, and elevated cholestatic enzymes may be due to other causes of bile duct damage. Histology is usually required, and detection of granulomatous cholangitis is mandatory for diagnosis of recurrent PBC. Histological features of recurrent disease can also include mononuclear cell portal inflammatory infiltrates, portal lymphoid aggregates, bile duct damage, ductopenia, ductular proliferation, portal fibrosis, and copper-associated protein deposition.

However, differentiation between recurrent PBC and other causes of bile duct damage in the allograft, such as allograft rejection, infection and drug exposure, may be difficult. Some investigators found that the immunosuppressive regimen influences timing of recurrence, suggesting that cyclosporin has a beneficial effect over tacrolimus[18,22]. Recently it has been suggested that immunosuppressive therapy including azathioprine decreases the incidence of recurrence in PBC. Sufficient data concerning the impact of UDCA treatment after LT on the rate of disease recurrence are not yet available. While matching is considered important for kidney transplantation, the significance of HLA testing in the liver transplant setting has often been questioned. Data from a large study at the University of Pittsburgh including 3261 transplant patients have been presented at the American Transplant Congress, Transplant 2002, in Washington, DC, and suggested that a mismatch between donor and recipient decreases the risk of disease recurrence in PBC patients. This study found that 35% of patients with two HLA-DR matches had disease recurrence as compared to 10% of PBC patients with only one match or complete mismatching. A similar tendency has been observed in a recent study by Hashimoto et al. in the living-related liver transplant setting[23].

In conclusion, survival rates of PBC patients undergoing LT have been shown to be excellent. PBC may recur in the allograft in some patients, but does not seem to have any impact on medium-term graft survival.

References

1. Poupon RE, Bonnand A-M, Chretien Y, Poupon R. Ten-year survival in ursodeoxycholic acid-treated patients with primary biliary cirrhosis. Hepatology. 1999;29:1668–71.
2. Kaczynski J, Hansson G, Wallerstedt S. Incidence of primary liver cancer and aetological aspects: a study of a defined population from a low-endemicity area. Br J Cancer. 1996;73: 1225–30.
3. Jones DE, Metcalf JV, Collier JD, Bassendine MF, James OF. Hepatocellular carcinoma in primary biliary cirrhosis and its impact on outcomes. Hepatology. 1997;26:1138–42.
4. Christensen E. Individual therapy-dependent prognosis based on data from controlled clinical trials in chronic liver disease. Dan Med Bull. 1988;35:167–82.
5. Grambsch PM, Dickson ER, Wiesner RH, Langworthy A. Application of the Mayo primary biliary cirrhosis survival model to Mayo liver transplant patients. Mayo Clin Proc. 1989;64: 699–704.

6. Goudie BM, Burt AD, Macfarlane GJ et al. Risk factors and prognosis in primary biliary cirrhosis. Am J Gastroenterol. 1989;84:713–16.

7. Russell H. Wiesner MD. Liver transplantation for primary biliary cirrhosis and primary sclerosing cholangitis: predicting outcomes with natural history models. Mayo Clin Proc. 1998;73: 575–88.

8. Markus BH, Dickson ER, Grambsch PM et al. Efficacy of liver transplantation in patients with primary biliary cirrhosis. N Engl J Med. 1989;320:1709–13.

9. Wiesner RH, Porayko MK, Dickson ER et al. Selection and timing of liver transplantation in primary biliary cirrhosis and primary sclerosing cholangitis. Hepatology. 1992;16:1290–9.

10. van Dam GM, Verbaan BW, Therneau TM et al. Primary biliary cirrhosis: Dutch application of the Mayo Model before and after orthotopic liver transplantation. Hepatogastroenterology. 1997; 44:732–43.

11. Shiomi S, Sasaki N, Tamori A et al. Use of scintigraphy with 99m technetium galactosyl human serum albumin for staging of primary biliary cirrhosis and assessment of prognosis. J Gastroenterol Hepatol. 1999;14:566–71.

12. Bonsel GJ, Klompmaker IJ, van't Veer F, Habbema JD, Slooff MJ. Use of prognostic models for assessment of value of liver transplantation in primary biliary cirrhosis. Lancet. 1990;335:493–7.

13. Liermann Garcia RF, Evangelista Garcia C, McMaster P, Neuberger J. Transplantation for primary biliary cirrhosis: retrospective analysis of 400 patients in a single center. Hepatology. 2001;33:22–7.

14. Rust C, Rau H, Gerbes AL et al. Liver transplantation in primary biliary cirrhosis: risk assessment and 11-year follow-up. Digestion. 2000;62:38–43.

15. Farges O, Saliba F, Farhamant H et al. Incidence of rejection and infection after liver transplantation as a function of primary disease: possible influence of alcohol and polyclonal immunoglobulins. Hepatology. 1996;23:240–8.

16. Adams DH, Hubscher SG, Neuberger JM, McMaster P, Elias E, Buckels JA. Reduced incidence of rejection in patients undergoing liver transplantation for chronic hepatitis B. Transplant Proc. 1991;23:1436–7.

17. Gross CR, Malinchoc M, Kim WR et al. Quality of life before and after liver transplantation for cholestatic liver disease. Hepatology. 1999;29:356–64.

18. Dmitrewski J, Hubscher SG, Mayer AD, Neuberger JM. Recurrence of primary biliary cirrhosis in the liver allograft: the effect of immunosuppression. J Hepatol. 1996;24:253–7.

19. Sebagh M, Farges O, Dubel L, Samuel D, Bismuth H, Reynes M. Histological features predictive of recurrence of primary biliary cirrhosis after liver transplantation. Transplantation. 1998; 65:1328–33.

20. Neuberger J. Recurrent primary biliary cirrhosis. Liver Transplant. 2003;9:539–46.

21. Balan V, Batts KP, Potayko MK, Krom RA, Ludwig J, Wiesner RH. Histological evidence for recurrence of primary biliary cirrhosis after liver transplantation. Hepatology. 1993;18:1392–8.

22. Wong PY, Portmann B, O'Grady JG et al. Recurrence of primary biliary cirrhosis after liver transplantation following FK506-based immunosuppression. J Hepatol. 1993;17:284–7.

23. Hashimoto E, Shimada M, Noguchi S et al. Disease recurrence after living liver transplantation for primary biliary cirrhosis: a clinical and histological follow-up study. Liver Transplant. 2001; 7:588–95.

Section VI
Diagnosis, epidemiology and prognosis of primary sclerosing cholangitis

20
Primary sclerosing cholangitis: diagnosis and differential diagnosis

K. M. BOBERG, O. P. F. CLAUSEN and E. SCHRUMPF

INTRODUCTION

Primary sclerosing cholangitis (PSC) is a chronic cholestatic disease that involves both intrahepatic and extrahepatic bile ducts. It is characterized by an inflammatory and fibrotic process that leads to irregular bile duct obliteration and formation of multiple bile duct strictures[1–7]. The clinical course of PSC varies considerably between patients, but in general it is a progressive disease with eventual development of cirrhosis and liver failure. According to several studies the median survival of PSC patients from time of diagnosis until liver transplantation or death is approximately 12 years[8–11]. Delbet[1] reported the first case of sclerosing cholangitis in 1924. In the early descriptions of PSC the diagnosis was based on findings at laparotomy, consisting of pathological bile ducts with thickening of the bile duct wall due to a diffuse sclerosing and stenotic process[2–5]. Intraoperative cholangiograms demonstrated irregularities, narrowing and strictures of the extrahepatic as well as the intrahepatic bile ducts[5]. When endoscopic retrograde cholangiography (ERC) was introduced, in the early 1970s, visualization of the bile duct tree became more accessible, and PSC could be diagnosed without surgery. It was then recognized that PSC was more common than previously believed. ERC has since been the major diagnostic tool in PSC[6,7]. During recent years magnetic resonance cholangiography (MRC) has also been used in the diagnosis of PSC[12–14]. PSC is strongly associated with inflammatory bowel disease (IBD)[15–17]. Investigation of abnormal liver tests detected during routine follow-up of IBD patients has contributed to diagnosis of an increased number of PSC cases[17]. Since the diagnosis has had to be confirmed by an invasive method (ERC or percutaneous transhepatic cholangiography (PTC)) with a certain complication risk, PSC is probably still an underdiagnosed condition.

PSC must be distinguished from secondary sclerosing cholangitis due to other disorders. In addition to findings of generalized sclerosis and stenosis of the bile

Table 1 Bases for diagnosis of PSC

Patient history and clinical findings
Biochemical and serological findings
Liver histology
Cholangiography

ducts, the traditional criteria for the diagnosis of PSC included: (1) absence of previous biliary surgery; (2) absence of cholelithiasis; and (3) exclusion of carcinoma of the bile ducts[3,4]. However, the experience that PSC patients are predisposed to development of biliary tract calculi[18], as well as cholangiocarcinoma[19–22], must be taken into consideration. Rather than being exclusion criteria for diagnosis of PSC, it is recognized that cholelithiasis or cholangiocarcinoma in some cases are complications of pre-existing PSC.

The diagnosis of PSC is based on clinical, biochemical, and histological data, in combination with the typical cholangiographic findings (Table 1).

DIAGNOSIS OF PSC

Patient history and clinical features

Males are more susceptible than females to develop PSC, with a male to female ratio of approximately 2:1[20,21]. The explanation for this sex difference is unknown. Mean age at diagnosis is around 40 years[8–11,20–23]. PSC can also be diagnosed in children[24,25] and in the elderly[10]. Quite often there is a delay of several years from the first biochemical sign or symptom of liver disease until PSC is diagnosed[10,22,26]. In a group of 305 Swedish patients the median age at diagnosis was 39 years (range 5–80), with a median 52 months (range 0–451) after the first biochemical or clinical sign compatible with PSC[10].

The clinical history of patients before diagnosis of PSC is quite variable. Some patients are asymptomatic and referred to investigation due to increased serum alkaline phosphatase (ALP) levels, most often in the presence of concomitant IBD[17]. Other patients present with symptoms of liver disease, ranging from mild to severe, with signs of liver cirrhosis and portal hypertension[17]. In a few cases the PSC patient even presents with cholangiocarcinoma[17,26–28]. The proportion of asymptomatic patients at diagnosis varies between studies from 10–25%[9,20,21,29] up to 44%[10,22]. This variation can partly be explained by differences in patient selection, but it can also be attributed to differences in definition of symptoms[10]. The most frequent symptoms are jaundice, pruritus, and right upper abdominal pain[17]. More unspecific symptoms such as weight loss, fever, and fatigue are also reported. Some patients have had episodes of acute cholangitis[20]. Signs of portal hypertension with ascites and variceal haemorrhage may occur, but are less frequent at the time of diagnosis. Physical examination at diagnosis was abnormal in 50% of the patients investigated by Wiesner and LaRusso[21], with jaundice, hepatomegaly and splenomegaly being the most prevalent findings.

PSC often has a variable course with intermittent periods of exacerbation of symptoms, followed by prolonged periods of remission. The patients frequently present, and are diagnosed, during episodes of exacerbations. Patients who initially are symptomatic may be asymptomatic at a later investigation. One general problem of prognostic models that are based on patient status at diagnosis in PSC is that they tend to overestimate survival when applied to follow-up data[11]. In the study by Schrumpf et al.[22] 21 of 43 symptomatic patients were asymptomatic at follow-up at a median 6.2 years after the diagnosis. Some patients remain asymptomatic for several years[22,29–31]. Some authors describe a more benign disease course with a prolonged survival in the asymptomatic patients compared with the symptomatic group[10,29]. In other studies there is no significant difference in the prognosis between asymptomatic and symptomatic patients[8,9,22], underlining the generally progressive nature of PSC.

Biochemical and serological tests

Biochemical tests in PSC patients usually show a cholestatic pattern. ALP activity is elevated in the majority of patients, often to a level at least three times the upper limit of normal[17]. On the other hand an elevated ALP level is not a prerequisite for the diagnosis. Up to 8.5% of PSC patients in large studies have had normal ALP levels at diagnosis[10]. In a group of 12 PSC patients with normal ALP activity at diagnosis, advanced cholangiographic and histological changes were present in four cases[32]. The ALP activity can fluctuate and return to normal during periods of the disease course[32]. Normal ALP values therefore should not preclude further steps to diagnose PSC if suspected on clinical basis.

Transaminase levels are elevated at diagnosis in the majority of PSC patients, often to levels about 2–3 times upper normal values. Serum bilirubin concentration is within normal limits in up to 60% of patients[10,23,29,30]. Bilirubin levels usually increase gradually with disease progression, but can also fluctuate due to bile duct sludge and calculi or episodes of bacterial cholangitis. Liver synthesis function is preserved in the majority of PSC patients at time of diagnosis, with normal serum levels of albumin and coagulation factors[17].

Increased levels of circulating immunoglobulins and positive titres of autoantibodies are frequently observed in PSC patients[17,20,21]. In a study of 114 patients the IgG concentration was elevated above the upper normal limit in 61%[33]. In the majority of cases (44%) the IgG level was up to 1.5 times the upper limit of normal, but in a few patients (5%) the IgG concentration was more than twice the upper limit of normal. Increased IgM levels have been observed in 20–45% of PSC patients[15,20]. Antinuclear antibodies (ANA) and smooth muscle antibodies (SMA) can be detected, but less frequently and in lower titres than in autoimmune hepatitis (AIH)[15,20,33,34]. Antimitochondrial antibodies (AMA) are rare in PSC[21,33]. PSC in childhood is also associated with elevated levels of immunoglobulins and positive titres of ANA and SMA[25,35,36]. Perinuclear antineutrophil cytoplasmic antibodies (pANCA) are present in serum in up to 88% of PSC patients[37–39]. Autoantibodies that are specific for PSC have not been detected.

Liver histology in PSC

The most prominent histological changes in liver biopsies from PSC patients are located in the portal tracts (Figure 1) featuring inflammation, periductal fibrosis, ductal obliteration, bile duct proliferation, or loss of bile ducts in later

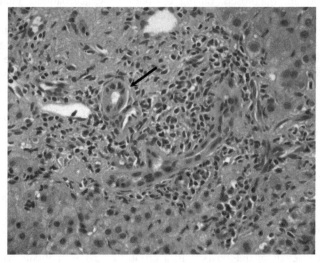

Figure 1 Liver biopsy from a PSC patient showing a somewhat expanded portal tract with inflammation with some interphase activity. An affected biliary duct is seen that on cross-section (arrow) shows variations in nuclear size and in the shape of epithelial cells

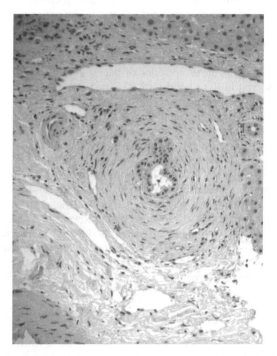

Figure 2 Liver biopsy from a PSC patient showing a septal area with typical concentric periductal fibrosis. This is not a common finding in biopsies from PSC patients, but it is highly suggestive of PSC

stages[40,41]. Parenchymal changes with piecemeal necrosis, focal necrosis, focal inflammation, Kupffer cell hyperplasia, and perilobular fibrosis can also be observed[20,30,40]. Four histological stages have been defined[40].

Stage 1 (portal stage) is characterized by portal oedema, mild portal hepatitis, and ductal proliferation. There is a mild, non-destructive cholangitis with infiltration of lymphocytes in the bile ducts. Parenchymal changes tend to be mild or absent[40]. In stage 2 (periportal stage or stage of portal enlargement) the lesion extends to involve periportal fibrosis and inflammation, sometimes with piecemeal necrosis of periportal hepatocytes. The portal tracts are often enlarged. There may be ductular proliferation, periductal fibrosis, and fibrous–obliterative cholangitis. Periductular fibrosis is considered highly suggestive of PSC[40] (Figure 2). Development of portal to portal fibrous septa characterizes the stage 3 lesion (septal stage). Bile ducts degenerate and disappear. Stage 4 is the cirrhotic end-stage showing regenerative nodules, often accompanied by ductular proliferation and oedema in the periphery[40].

None of the histological findings in PSC is pathognomonic, and a definite diagnosis must be established by cholangiography.

Cholangiography

Characteristic cholangiographic findings including bile duct mural irregularities and diffusely distributed multifocal strictures are essential to confirm the diagnosis of PSC[6,7] (Figure 3). The bile ducts are most commonly visualized by ERC,

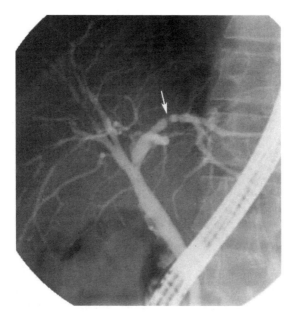

Figure 3 Endoscopic retrograde cholangiography in a PSC patient, showing intrahepatic bile duct irregularities. The alternating stenoses and dilations of the left hepatic duct are marked (arrow) for comparison with the magnetic resonance cholangiography findings in the same patient (Figure 4)

but PTC is an alternative approach. Recently, the non-invasive MRC technique has also been introduced. The majority of patients have combined intrahepatic and extrahepatic bile duct involvement[10,17]. Isolated intrahepatic changes are found in 20–30% of cases, whereas isolated extrahepatic PSC is rare[10,17]. Efforts should be made to visualize the intrahepatic bile ducts adequately. Since intrahepatic bile duct abnormalities can also be seen in other chronic liver disease, one must be cautious when diagnosing PSC in the presence of intrahepatic changes only.

The bile duct strictures in PSC typically are short and annular with intervening normal or dilated segments, resulting in a pattern of 'beading'. Sometimes the dilations can have a diverticular appearance[7]. Long, confluent strictures can be seen with more advanced disease. Development of cirrhosis results in approximation and tortuosity or a stretched and displaced appearance of the intrahepatic bile ducts[7]. The gall bladder and cystic duct are involved in about 15% of cases[42]. Abnormalities of the pancreatic duct resembling those of chronic pancreatitis are visualized in a variable number of PSC patients[7,43,44].

MRC is a relatively new imaging modality that is a non-invasive alternative to direct cholangiography in diagnosis of biliary tract disease (Figure 4). The bile itself provides a signal that contrasts to the surrounding structures. High sensitivity and specificity of MRC in diagnosing PSC have been described[12–14]. In a study comprising 150 patients with symptoms or signs of cholestasis, including 34 PSC patients, the sensitivity and specificity of MRC for diagnosing PSC were 88% and 99%, respectively[14]. More bile duct stenoses and pruning were seen with ERC and more skip dilations with MRC[14]. In general, MRC has the ability to perform better than ERC in visualizing dilated bile ducts peripherally to strictures. In a recent study MRC was superior to ERC for visualization of the intrahepatic bile ducts in

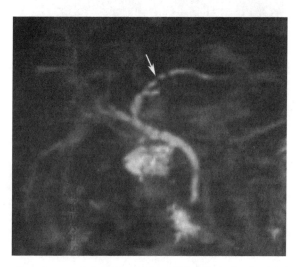

Figure 4 Magnetic resonance cholangiography in a PSC patient, showing intrahepatic bile duct irregularities. The alternating stenoses and dilations of the left hepatic duct are marked (arrow) for comparison with the endoscopic retrograde cholangiography findings in the same patient (Figure 3)

PSC[13]. On the other hand mild PSC without significant bile duct dilation on ERC gave rise to false-negative results by MRC[12]. In our experience MRC has missed cases of intrahepatic PSC (unpublished results). One should be cautious to exclude early PSC based on a normal MRC. PSC with cirrhosis is probably also more precisely diagnosed by ERC. With improved technology, MRC can be expected to diagnose PSC in a majority of cases. Another advantage of the MRC technique is that it provides additional information on periductal tissue and other organs. ERC will still be required when therapeutic intervention or invasive diagnostic procedures such as brush cytology are anticipated.

DIFFERENTIAL DIAGNOSIS IN PSC

PSC must be distinguished from other hepatobiliary disorders that can present with cholestasis and ductopenia in liver biopsies, e.g. primary biliary cirrhosis (PBC), drug-induced reactions, sarcoidosis, liver allograft rejection, and chronic graft-versus-host disease[17]. In some cases autoimmune hepatitis (AIH), alcoholic hepatitis, or viral hepatitis can also present with a cholestatic biochemical pattern[45]. Cholangiographic features resembling those of PSC have been reported in immunodeficiency disorders, such as the acquired immunodeficiency syndrome, and in association with certain viral infections, e.g. cytomegalovirus infection[46]. Ischaemia secondary to hepatic artery injury or injection of toxic substances can result in fibrosis and strictures of the bile ducts[47,48]. Bile duct obstruction caused by choledocholithiasis, tumours, or surgical trauma must be excluded as causes of secondary sclerosing cholangitis (Table 2). In most cases patient history, serological and virological tests, and liver histology will contribute to the correct diagnosis.

Some important differential diagnostic problems will be discussed (Table 3).

Hepatobiliary disorders in ulcerative colitis

PSC is associated with IBD in up to 80–90% of cases[49]. The majority (80%) of PSC patients with IBD have ulcerative colitis, but there is also an association with

Table 2   Reasons for distinguishing secondary sclerosing cholangitis from PSC

Previous biliary surgery	Viral infections
Cholelithiasis	Ischaemia
Tumours of the bile ducts	Exposure to biliary toxins
Immunodeficiency disorders	

Table 3   Important differential diagnoses when PSC is suspected

Other hepatobiliary disorders in ulcerative colitis
Autoimmune hepatitis
Primary biliary cirrhosis
Cirrhosis
Cholangiocarcinoma

Crohn's colitis[49]. Evidence of hepatobiliary disorders has been reported in 3–15% of patients with ulcerative colitis[16,50–53]. PSC is the single most frequent hepatobiliary lesion in ulcerative colitis and is diagnosed in 2.1–4% of cases. In selected patient groups the prevalence of PSC in ulcerative colitis is as high as 7.5%[53]. Liver biopsies from patients with ulcerative colitis feature a spectrum of histological abnormalities including fatty changes, portal inflammation and fibrosis, pericholangitis, chronic active hepatitis, cirrhosis, and cholangiocarcinoma[16,54,55]. The cholangiographic findings in ulcerative colitis also vary[56]. Pericholangitis has been described with or without concomitant typical cholangiographic findings of PSC.

A subgroup of patients, usually with IBD, present with clinical, biochemical and liver histology compatible with PSC but have normal findings on cholangiography. Wee and Ludwig suggested the term *small duct PSC* for this entity[55,57]. Small duct PSC was later described from several centres[58–61]. The definition of small duct PSC has varied. Some authors have included only patients with IBD[58,59], whereas in other studies IBD has been diagnosed in from 50%[60] to 88%[61] of the patients. One study also included patients with minor involvement of the intrahepatic bile ducts, judged to be different from those of classical PSC[58]. Small duct PSC and classical PSC most likely represent different aspects of the same disease spectrum. Even though it has been suggested that small duct PSC is a distinct clinical entity[62], it is possible that small duct PSC represents an early-stage PSC that can progress to classical PSC[59,61]. Differential diagnosis between small duct PSC and intrahepatic PSC progressing to cirrhosis will be a particular challenge.

Autoimmune hepatitis

PSC patients sometimes have biochemical, histological, and clinical features resembling those of AIH[15,20,21,40]. The concurrence of PSC and AIH in the same

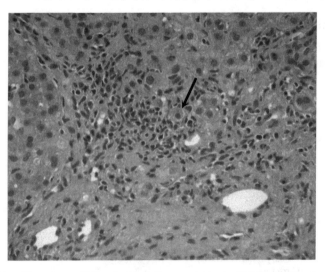

Figure 5 Liver biopsy from a PSC patient including a portal tract with inflammation clearly showing interphase activity (arrow) that may cause difficulties in distinguishing PSC from autoimmune hepatitis

patient has even been suggested[63–65]. Elevated levels of circulating immunoglobulins and non-organ-specific autoantibodies, and the presence of interface hepatitis in liver biopsies in some patients, can be difficult to differentiate from the findings in AIH (Figure 5). Treatment with corticosteroids may at least temporarily induce biochemical and clinical improvement in selected cases[33]. A markedly increased serum transaminase activity and less prominent ALP elevation, together with a sustained response to immunosuppressive therapy, would favour a diagnosis of AIH. When 114 PSC patients were assessed according to a scoring system for the diagnosis of AIH[66], 2% of the patients could be classified as 'definite' AIH and 33% as 'probable' AIH[33]. Among the 114 PSC patients, five carried a diagnosis of AIH for several years before PSC was diagnosed by ERC. In particular in patients with IBD, one should be reluctant to diagnose AIH until ERC has excluded PSC[53]. PSC patients presenting with features of AIH are sometimes considered to have a PSC/AIH overlap syndrome[67]. Diagnostic criteria for overlap syndromes remain to be defined.

Primary biliary cirrhosis

Patients with PBC also present with cholestasis and can clinically be difficult to differentiate from PSC[68]. The diagnosis of PBC is usually confirmed by the presence of AMA and typical histological features with chronic, destructive cholangitis of the small intrahepatic bile ducts[69]. Histological findings may sometimes be difficult to distinguish from those of PSC, in particular in late disease stages[70]. AMA-positivity supports the diagnosis of PBC in such cases, since this finding is far less frequent in PSC[33]. About 5–10% of patients with biochemical and histological features of PBC lack AMA[69,70]. The majority of the AMA-negative patients are positive for ANA (often in high titres)[71]. They are also more frequently SMA-positive, but have significantly lower IgM levels than the AMA-positive patients. The terms autoimmune cholangitis or autoimmune cholangiopathy have been proposed to denote this patient category[71–73]. ERC should be carried out to confirm PSC when this remains a possibility. In patients with normal cholangiograms, small duct PSC remains a possible diagnosis. Distinction between small duct PSC and AMA-negative PBC can be difficult or even impossible.

Cirrhosis

Development of cirrhosis in PSC leads to cholangiographic changes of the intrahepatic bile ducts similar to those of cirrhosis of any aetiology[40]. In the absence of extrahepatic duct changes it can be impossible on the basis of cholangiography to determine whether cirrhosis developed due to small duct PSC, large duct PSC with intrahepatic involvement only, or other chronic liver disorders.

Cholangiocarcinoma

PSC patients are predisposed to cholangiocarcinoma development, which is seen in up to 20% of patients[9,10,19–22,26,74–76]. In the majority of cases cholangiocarcinoma develops in a patient with a known diagnosis of PSC, but simultaneous diagnosis of PSC and cholangiocarcinoma has been reported[19,26–28].

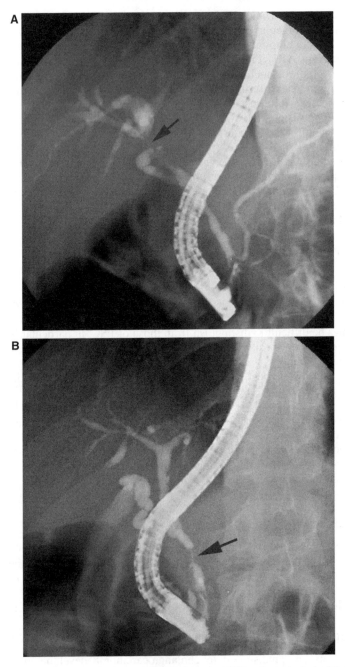

Figure 6 Endoscopic retrograde cholangiography from **A**: a PSC patient who had a hilar stricture (arrow) that proved to be a cholangiocarcinoma and **B**: a PSC patient who had a benign stricture of the common bile duct (arrow)

Up to 30–50% of cases of cholangiocarcinoma are diagnosed during the first year from diagnosis of PSC[10,26,27]. There is an inherent problem in diagnosing PSC in the presence of cholangiocarcinoma; it could be argued that the cholangiographic changes are solely secondary to cholangiocarcinoma. In such cases factors such as the distribution of the cholangiographic abnormalities relative to the localization of the tumour, as well as a history of pathological liver tests, and presence of IBD, have to be considered[26,78,79].

The clinical differentiation between PSC alone and PSC complicated by cholangiocarcinoma may be extremely difficult, and represents a challenge. Cholangiocarcinoma is not detected until laparotomy in connection with intended liver transplantation or at autopsy in up to 37% of cases[26]. Cholangiographic features such as markedly dilated bile duct segments, polypoid masses within the bile duct, and progressive stricture formation on serial investigations are suggestive of cholangiocarcinoma[7]. Most often it is impossible to differentiate malignant from the benign strictures of PSC by cholangiography (Figure 6). It is advisable to combine several additional radiological modalities, e.g. computed tomography scans, ultrasonography, and MRC, when cholangiocarcinoma in PSC is suspected[26,80]. The sensitivity of brush cytology sampling from bile duct strictures in detection of cholangiocarcinoma is only 40–70%[81,82]. Specificity can approach 100%[82], but a risk of false-positive results remains[83]. Bile duct epithelial dysplasia in liver biopsy specimens have been associated with development of cholangiocarcinoma[84], but its significance has to be further investigated.

High levels of the tumour-associated antigen CA19-9 in serum are present in up to 80–90% of PSC patients with concurrent cholangiocarcinomas, and CA19-9 has been suggested as a diagnostic marker of malignancy, alone or in combination with carcinoembryonic antigen[85,86]. CA19-9 is not specific since it may also be increased in patients with benign disease[87].

CONCLUSION

The 'typical' PSC patient is a 30–40-year-old male who has IBD and presents with cholestatic biochemical tests. If PSC is suspected, and ERC is performed, the diagnosis is easily established in most cases. MRC is increasingly used in diagnosis of PSC, but this method still appears less sensitive than ERC. In a small proportion of patients the differentiation between PSC and closely related disorders can be particularly difficult, and in some cases impossible. Specific diagnostic tests for PSC, either in bioptical specimens or in blood samples, are needed.

Acknowledgements

We thank Professor Hans-Jørgen Smith, Department of Radiology, Rikshospitalet, Oslo, Norway, for assistance with figures.

References

1. Delbet MP. Rétrécissement du cholédoque. Cholécysto-duodenostomie. Bull Mem Soc Nat Chir. 1924;50:11446.

2. Schwartz SI, Dale WA. Primary sclerosing cholangitis. Review and report of six cases. AMA Arch Surg. 1958;77:439–51.
3. Holubitsky IB, McKenzie AD. Primary sclerosing cholangitis of the extrahepatic bile ducts. Can J Surg. 1964;7:277–83.
4. Warren KW, Athanassiades S, Monge JI. Primary sclerosing cholangitis. A study of forty-two cases. Am J Surg. 1966;111:23–38.
5. Thorpe MEC, Scheuer PJ, Sherlock S. Primary sclerosing cholangitis, the biliary tree, and ulcerative colitis. Gut. 1967;8:435–48.
6. Ayoola EA, Vennes JA, Silvis SE, Rohrmann CA, Ansel HJ. Endoscopic retrograde intrahepatic cholangiography in liver diseases. Gastrointest Endosc. 1976;22:156–9.
7. MacCarty RL, LaRusso NF, Wiesner RH, Ludwig J. Primary sclerosing cholangitis: findings on cholangiography and pancreatography. Radiology. 1983;149:39–44.
8. Wiesner RH, Grambsch PM, Dickson ER et al. Primary sclerosing cholangitis: natural history, prognostic factors and survival analysis. Hepatology. 1989;10:430–6.
9. Farrant JM, Hayllar KM, Wilkinson ML et al. Natural history and prognostic variables in primary sclerosing cholangitis. Gastroenterology. 1991;100:1710–17.
10. Broomé U, Olsson R, Lööf L et al. Natural history and prognostic factors in 305 Swedish patients with primary sclerosing cholangitis. Gut. 1996;38:610–15.
11. Boberg KM, Rocca G, Egeland T et al. Time-dependent Cox regression model is superior in prediction of prognosis in primary sclerosing cholangitis. Hepatology. 2002;35:652–7.
12. Angulo P, Pearce DH, Johnson CD et al. Magnetic resonance cholangiography in patients with biliary disease: its role in primary sclerosing cholangitis. J Hepatol. 2000;33:520–7.
13. Vitellas KM, Enns RA, Keogan MT et al. Comparison of MR cholangiopancreatographic techniques with contrast-enhanced cholangiography in the evaluation of sclerosing cholangitis. Am J Roentgenol. 2002;178:327–34.
14. Textor HJ, Flacke S, Pauleit D et al. Three-dimensional magnetic resonance cholangiopancreatography with respiratory triggering in the diagnosis of primary sclerosing cholangitis: comparison with endoscopic retrograde cholangiography. Endoscopy. 2002;34:984–90.
15. Schrumpf E, Fausa O, Kolmannskog F, Elgjo K, Ritland S, Gjone E. Sclerosing cholangitis in ulcerative colitis. A follow-up study. Scand J Gastroenterol. 1982;17:33–9.
16. Schrumpf E, Elgjo K, Fausa O, Gjone E, Kolmannskog F, Ritland S. Sclerosing cholangitis in ulcerative colitis. Scand J Gastroenterol. 1980;15:689–97.
17. Wiesner RH. Diagnostic criteria, clinical manifestations and natural history of primary sclerosing cholangitis. In: Krawitt EL, Wiesner RH, Nishioka M, editors. Autoimmune Liver Diseases, 2nd edn. Amsterdam: Elsevier, 1998:381–412.
18. Kaw M, Silverman WB, Raninovitz M, Schade RR. Biliary tract calculi in primary sclerosing cholangitis. Am J Gastroenterol. 1995;90:72–5.
19. Rosen C, Nagorney DM, Wiesner RH, Coffey RJ, LaRusso NF. Cholangiocarcinoma complicating primary sclerosing cholangitis. Ann Surg. 1991;213:21–5.
20. Chapman RWG, Arborgh BÅM, Rhodes JM et al. Primary sclerosing cholangitis: a review of its clinical features, cholangiography, and hepatic histology. Gut. 1980;21:870–7.
21. Wiesner RH, LaRusso NF. Clinicopathological features of the syndrome of primary sclerosing cholangitis. Gastroenterology. 1980;79:200–6.
22. Schrumpf E, Abdelnoor M, Fausa O, Elgjo K, Jenssen E, Kolmannskog F. Risk factors in primary sclerosing cholangitis. J Hepatol. 1994;21:1061–6.
23. Okolicsanyi L, Fabris L, Viaggi S et al. Primary sclerosing cholangitis: clinical presentation, natural history and prognostic variables: an Italian multicenter study. Eur J Gastroenterol Hepatol. 1996;8:685–91.
24. Wilschanski M, Chait P, Wade JA et al. Primary sclerosing cholangitis in 32 children: clinical, laboratory, and radiographic features, with survival analysis. Hepatology. 1995;22:1415–22.
25. Gregorio GV, Portmann B, Karani J et al. Autoimmune hepatitis/sclerosing cholangitis overlap syndrome in childhood: a 16-year prospective study. Hepatology. 2002;33:544–53.
26. Boberg KM, Bergquist A, Mitchell S et al. Cholangiocarcinoma in primary sclerosing cholangitis: risk factors and clinical presentation. Scand J Gastroenterol. 2002;37:1205–11.
27. Ahrendt SA, Pitt HA, Nakeeb A et al. Diagnosis and management of cholangiocarcinoma in primary sclerosing cholangitis. J Gastrointest Surg. 1999;3:357–68.
28. Kaya M, de Groen PC, Angulo P et al. Treatment of cholangiocarcinoma complicating primary sclerosing cholangitis: the Mayo clinic experience. Am J Gastroenterol. 2001;96:1164–9.

29. Helzberg JH, Petersen JM, Boyer JL. Improved survival with primary sclerosing cholangitis. A review of clinicopathologic features and comparison of symptomatic and asymptomatic patients. Gastroenterology. 1987;92:1869–75.
30. Aadland E, Schrumpf E, Fausa O et al. Primary sclerosing cholangitis: a long-term follow-up study. Scand J Gastroenterol. 1987;22:655–64.
31. Chapman RWG, Burroughs AK, Bass MN, Sherlock S. Long-standing asymptomatic primary sclerosing cholangitis: report of three cases. Dig Dis Sci. 1981;26:778–82.
32. Balasubramaniam K, Wiesner RH, LaRusso NF. Primary sclerosing cholangitis with normal serum alkaline phosphatase activity. Gastroenterology. 1988;95:1395–8.
33. Boberg KM, Fausa O, Haaland T et al. Features of autoimmune hepatitis in primary sclerosing cholangitis: an evaluation of 114 primary sclerosing cholangitis patients according to a scoring system for the diagnosis of autoimmune hepatitis. Hepatology. 1996;23:1369–76.
34. Zauli D, Schrumpf E, Crespi C, Cassani F, Fausa O, Aadland E. An autoantibody profile in primary sclerosing cholangitis. J Hepatol. 1987;5:14–18.
35. El-Shabrawi M, Wilkinson ML, Portmann B et al. Primary sclerosing cholangitis in childhood. Gastroenterology. 1987;92:1226–35.
36. Mieli-Vergani G, Lobo-Yeo A, McFarlane BM, McFarlane IG, Mowat AP, Vergani D. Different immune mechanisms leading to autoimmunity in primary sclerosing cholangitis and autoimmune chronic active hepatitis of childhood. Hepatology. 1989;9:198–203.
37. Duerr RH, Targan SR, Landers CJ et al. Neutrophil cytoplasmic antibodies: a link between primary sclerosing cholangitis and ulcerative colitis. Gastroenterology. 1991;100:1385–91.
38. Seibold F, Weber P, Klein R, Berg PA, Wiedmann KH. Clinical significance of antibodies against neutrophils in patients with inflammatory bowel disease and primary sclerosing cholangitis. Gut. 1992;33:657–62.
39. Bansi DS, Bauducci M, Bergqvist A et al. Detection of antineutrophil cytoplasmic antibodies in primary sclerosing cholangitis: a comparison of the alkaline phosphatase and immunofluorescent techniques. Eur J Gastroenterol Hepatol. 1997;9:575–80.
40. Ludwig J, LaRusso NF, Wiesner RH. Primary sclerosing cholangitis. In: Peters RL, Craig JR, editors. Liver Pathology. New York: Churchill Livingstone, 1986:193–213.
41. Barbatis C, Grases P, Shepherd HA et al. Histological features of sclerosing cholangitis in patients with chronic ulcerative colitis. J Clin Pathol. 1985;38:778–83.
42. Brandt DJ, MacCarty RL, Charboneau JW, LaRusso NF, Wiesner RH, Ludwig J. Gallbladder disease in patients with primary sclerosing cholangitis. Am J Roentgenol. 1988;150:571–4.
43. Epstein O, Chapman RWG, Lake-Bakaar G, Foo AV, Rosalki SB, Sherlock S. The pancreas in primary biliary cirrhosis and primary sclerosing cholangitis. Gastroenterology. 1982;83:1177–82.
44. Børkje B, Vetvik K, Ødegaard S, Schrumpf E, Larssen TB, Kolmannskog F. Chronic pancreatitis in patients with sclerosing cholangitis and ulcerative colitis. Scand J Gastroenterol. 1985;20:539–42.
45. Harnois DM, Lindor KD. Primary sclerosing cholangitis: evolving concepts in diagnosis and treatment. Dig Dis. 1997;15:23–41.
46. Sherlock S. Pathogenesis of sclerosing cholangitis: the role of nonimmune factors. Semin Liver Dis. 1991;11:5–10.
47. Terblanche J, Allison HF, Northover JMA. An ischemic basis for biliary strictures. Surgery. 1983;94:52–7.
48. Kemeny M, Battifora H, Blayney DW et al. Sclerosing cholangitis after continuous hepatic artery infusion of FUDR. Ann Surg. 1985;202:176–81.
49. Fausa O, Schrumpf E, Elgjo K. Relationship of inflammatory bowel disease and primary sclerosing cholangitis. Semin Liver Dis. 1991;11:31–9.
50. Dew MJ, Thompson H, Allan RN. The spectrum of hepatic dysfunction in inflammatory bowel disease. Q J Med. 1979;189:113–35.
51. Olsson R, Danielsson Å, Järnerot G et al. Prevalence of primary sclerosing cholangitis in patients with ulcerative colitis. Gastroenterology. 1991;100:1319–23.
52. Broomé U, Glaumann H, Hellers G, Nilsson B, Sörstad J, Hultcrantz R. Liver disease in ulcerative colitis: an epidemiological and follow up study in the county of Stockholm. Gut. 1994;35:84–9.
53. Schrumpf E, Fausa O, Elgjo K, Kolmannskog F. Hepatobiliary complications of inflammatory bowel disease. Semin Liver Dis. 1988;8:201–9.

54. Eade MN. Liver disease in ulcerative colitis. I. Analysis of operative liver biopsy in 138 consecutive patients having colectomy. Ann Intern Med. 1970;72:475–87.

55. Wee A, Ludwig J. Pericholangitis in chronic ulcerative colitis: primary sclerosing cholangitis of the small bile ducts? Ann Intern Med. 1985;102:581–7.

56. Kolmannskog F, Aakhus T, Fausa O et al. Cholangiographic findings in ulcerative colitis. Acta Radiol (Diagn). 1981;22:151–7.

57. Ludwig J. Small-duct primary sclerosing cholangitis. Semin Liver Dis. 1991;11:11–17.

58. Boberg KM, Schrumpf E, Fausa O et al. Hepatobiliary disease in ulcerative colitis. An analysis of 18 patients with hepatobiliary lesions classified as small-duct primary sclerosing cholangitis. Scand J Gastroenterol. 1994;29:744–52.

59. Angulo P, Maor-Kendler Y, Lindor KD. Small-duct primary sclerosing cholangitis: a long-term follow-up study. Hepatology. 2002;35:1494–500.

60. Broomé U, Glaumann H, Lindström E et al. Natural history and outcome in 32 Swedish patients with small duct primary sclerosing cholangitis (PSC). J Hepatol. 2002;36:586–9.

61. Björnsson E, Boberg KM, Cullen S et al. Patients with small duct primary sclerosing cholangitis have a favourable long term prognosis. Gut. 2002;51:731–5.

62. Chapman RW. Small duct primary sclerosing cholangitis. J Hepatol. 2002;36:692–4.

63. Minuk GY, Sutherland LR, Pappas SC, Kelly JK, Martin SE. Autoimmune chronic active hepatitis (lupoid hepatitis) and primary sclerosing cholangitis in two young adult females. Can J Gastroenterol. 1988;2:22–7.

64. Rabinovitz M, Demetris AJ, Bou-Abboud CH, Van Thiel DH. Simultaneous occurrence of primary sclerosing cholangitis and autoimmue chronic active hepatitis in a patient with ulcerative colitis. Dig Dis Sci. 1992;37:1606–11.

65. Lawrence SP, Sherman KE, Lawson JM, Goodman ZD. A 39 year old man with chronic hepatitis. Semin Liver Dis. 1994;14:97–105.

66. Johnson PJ, McFarlane IG. Meeting report: International Autoimmune Hepatitis Group. Hepatology. 1993;18:998–1005.

67. Heathcote J. Overlap syndromes of autoimmune hepatitis, primary biliary cirrhosis and primary sclersoing cholangitis. In: Krawitt EL, Wiesner RH, Nishioka M, editors. Autoimmune Liver Diseases, 2nd edn. Amsterdam: Elsevier, 1998:449–56.

68. Wiesner RH, LaRusso NF, Ludwig J, Dickson ER. Comparison of the clinicopathologic features of primary sclerosing cholangitis and primary biliary cirrhosis. Gastroenterology. 1985;88:108–14.

69. Sherlock S, Scheuer PJ. The presentation and diagnosis of 100 patients with primary biliary cirrhosis. N Engl J Med. 1973;289:674–8.

70. Batts KP, Ludwig J. Histopathology of autoimmune chronic active hepatitis, primary biliary cirrhosis, and primary sclerosing cholangitis. In: Krawitt EL, Wiesner RH, editors. Autoimmune Liver Diseases. New York: Raven Press, 1991:75–92.

71. Michieletti P, Wanless IR, Katz A et al. Antimitochondrial antibody negative primary biliary cirrhosis: a distinct syndrome of autoimmune cholangitis. Gut. 1994;35:260–5.

72. Ben-Ari Z, Dhillon AP, Sherlock S. Autoimmune cholangiopathy: part of the spectrum of autoimmune chronic active hepatitis. Hepatology. 1993;18:10–15.

73. Heathcote J. Autoimmune cholangitis. Gut. 1997;40:440–2.

74. Bergquist A, Ekbom A, Olsson R et al. Hepatic and extrahepatic malignancies in primary sclerosing cholangitis. J Hepatol. 2002;36:321–7.

75. Abu-Elmagd KM, Selby R, Iwatsuki S et al. Cholangiocarcinoma and sclerosing cholangitis: clinical characteristics and effect on survival after liver transplantation. Transplant Proc. 1993;25:1124–5.

76. Farges O, Malassagne B, Sebagh M, Bismuth H. Primary sclerosing cholangitis: liver transplantation or biliary surgery. Surgery. 1995;117:146–55.

77. Wee A, Ludwig J, Coffey RJ Jr, LaRusso NF, Wiesner RH. Hepatobiliary carcinoma associated with primary sclerosing cholangitis and chronic ulcerative colitis. Hum Pathol. 1985;16:719–26.

78. Mir-Madjlessi SH, Farmer RG, Sivak MV. Bile duct carcinoma in patients with ulcerative colitis. Relationship to sclerosing cholangitis: report of six cases and review of the literature. Dig Dis Sci. 1987;32:145–54.

79. MacCarty RL, LaRusso NF, May GR et al. Cholangiocarcinoma complicating primary sclerosing cholangitis: cholangiographic appearances. Radiology. 1985;156:43–6.

80. Campbell WL, Ferris JV, Holbert BL, Thaete FL, Baron RL. Biliary tract carcinoma complicating primary sclerosing cholangitis: evaluation with CT, cholangiography, US, and MR imaging. Radiology. 1998;207:41–50.
81. Rabinowitz M, Zajko AB, Hassanein T et al. Diagnostic value of brush cytology in the diagnosis of bile duct carcinoma: a study in 65 patients with bile duct strictures. Hepatology. 1990; 12:747–52.
82. Lindberg B, Arnelo U, Bergquist A et al. Diagnosis of biliary strictures in conjunction with endoscopic retrograde cholangiopancreaticography, with special reference to patients with primary sclerosing cholangitis. Endoscopy. 2002;34:909–16.
83. Ponsioen CY, Lam K, van Milligen de Wit AWM et al. Four years experience with short term stenting in primary sclerosing cholangitis. Am J Gastroenterol. 1999;94:2403–7.
84. Fleming KA, Boberg KM, Glaumann H, Bergquist A, Smith D, Clausen OPF. Biliary dysplasia as a marker of cholangiocarcinoma in primary sclerosing cholangitis. J Hepatol. 2001;34:360–5.
85. Nichols JC, Gores GJ, LaRusso NF, Wiesner RH, Nagorney DM, Ritts RE. Diagnostic role of serum CA 19-9 for cholangiocarcinoma in patients with primary sclerosing cholangitis. Mayo Clin Proc. 1993;68:874–9.
86. Ramage JK, Donaghy A, Farrant JM, Iorns R, Williams R. Serum tumor markers for the diagnosis of cholangiocarcinoma in primary sclerosing cholangitis. Gastroenterology. 1995;108:865–9.
87. Albert MB, Steinberg WM, Henry JP. Elevated serum levels of tumor marker CA 19-9 in acute cholangitis. Dig Dis Sci. 1988;33:1223–5.

21
Incidence and prevalence of primary sclerosing cholangitis around the world

C. Y. PONSIOEN

INTRODUCTION

Many aspects of primary sclerosing cholangitis (PSC) are still unresolved; its aetiology is unknown and the pathogenesis poorly understood. Treatment is largely supportive and aimed at alleviating complications such as dominant strictures and terminal liver failure.

The reasons for our lack of understanding are probably twofold: (1) PSC is a rare disease, and (2) the pathology is hidden deep in the body and thus not readily accessible for investigation and study.

As for the epidemiology of PSC, only a handful of papers with reliable population-based data exist. Nonetheless, improving our understanding of the prevalence of PSC among different populations is important, above all because insight in the worldwide distribution may give us valuable information regarding the still-elusive aetiology. The median survival of large duct PSC in terms of death or liver transplantation is currently estimated to be 12–18 years[1–4]. End-stage PSC now ranks among the five main indications for liver transplantation in several countries[5–7]. Proper incidence and prevalence rates can be of importance to health-care officials in planning future facilities for liver transplantation.

This chapter attempts to give an overview of the literature from 1980 onwards regarding the epidemiology of this elusive disease.

INCIDENCE AND PREVALENCE OF PSC

Since the first published documented case of PSC, by Delbet in 1924, many descriptive series have been published[8]; however, almost all papers are case-series and focus on the natural history or the association with inflammatory

Table 1 Population-based studies on incidence and prevalence of PSC

Region	Period	References	No. of patients	Population defined*	Incidence $(\times 10^{-5})$	Prevalence $(\times 10^{-5})$
Alaska	1983–2000	9	100 312	+++	–	0
Singapore	1989–1998	10	750 000	++	–	1.3
Oslo, Norway	1986–1995	11	130 000	+++	1.3	8.5
Manitoba, Canada	1987–1994	12	650 000	++	–	6.5
Spain	1984–1988	13	19 200 000	+	0.07	0.22

* Degree of proper delineation of population studied; + = poor, ++ = medium, +++ = good.

bowel disease (IBD). From these largely European and North American studies a fairly uniform picture emerges. The median age at diagnosis is approximately 39 years, there is a male predominance of 60–70%, and 70–80% of PSC patients have or will develop IBD[1–4].

There are only a handful of population-based studies assessing the epidemiology of PSC. All these stem from highly developed countries in Europe and North America, with the exception of one study from Singapore[9–13]. Some key data from these studies are summarized in Table 1. In short, the prevalence ranges from 0 to 8.5 × 10⁻⁵.

There are more data available regarding the association between PSC and IBD. As early as 1959 it was observed that PSC often occurred in relation to IBD, notably ulcerative colitis (UC); indeed most series on PSC mention this association[14]. Table 2 shows some key figures from the most relevant studies from 1980 onwards. In summary, clinical overt IBD, mostly UC, is encountered in 47–79% of PSC cases in Europe and North America. In East Asia IBD is seen only in a minority (±20%) of PSC patients. Conversely, IBD patients, UC and (colonic) Crohn's disease (CD) alike, develop PSC in about 3.4%, again according to series from Western countries. As for PSC in children, only a few small series have been published. Concomitant IBD seems to occur as frequently as in adult PSC[15,16].

Now that coexisting IBD is no longer a prerequisite for a diagnosis of small duct PSC, UC and CD seem to occur as often as in large duct PSC[26].

A crude estimate of the annual incidence of PSC can be inferred by multiplying the known annual incidence of UC by 100/70 × 0.034. Table 3 shows an estimate of the annual incidence of PSC in some countries.

DISCUSSION

The main conclusion that can be drawn from this literature overview is that the paucity of population-based data precludes a reliable global assessment of the epidemiology of PSC. If at all, PSC seems to be a disease of the Western world. In Europe PSC seems to be more prevalent in northern parts.

In most epidemiological studies on PSC, case definition is largely based on the typical cholangiographic abnormalities. This implies that small duct PSC, an

Table 2 PSC and concomitant IBD and vice-versa

Region	References	Period	No. of patients	Percentage UC in PSC	Percentage CD in PSC	Percentage IBD in PSC	Percentage PSC in UC	Percentage PSC in CD	Population defined*
Sweden	17	1965–1989	55				3.9		+++
Sweden	18	1970–1998	604			79			++
Oslo, Norway	11	1986–1995	17			71			+++
Aalborg, Denmark	19	1976–1987	11				3.6		++
Aalborg, Denmark	20	1976–1991	9					3.4	++
London, UK	2	1972–1989	126	71	2				+
Italy	21	1980–1992	117	36	10	54			+
Spain	13	1984–1988	43	44	2.5				+
Turkey	22	1993–2000	18	50	22		2.3	3.6	+
USA (Mayo)	1	1970–1986	174			71			+
USA (Mayo)†	15	1975–1999	52			84			+
Toronto, Canada†	16	1986–1994	32	44	9				+
Manitoba, Canada	24	1984–1996	–				2	0.4	+++
Chandigarh, India	23	1984–1994	18			50			+
Singapore	10	1989–1998	10	0	20				+
Japan	25	–	192	20	1				+

* Degree of proper delineation of population studied; + = poor, ++ = medium, +++ = good.
† Series in children.

Percentage UC in PSC = proportion of PSC patients with coexisting ulcerative colitis. Percentage CD in PSC = proportion of PSC patients with coexisting Crohn's disease. Percentage IBD in PSC = proportion of PSC patients with coexisting unspecified inflammatory bowel disease. Percentage PSC in UC = proportion of ulcerative colitis patients with PSC. Percentage PSC in CD = proportion of Crohn's disease patients with PSC.

220

Table 3 Crude estimate of annual incidence of PSC inferred from UC

Country	Annual incidence of UC ($\times 10^{-5}$)*	Inferred annual incidence of PSC ($\times 10^{-5}$)
UK	4–15	0.19–0.73
USA	3–7	0.15–0.34
Scandinavia	4–15	0.19–0.73

* From ref. 27.

entity first introduced by the Mayo group in 1985, is not accounted for[28]. The diagnosis of small duct PSC was originally defined as: (a) typical liver biopsy findings, (b) biochemical profile as in large duct PSC, and (c) the presence of IBD. Recently several groups have looked at the clinical course of small duct PSC in their cohorts[26,29,30]. Small duct PSC represented 4.3–10% in these cohorts. Among small duct PSC patients, none developed cholangiocarcinoma, and survival free of liver transplantation was significantly better. Although small duct PSC seems to run a more favourable course than classic PSC, it probably represents an earlier stage or one end of the disease spectrum. Indeed, small duct PSC was shown to progress to large duct PSC in approximately 15% of cases[26,29,30]. Therefore, both variants of PSC should probably be regarded as one disease entity. Consequently, most of the published epidemiological data may underestimate the true prevalence of small and large duct PSC together.

One of the striking notions from this literature overview is the virtual lack of data from South America, Africa, and Australia. As far as the last continent is concerned, PSC is prevalent in Australia. From papers on transplantation series it can be deduced that PSC does occur, and probably more or less to the same extent as in Europe and North America[5,6].

What about Latin America and Africa? Is PSC extremely rare, does it go unnoticed, or is there a lack of interest from research groups?

Making a diagnosis of PSC can be difficult. A reliable and readily applicable diagnostic test such as the antimitochondrial antibody assay for primary biliary cirrhosis is still lacking. The diagnosis still relies on cholangiography and/or liver histology, but pathognomonic findings are infrequently encountered. Moreover, PSC must be distinguished from several other diseases including complicated cholelithiasis, primary cholangiocarcinoma, AIDS-related cholangiopathy, ischaemia, etc.[31–33]. Facilities for cholangiography and liver histology expertise are scant in some parts of the developing world, so it is conceivable that quite a number of PSC patients are not recognized. Alternatively, medical scientists in large parts of South America and Africa, where health care is primarily directed at coping with the vast burden of infectious diseases, may simply lack sufficient interest in a rare and elusive biliary disease. Yet PSC may indeed be very rare in Latin America and Africa. If this were true it would emphasize the pattern that PSC is mainly a disease of the industrialized northern hemisphere. Putative aetiological factors involved in such a geographical distribution could be of racial, ethnic, environmental, or behavioural origin.

If race does play a role the available geographical data suggest that being from Caucasian white origin would predispose to PSC. In favour of such a hypothesis is the well-designed population-based survey in over 100 000 non-white Alaskan natives[9]. This study found no case of PSC. To my knowledge there are only two reports that specifically described PSC in patients from African genetic origin[34,35]. Although small series, both found that African origin was associated with an increased odds ratio for PSC.

It is generally believed that immunogenetics play a role in the aetiopathogenesis of PSC. Five HLA haplotypes and two non-MHC genes have so far been linked with PSC[36]. Unfortunately, almost all published data on immunogenetics in PSC come from a single racial group, namely European Caucasians. Therefore, it remains to be seen whether putative racial differences in the prevalence of PSC can be accounted for by racial differences in the distribution of these immunogenetic factors.

Another attractive candidate hypothesis to explain the north–south gradient comes from the strong link between PSC and IBD. Both UC and Crohn's disease appear to be more common in industrialized countries such as Scandinavia, the United Kingdom, and North America, and less common in southern Europe, Asia, and Africa[37,38]. Some authors reported that, when meticulously screened for, all PSC patients have concomitant IBD, or will develop IBD in the future[39]. If IBD did constitute a prerequisite for the development of PSC, the geographical differences in the prevalence of PSC would merely reflect the global distribution of IBD. As far as environmental and behavioural factors are concerned, only the influence of smoking has been studied to a limited extent. Smoking seems to confer some degree of protection against PSC[40,41]. Though this would not be in line with the male predominance in PSC, it may offer some explanation for the difference in prevalence between northern and southern Europe. Again, it should be emphasized that all these considerations remain speculative, as long as there are so many blank spots on the globe. There is an obvious need for more reliable population-based epidemiological data, especially from non-industrialized countries. Better diagnostic tools such as a serological test would greatly augment proper data collection.

References

1. Wiesner RH, Grambsch PM, Dickson ER et al. Primary sclerosing cholangitis: natural history, prognostic factors and survival analysis. Hepatology. 1989;10:430–6.
2. Farrant JM, Hayllar KM, Wilkinson ML et al. Natural history and prognostic variables in primary sclerosing cholangitis. Gastroenterology. 1991;100:1710–17.
3. Broome U, Olsson R, Loof L et al. Natural history and prognostic factors in 305 Swedish patients with primary sclerosing cholangitis. Gut. 1996;38:610–15.
4. Ponsioen CY, Vrouenraets SME, Prawirodirdjo W et al. Natural history of primary sclerosing cholangitis and prognostic value of cholangiography in a Dutch population. Gut. 2002;51:562–6.
5. Kilpe VE, Krakauer H, Wren RE. An analysis of liver transplant experience from 37 transplant centers as reported to medicare. Transplantation. 1993;56:554–61.
6. Sheil AG, McCaughan GW, Thompson JF, Dorney SF, Stephen MS, Bookallil MJ. The first five years' clinical experience of the Australian National liver transplantation unit. Med J Aust. 1992;156:9–16.
7. Bjoro K, Friman S, Hockerstedt K et al. Liver transplantation in the Nordic countries, 1982–1998: changes of indications and improving results. Scand J Gastroenterol. 1999;34:714–22.
8. Delbet MP. Retrecissement du coledoque. Cholecysto-duodenostomie. Bull Mem Soc Chirurg Paris. 1924;50:1144–6.

9. Hurlburt KJ, McMahon BJ, Deubner H, Hsu-Trawinski B, Williams JL, Kowdley KV. Prevalence of autoimmune liver disease in Alaska natives. Am J Gastroenterol. 2002;97:2402–7.
10. Ang TL, Fock KM, Ng TM, Teo EK, Chua TS, Tan JY. Clinical profile of primary sclerosing cholangitis in Singapore. J Gastroenterol Hepatol. 2002;17:908–13.
11. Boberg KM, Aadland E, Jahnsen J, Raknerud N, Stiris M, Bell H. Incidence and prevalence of primary biliary cirrhosis, primary sclerosing cholangitis, and autoimmune hepatitis in a Norwegian population. Scand J Gastroenterol. 1998;33:99–103.
12. Byron D, Minuk GY. Clinical hepatology: profile of an urban, hospital-based practice. Hepatology. 1996;24:813–15.
13. Escorsell A, Pares A, Rodes J, Solis-Herruzo JA, Miras M, de la Morena E. Epidemiology of primary sclerosing cholangitis in Spain. Spanish Association for the Study of the Liver. J Hepatol. 1994;21:787–91.
14. Boden RW, Rankin JG, Goulston SJM et al. The liver in ulcerative colitis. Lancet. 1959;2:245–8.
15. Faubion WA, Loftus EV, Sandborn WJ, Freese DK, Perrault J. Pediatric 'PSC–IBD': a descriptive report of associated inflammatory bowel disease among pediatric patients with PSC. J Pediatr Gastroenterol Nutr. 2001;33:296–300.
16. Wilschanski M, Chait P, Wade JA et al. Primary sclerosing cholangitis in 32 children: clinical, laboratory, and radiographic features, with survival analysis. Hepatology. 1995;22:1415–22.
17. Olsson R, Danielsson A, Jarnerot G et al. Prevalence of primary sclerosing cholangitis in patients with ulcerative colitis. Gastroenterology. 1991;100:1319–23.
18. Bergquist A, Ekbom A, Olsson R et al. Hepatic and extrahepatic malignancies in primary sclerosing cholangitis. J Hepatol. 2002;36:321–7.
19. Rasmussen HH, Fallingborg JF, Mortensen PB et al. Skleroserende cholangitis og colitis ulcerosa. Ugeskr Laeger. 1994;156:179–82.
20. Rasmussen HH, Fallingborg JF, Mortensen PB, Vyberg M, Tage-Jensen U, Rasmussen SN. Hepatobiliary dysfunction and primary sclerosing cholangitis in patients with Crohn's disease. Scand J Gastroenterol. 1997;32:604–10.
21. Okolicsanyi L, Fabris L, Viaggi S et al. Primary sclerosing cholangitis: clinical presentation, natural history and prognostic variables: an Italian multicentre study. Eur J Gastroenterol Hepatol. 1996;8:685–91.
22. Parlak E, Kosar Y, Ulker A, Dagli U, Alkim C, Sahin B. Primary sclerosing cholangitis in patients with inflammatory bowel disease in Turkey. J Clin Gastroenterol. 2001;33:299–301.
23. Kochhar R, Goenka MK, Das K et al. Primary sclerosing cholangitis: an experience from India. J Gastroenterol Hepatol. 1996;11:429–33.
24. Bernstein CN, Blanchard JF, Rawsthorne P, Yu N. The prevalence of extraintestinal diseases in inflammatory bowel disease: a population-based study. Am J Gastroenterol. 2001;96:1116–22.
25. Takikawa H, Manabe T. Primary sclerosing cholangitis in Japan – analysis of 192 cases. J Gastroenterol. 1997;32:134–7.
26. Bjornsson E, Boberg KM, Cullen S et al. Patients with small duct primary sclerosing cholangitis have a favourable long term prognosis. Gut. 2002;51:731–5.
27. Mayberry JF. Some aspects of the epidemiology of ulcerative colitis. Gut. 1985;26:968–74.
28. Wee A, Ludwig J. Pericholangitis in chronic ulcerative colitis: primary sclerosing cholangitis of the small bile ducts? Ann Intern Med. 1985;102:581–7.
29. Angulo P, Maor-Kendler Y, Lindor K. Small-duct primary sclerosing cholangitis: a long-term follow-up study. Hepatology. 2002;35:1494–500.
30. Broome U, Glaumann H, Lindstrom E et al. Natural history and outcome in 32 Swedish patients with small duct primary sclerosing cholangitis (PSC). J Hepatol. 2002;36:586–9.
31. Porayko MK, LaRusso NF, Wiesner RH. Primary sclerosing cholangitis: a progressive disease? [review]. Semin Liver Dis. 1991;11:18–25.
32. Cello JP. Acquired immunodeficiency syndrome cholangiopathy: spectrum of disease. Am J Med. 1989;86:539–46.
33. Shea WJ, Demas BE, Goldberg HI et al. Sclerosing cholangitis associated with hepatic arterial FUDR chemotherapy: radiographic–histologic correlation. Am J Roentgenol. 1986;146:717–21.
34. Simsek H, Schuman BM. Inflammatory bowel disease in 64 black patients: analysis of course, complications, and surgery. J Clin Gastroenterol. 1989;11:294–8.
35. Kelly P, Patchett S, McCloskey D, Alstead E, Farthing M, Fairclough P. Sclerosing cholangitis, race and sex. Gut. 1997;41:688–9.
36. Donaldson PT, Norris S. Immunogenetics in PSC. Best Pract Clin Gastroenterol. 2001;15:611–27.

37. Farrokhyar F, Swarbrick ET, Irvine EJ. A critical review of epidemiological studies in inflammatory bowel disease. Scand J Gastroenterol. 2001;36:2–15.
38. Karlinger K, Gyorke T, Mako E, Mester A, Tarjan Z. The epidemiology and the pathogenesis of inflammatory bowel disease. Eur J Radiol. 2000;35:154–67.
39. Aadland E, Schrumpf E, Fausa O et al. Primary sclerosing cholangitis: a long-term follow-up study. Scand J Gastroenterol. 1987;22:655–64.
40. Loftus EV, Sandborn WJ, Tremaine WJ et al. Primary sclerosing cholangitis is associated with nonsmoking: a case–control study. Gastroenterology. 1996;110:1496–502.
41. Erpecum v KJ, Smits SJ, Meeberg vd PC et al. Risk of primary sclerosing cholangitis is associated with nonsmoking behaviour. Gastroenterology. 1996;110:1658–62.

22
Small duct primary sclerosing cholangitis: a separate disease?

R. OLSSON

INTRODUCTION

The term 'small duct primary sclerosing cholangitis' (SD-PSC) was coined by Wee and Ludwig in 1985[1] for patients with 'chronic hepatobiliary disease associated with chronic ulcerative colitis' who 'morphologically had shown hepatic changes similar to those of classic or large duct primary sclerosing cholangitis' but with 'no confirmatory evidence of large duct disease'.

Even though cholangiographic follow-up was not performed in the 37 patients, 'later clinical and laboratory data' in five patients 'suggested that they had developed large-duct involvement'. The true natural history of SD-PSC remained unknown until 2002, when three groups reported their experience with this entity, based on a material of a total of 83 patients[2–4].

Before discussing the findings in these publications I will discuss some issues regarding the identification of cases with SD-PSC, as well as the diagnostic accuracy of this entity.

DIAGNOSTIC PROBLEMS

First, as to the requirement that 'the chronic hepatobiliary disease' should be associated with 'chronic ulcerative colitis', a strict adherence to this requirement implies that an unknown number of patients who in other respects fulfil the criteria for SD-PSC will not be diagnosed to have this disease. This may be unfortunate in view of the well-known fact that all patients with classical large duct PSC do not have inflammatory bowel disease, at least when the PSC is diagnosed. In some cases the PSC may precede inflammatory bowel disease by several years, other patients may not have chronic ulcerative colitis but Crohn colitis or non-specific colitis.

Second, the requirement that patients with SD-PSC should have morphological changes 'similar to those of classic or large duct' PSC is of course mandatory. However, even in this respect there is a risk that the criteria will leave many cases undiagnosed. This risk is a consequence of the high sampling variability for histological changes in PSC. In the SILK study of colchicine treatment of PSC[5] we made duplicate liver biopsies in 56 biopsy occasions (=112 biopsy samples) in 44 of the patients. A PSC diagnosis based on the presence of periductal fibrosis and/or bile duct destruction was made in only 14% – in spite of clear radiological evidence for large duct PSC. This low sensitivity of liver biopsy for the diagnosis of PSC may to a large extent be explained by sampling error, for in the duplicate biopsies periductal fibrosis was missed in the one sample in 50%. Similarly, bile duct destruction was missed in 70%[6].

Third, the requirement that there should be 'no confirmatory evidence of large-duct disease' is a source of under- as well as over-diagnosis of SD-PSC. Besides the risk of diagnosing SD-PSC because of underfilling of the biliary tree at ERC, there is to my knowledge no study of inter-observer agreement in low-grade PSC. Furthermore, even if there are a number of studies demonstrating good agreement of ERC and MRC in the diagnosis of PSC[7–12], these studies were not specifically addressed to investigate the usefulness of MRC in differentiating low grade from small duct PSC.

SD-PSC – CLINICAL FEATURES

In all the three recent studies of SD-PSC the diagnosis of SD-PSC was based on cholestatic liver tests not explained by other liver disease, a normal cholangiogram, and a histological picture consistent with PSC. A diagnosis of IBD was compulsory in one study[4]; in the other two studies 50–88% of the patients had IBD. In the Mayo Clinic study 18 SD-PSC patients were compared with 36 patients with 'classic PSC and IBD', blindly matched by age and sex[4]. In the Oxford–Oslo study 33 SD-PSC patients were compared with 100 large duct PSC patients from each of the two centres[5]. In the Swedish multicentre study, performed by the Swedish Internal Medicine Liver Club (SILK), there was no direct comparison with large-duct PSC, but I will compare these with the 305 large-duct PSC patients previously reported by the same group[13].

In the three studies the male/female ratio (1.4–1.7) was very similar to the ratio in large duct PSC, as was the age at diagnosis (38–39 years), the liver tests at diagnosis, and the prevalence of symptoms classically associated with large duct PSC (Figure 1). The classical PSC-related symptoms of fever, pruritus, right upper quadrant abdominal pain, and jaundice were encountered in roughly the same frequency in SD-PSC as in large duct PSC, being significantly more frequent in large duct PSC only in the Oxford–Oslo study. Liver biopsy at the time of diagnosis was available in all Swedish[2] and US[4] patients, and in 29/33 British–Norwegian patients, showing stage 3 or 4 according to Ludwig in 10–29%. The histological stage of the disease did not differ significantly from that in an age- and sex-matched group of patients with large duct PSC in the US study[4] (Figure 2).

226

SMALL DUCT PSC

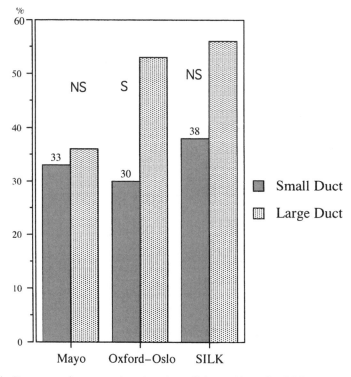

Figure 1 Percentage of symptomatic patients in small duct and large duct PSC

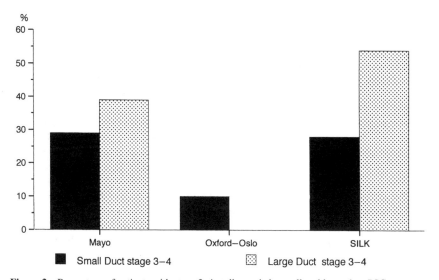

Figure 2 Percentage of patients with stage 3–4 at diagnosis in small and large duct PSC

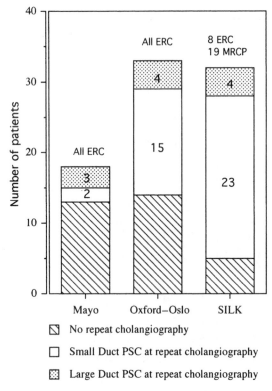

Figure 3 Progression of small duct PSC to large duct PSC after 2–21 years in patients subjected to subsequent cholangiography during follow-up

SD-PSC – NATURAL HISTORY

Mean follow-up time varied between 5.5 and 10.5 years with maximum follow-up times varying between 16 and 32 years. Subsequent cholangiograms were performed in 27 of the 32 Swedish patients, demonstrating large duct PSC in four, after 4–15 years[2] (Figure 3). Subsequent cholangiograms were furthermore performed in 19 of the 33 British–Norwegian patients, showing large duct PSC in four[3], and in five of the 18 US patients, displaying large duct PSC in three patients, after 4–21 years[4]. Thus, roughly 15% developed large duct PSC.

In total, five patients (6%) were transplanted and two died from liver-related complications (Figure 4). One patient developed hepatocellular carcinoma, but none developed cholangiocarcinoma. Compared to patients with large duct PSC, survival without liver transplantation was substantially better in SD-PSC.

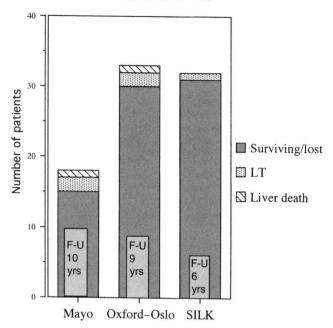

Figure 4 Small duct PSC – survival data

CONCLUSION

To conclude, SD-PSC may not be a separate disease, since it sometimes progresses to large duct PSC. The very similar age and histological stage at diagnosis argue against SD-PSC being diagnosed only at an early stage of large duct PSC. Rather, the data are consistent with SD-PSC being a more benign and slowly progressive form of PSC.

References

1. Wee A, Ludwig J. Pericholangitis in chronic ulcerative colitis; primary sclerosing cholangitis of the small ducts? Ann Intern Med. 1985;102:581–7.
2. Broomé U, Glaumann H, Lindström E et al. Natural history and outcome in 32 Swedish patients with small duct primary sclerosing cholangitis (PSC). J Hepatol. 2002;36:586–9.
3. Björnsson E, Boberg KM, Cullen S et al. Patients with small duct primary sclerosing cholangitis have a favourable long term prognosis. Gut. 2002;51:731–5.
4. Angulo P, Maor-Kendler Y, Lindor K. Small-duct primary sclerosing cholangitis: a long-term follow-up study. Hepatology. 2002;35:1494–500.
5. Olsson R, Broome U, Danielsson A et al. Colchicine treatment of primary sclerosing cholangitis. Gastroenterology. 1995;108:1199–203.
6. Olsson R, Hagerstrand I, Broome U et al. Sampling variability of percutaneous liver biopsy in primary sclerosing cholangitis. J Clin Pathol. 1995;48:933–5.

7. Oberholzer K, Lohse AW, Mildenberger P et al. [Diagnosis of primary sclerosing cholangitis: prospective comparison of MR cholangiography with endoscopic retrograde cholangiography]. Rofo Fortschr Geb Rontgenstr Neuen Bildgeb Verfahr. 1998;169:622–6.

8. Angulo P, Pearce DH, Johnson CD et al. Magnetic resonance cholangiography in patients with biliary disease: its role in primary sclerosing cholangitis. J Hepatol. 2000;33:520–7.

9. Fulcher AS, Turner MA, Franklin KJ et al. Primary sclerosing cholangitis: evaluation with MR cholangiography – a case–control study. Radiology. 2000;215:71–80.

10. Ferrara C, Valeri G, Salvolini L, Giovagnoni A. Magnetic resonance cholangiopancreatography in primary sclerosing cholangitis in children. Pediatr Radiol. 2002;32:413–17.

11. Textor HJ, Flacke S, Pauleit D et al. Three-dimensional magnetic resonance cholangiopancreatography with respiratory triggering in the diagnosis of primary sclerosing cholangitis: comparison with endoscopic retrograde cholangiography. Endoscopy. 2002;34:984–90.

12. Weber C, Krupski G, Lorenzen J et al. [MRCP in primary sclerosing cholangitis]. Rofo Fortschr Geb Rontgenstr Neuen Bildgeb Verfahr. 2003;175:203–10.

13. Broome U, Olsson R, Loof L et al. Natural history and prognostic factors in 305 Swedish patients with primary sclerosing cholangitis. Gut. 1996;38:610–15.

23
Prognosis of untreated primary sclerosing cholangitis

E. CHRISTENSEN

INTRODUCTION

Primary sclerosing cholangitis (PSC) is a chronic cholestatic liver disease characterized by inflammation and fibrosis of the intra- and extrahepatic bile ducts. Although immunological and genetic factors seem to be involved in the pathogenesis, the aetiology of PSC remains unknown.

Long-term studies have established PSC as a progressive disease[1–8], which ultimately may lead to biliary cirrhosis, liver failure and death. The mean age at time of diagnosis is 35–40 years and two-thirds of patients are males. Up to half of patients are symptomatic at diagnosis, and the majority have associated inflammatory bowel disease, mainly ulcerative colitis. The initial presentation and the subsequent rate of disease progression are highly variable among patients. In most patients the rate of progression is relatively slow, with median survival being about 12 years; however, the development of cholangiocarcinoma, which occurs in about 10%, worsens the prognosis considerably[9,10]. Recently it has been demonstrated in more studies that patients with only small duct PSC – comprising about 10% of patients – have a much better prognosis and a much lower risk of developing cholangiocarcinoma than patients with large duct PSC[11–14].

Several large studies have described the natural history of PSC, including patient characteristics at diagnosis, survival and its association with variables describing the patients – most frequently at the time of diagnosis[15–24].

SURVIVAL

The median survival time has been found to be about 12 years in more of the larger studies; however, median survival times up to 18 years have been reported in a Dutch study[24]. In another smaller series of referred and probably highly selected patients a median survival of less than 1 year from referral was observed[17]. This shows the wide variation in course and outcome of the disease.

CHARACTERISTICS AT TIME OF DIAGNOSIS AND ASSOCIATION WITH PROGNOSIS

It is obvious that the course of disease, which can be observed, will be dependent on: (a) the time of diagnosis in relation to the start of the disease, i.e. the diagnostic delay; and (b) the rate of progression of the disease. Because of the insidious nature of the disease it may be difficult to determine the starting time. Although diagnosis of asymptomatic cases does occur, most frequently the diagnosis is made only following the occurrence of symptoms, which may occur after many years of asymptomatic disease. Even in the symptomatic phase the course may be irregular with phases of deterioration and improvement for many years. Furthermore, the rate of disease progression may differ considerably between patients even if they are at the same stage. In later phases of the disease the rate of progression may accelerate towards liver insufficiency over a short period of time (months). These characteristics of the disease explain the variability of the results obtained in regard to variables found to be associated with prognosis.

Tables 1–3 present a summary of the variables found to be associated with survival in univariate analysis in the published studies. In most of the reports a strong association between older age and a poorer survival has been found establishing age at diagnosis as a strong prognostic variable (Table 1).

In the study comprising referred patients[17] a long duration of history was strongly associated with a poor prognosis.

The same study found a worse survival in males. In other studies there have been only weak insignificant trends towards a poorer prognosis in males than in females; however, in one study there was a trend in the other direction[19].

The presence of symptoms and the association with inflammatory bowel disease have in some studies been found to be associated with poorer prognosis.

Some milder signs and symptoms, such as pruritus, fatigue, weight loss, fever and abdominal pain, have been reported in some studies to be associated with a poorer prognosis (Table 1); however, the symptoms and signs most frequently associated with poorer prognosis include features of advanced later-stage disease such as ascites, jaundice, varices, variceal bleeding, hepatomegaly and splenomegaly (Table 1).

The biochemical variables most frequently associated with a poorer prognosis (Table 2) include: (a) indicators of cholestasis, such as high bilirubin, high alkaline phosphatase, high cholesterol; (b) indicators of inflammatory activity and liver cell destruction such as high AST, high gamma-globulin; and (c) indicators of decreased liver cell function, portal hypertension and hypersplenism, such as low albumin, prolonged prothrombin time, low haemoglobin, and low platelet count.

Macroscopic structural variables being associated with poorer survival (Table 3) include presence of common bile duct stricture, extrahepatic PSC, and cholangiographic score with markedly abnormal cholangiogram in regard to both intrahepatic and extrahepatic strictures. The prognostic value of strictures

Table 1 Clinical variables associated with poorer prognosis in PSC in univariate analysis

	Study (main author) and ref.									
	Wiesner[15]	Farrant[16]	Ismail[17]	Dickson[18]	Schrumpf[19]	Broome[20]	Okolicsanyi[21]	Kim[22]	Boberg[23]	Ponsioen[24]
Year	1989	1991	1991	1992	1994	1996	1996	2000	2002	2002
Number of patients	174	126	48	426	77	305	117	405	330	174
Variables										
Older age	+++			+++	++	+++	++	++	+++	+++
Male gender			+					(+)		
Long duration of history			+++							
Presence of symptoms	++					+++				
Inflammatory bowel disease	+			+						
Pruritus						+++			++	
Fatigue									+++	
Weight loss									++	
Fever						+			+	
Abdominal pain						+			++	
Ascites	+++			+++		+++		++	+++	
Jaundice	+++			+++		+++			+++	
Varices		++							+++	
Variceal bleeding	+++	++		++				++	+++	
Hepatomegaly	+	++		+++				++	+++	
Splenomegaly	+++	++		+++				++	+	

+++, p < 0.001; ++, p < 0.01; +, p < 0.05; (+), p < 0.10.

233

Table 2 Biochemical variables associated with poorer prognosis in PSC in univariate analysis

	Study (main author) and ref.									
	Wiesner[15]	Farrant[16]	Ismail[17]	Dickson[18]	Schrumpf[19]	Broomé[20]	Okolicsanyi[21]	Kim[22]	Boberg[23]	Ponsioen[24]
Year	1989	1991	1991	1992	1994	1996	1996	2000	2002	2002
Number of patients	174	126	48	426	77	305	117	405	330	174
Variables										
High bilirubin	+++	+	++	+++	++	+++	++	++	+++	
High alkaline phosphatase		+		(+)		++	+	+	++	
High cholesterol							+++			
High AST	(+)			+++		++	++	++	(+)	
High gamma-globulin	+									
Low albumin	+++			+++	(+)	++	++	++	+++	
Prolonged prothrombin time								++	+++	
Low haemoglobin	+++			+++	(+)		++	++	+++	
Low platelet count	++				(+)			++	(+)	

+++, p < 0.001; ++, p < 0.01; +, p < 0.05; (+), p < 0.10.

234

Table 3 Histological and structural variables associated with poorer prognosis in PSC in univariate analysis

	Study (main author) and ref.									
	Wiesner[15]	Farrant[16]	Ismail[17]	Dickson[18]	Schrumpf[19]	Broomé[20]	Okolicsanyi[21]	Kim[22]	Boberg[23]	Ponsioen[24]
Year	1989	1991	1991	1992	1994	1996	1996	2000	2002	2002
Number of patients	174	126	48	426	77	305	117	405	330	174
Variables										
Common bile duct stricture		+								
Extrahepatic PSC						+++				
High cholangiographic score										+++
Ductopenia	++									
Cholestasis	+++	++								
Piecemeal necrosis	+++									
Portal fibrosis		++								
Advanced histological stage	+++	+++		+++		+++				
Cirrhosis			++							

+++, $p < 0.001$; ++, $p < 0.01$; +, $p < 0.05$; (+), $p < 0.10$.

235

on cholangiography, in particular intrahepatic strictures, is supported by other studies[25-26].

Microscopic structural variables being associated with poorer survival (Table 3) include early lesions such as ductopenia, cholestasis, and piecemeal necrosis, and later more advanced features such as portal fibrosis, advanced histological stage and cirrhosis.

Recently the intrahepatic or small duct form of PSC comprising about 10 percent of the patients was studied more closely[11-14]. Small duct PSC seems to have a more benign course with a better survival and less risk of cholangiocarcinoma.

Over the years less emphasis has been put on liver biopsy findings as a source of prognostic information. No study after 1996 includes histological variables among the prognostic indicators.

PROGNOSTIC MODELS

Prognostic variables have been combined into prognostic models mainly using the Cox model for proportional hazards[27]. In such models each included variable contributes in proportion to its independent association with survival. Since most of the variables recorded for the PSC patients are intercorrelated to a higher or lesser degree, only the strongest prognostic variables will be included in the prognostic models.

Table 4 gives an outline of the variables included in various prognostic models. The models differ markedly, reflecting differences in the patient samples from which they have been developed. Beyond the differences in distribution of types and stages of PSC the variables recorded and analysed at baseline vary considerably between the studies. The most important indicator of a poor prognosis is a high serum bilirubin, this variable being included in nearly all the models. Other important independent predictors of a poor prognosis include high age, low albumin and advanced histological stage. However, variables such as hepatomegaly, splenomegaly, variceal bleeding, inflammatory bowel disease, low haemoglobin, high alkaline phosphatase, high AST, high cholesterol, and a high cholangiographic score are also included in some models as independent indicators of a poor prognosis.

The Child–Pugh score is inferior to the prognostic models specific for PSC[8,28].

TIME-DEPENDENT PROGNOSTIC MODEL

The time-fixed models referred to above utilize only the baseline data. This limits the applicability of the models because the stage and activity of the disease may change soon after baseline and thus change the prognosis. Generally the time-fixed models cannot predict reliably more than a few years ahead, and even then the prognostic estimates may not be very precise.

In one study, by Boberg et al.[23], follow-up data have been utilized to develop a so-called time-dependent Cox regression model[27]. In utilizing the follow-up data this model is based on a much larger amount of data being related to subsequent survival. This means that the resulting model can give more precise predictive estimates. The time-dependent model is well suited for monitoring of patients.

Table 4 Variables with independent association with poorer prognosis in PSC (multivariate analysis)

	Study (main author) and ref.									
	Wiesner[15]	Farrant[16]	Ismail[17]	Dickson[18]	Schrumpf[19]	Broomé[20]	Okolicsanyi[21]	Kim[22]	Boberg[23]	Ponsioen[24]
Year	1989	1991	1991	1992	1994	1996	1996	2000	2002	2002
Number of patients	174	126	48	426	77	305	117	405	330	174
Variables										
Older age	+++	++		+++	++	+		++	+++	(+)
Long duration of history			(+)							
Hepatomegaly		++		++						
Splenomegaly		+								
Variceal bleeding								++		
Inflammatory bowel disease	+++									
High bilirubin	+++		+++	+++	++	+++	(+)	++	+++	
Low albumin							+	++	+++	
Low haemoglobin	+++									
High alkaline phosphatase		++					+			
High AST								++		
High cholesterol							+++			
Advanced histological stage	+++	+		+++		++				
High cholangiographic score										+++

+++, p < 0.001; ++, p < 0.01; +, p < 0.05; (+), p < 0.10.

Whenever changes occur during the course of the disease a new updated short-term prognostic estimate can be made for the next time period by applying the current values of the prognostic variables in the model.

Boberg et al.[23] performed both a time-fixed analysis and a time-dependent analysis on their series of 330 patients from five European centres followed for a median of 8.4 years after diagnosis. Both analyses identified age, bilirubin and albumin as independent predictors of prognosis. However, the prognostic information of bilirubin and albumin was much stronger, i.e. the regression coefficients were numerically larger, in the time-dependent than in the time-fixed model. Accordingly, the 1-year survival probabilities estimated from the time-dependent model corresponded better with the observed survival than those estimated from the time-fixed model in 18 PSC patients dying within 1 year after diagnosis. Using an additive regression analysis the authors made the interesting observation that the influence of albumin was significant only in the first 5 years after diagnosis[23].

APPLICABILITY OF THE PROGNOSTIC MODELS

Generally the prognostic models 'explain' only a quite small part of the variation of the survival time seen in patients; the vast majority of the variation is not explained. This limits the applicability of the prognostic models[29]. Individual estimates of survival are imprecise, even if a time-dependent model is used. The confidence interval of the survival estimates will most often be very wide. Thus a prognostic estimate can serve only as a crude guide to prognosis, and thus only be a supplement to other relevant clinical information needed to decide if and when special therapeutic procedures will be needed. Of particular importance is the decision of if and when to perform liver transplantation[30,31], which may be necessary for end-stage PBC patients because of the inefficiency of medical and other conservative therapies[32]. The timing of liver transplantation is difficult[33,34] and a decision regarding the procedure should not be based on prognostic estimates alone. Instead the prognostic information should be considered together with all other clinically relevant data to ensure the best possible foundation for the decision.

PERSPECTIVES

Prognostic modelling for PSC is difficult for the following reasons: the disease is rather rare, accumulation of large databases requires close cooperation between many centres, the clinical course of the disease is very long, and the number of endpoints is limited. Furthermore, the course of the disease is not steadily progressing but will present short-term phases of improvement and deterioration. The transition from one stage to another (asymptomatic to symptomatic, symptomatic to decompensated, decompensated to terminal) is insidious and not well defined. The prognostic determinants may well differ in the various phases. This will complicate a useful description. In addition different medical and conservative therapies may modify the course in various ways.

At present a large number of rather different prognostic models are available. Probably their prognostic information is rather similar, although this has not been investigated. It would be desirable if general agreement could be obtained on a common prognostic model to be used for PSC[35,36]. To obtain such an agreement, cooperative studies on combined databases from all centres seem necessary.

Thus the challenge for the future in improving the description of the natural history and its determinants is substantial. A wider application of time-dependent Cox regression analysis, which can model both deterioration and improvement, may lead to some further progress. The pattern of intercorrelation between the descriptive variables at various phases during the course of the disease should be studied further to evaluate if interaction terms between variables should be included in the models. Furthermore, modelling of the course of the prognostic variables themselves may also result in some progress[35]. Close cooperation with qualified statisticians, to ensure the best quality of the analyses, is essential in this process[35,36]. In addition the search should continue for better descriptive variables, which characterize as precisely as possible the core problem(s) in the disease, preferably in molecular terms[37]. Such information will most likely improve the prognostication markedly compared to the current prognostic models, which are mainly based on peripheral epiphenomena secondary to the core problem(s) defining the disease.

References

1. Chapman RW, Arborgh BA, Rhodes JM et al. Primary sclerosing cholangitis: a review of its clinical features, cholangiography, and hepatic histology. Gut. 1980;21:870–7.
2. Aadland E, Schrumpf E, Fausa O et al. Primary sclerosing cholangitis: a long-term follow-up study. Scand J Gastroenterol. 1987;22:655–64.
3. Helzberg JH, Petersen JM, Boyer JL. Improved survival with primary sclerosing cholangitis. A review of clinicopathologic features and comparison of symptomatic and asymptomatic patients. Gastroenterology. 1987;92:1869–75.
4. Lebovics E, Palmer M, Woo J, Schaffner F. Outcome of primary sclerosing cholangitis. Analysis of long-term observation of 38 patients. Arch Intern Med. 1987;147:729–31.
5. Chapman RW. Aetiology and natural history of primary sclerosing cholangitis – a decade of progress? Gut. 1991;32:1433–5.
6. Floreani A, Zancan L, Melis A, Baragiotta A, Chiaramonte M. Primary sclerosing cholangitis (PSC): clinical, laboratory and survival analysis in children and adults. Liver. 1999;19:228–33.
7. Narayanan Menon KV, Wiesner RH. Etiology and natural history of primary sclerosing cholangitis. J Hepatobil Pancreat Surg. 1999;6:343–51.
8. Talwalkar JA, Lindor KD. Natural history and prognostic models in primary sclerosing cholangitis. Best Pract Res Clin Gastroenterol. 2001;15:563–75.
9. Bergquist A, Broomé U. Hepatobiliary and extra-hepatic malignancies in primary sclerosing cholangitis. Best Pract Res Clin Gastroenterol. 2001;15:643–56.
10. Boberg KM, Bergquist A, Mitchell S et al. Cholangiocarcinoma in primary sclerosing cholangitis: risk factors and clinical presentation. Scand J Gastroenterol. 2002;37:1205–11.
11. Björnsson E, Boberg KM, Cullen S et al. Patients with small duct primary sclerosing cholangitis have a favourable long term prognosis. Gut. 2002;51:731–5.
12. Angulo P, Maor-Kendler Y, Lindor KD. Small-duct primary sclerosing cholangitis: a long-term follow-up study. Hepatology. 2002;35:1494–500.
13. Broomé U, Glaumann H, Lindstom E et al. Natural history and outcome in 32 Swedish patients with small duct primary sclerosing cholangitis (PSC). J Hepatol. 2002;36:586–9.
14. Chapman RW. Small duct primary sclerosing cholangitis. J Hepatol. 2002;36:692–4.
15. Wiesner RH, Grambsch PM, Dickson ER et al. Primary sclerosing cholangitis: natural history, prognostic factors and survival analysis. Hepatology. 1989;10:430–6.

16. Farrant JM, Hayllar KM, Wilkinson ML et al. Natural history and prognostic variables in primary sclerosing cholangitis. Gastroenterology. 1991;100:1710–17.
17. Ismail T, Angrisani L, Powell JE et al. Primary sclerosing cholangitis: surgical options, prognostic variables and outcome. Br J Surg. 1991;78:564–7.
18. Dickson ER, Murtaugh PA, Wiesner RH et al. Primary sclerosing cholangitis: refinement and validation of survival models. Gastroenterology. 1992;103:1893–901.
19. Schrumpf E, Abdelnoor M, Fausa O, Elgjo K, Jenssen E, Kolmannskog F. Risk factors in primary sclerosing cholangitis. J Hepatol. 1994;21:1061–6.
20. Broomé U, Olsson R, Loof L et al. Natural history and prognostic factors in 305 Swedish patients with primary sclerosing cholangitis. Gut. 1996;38:610–15.
21. Okolicsanyi L, Fabris L, Viaggi S, Carulli N, Podda M, Ricci G. Primary sclerosing cholangitis: clinical presentation, natural history and prognostic variables: an Italian multicentre study. The Italian PSC Study Group. Eur J Gastroenterol Hepatol. 1996;8:685–91.
22. Kim WR, Therneau TM, Wiesner RH et al. A revised natural history model for primary sclerosing cholangitis. Mayo Clin Proc. 2000;75:688–94.
23. Boberg KM, Rocca G, Egeland T et al. Time-dependent Cox regression model is superior in prediction of prognosis in primary sclerosing cholangitis. Hepatology. 2002;35:652–7.
24. Ponsioen CY, Vrouenraets SM, Prawirodirdjo W et al. Natural history of primary sclerosing cholangitis and prognostic value of cholangiography in a Dutch population. Gut. 2002;51:562–6.
25. Craig DA, MacCarty RL, Wiesner RH, Grambsch PM, LaRusso NF. Primary sclerosing cholangitis: value of cholangiography in determining the prognosis. Am J Roentgenol. 1991;157:959–64.
26. Olsson RG, Asztely MS. Prognostic value of cholangiography in primary sclerosing cholangitis. Eur J Gastroenterol Hepatol. 1995;7:251–4.
27. Christensen E. Multivariate survival analysis using Cox's regression model. Hepatology. 1987;7:1346–58.
28. Shetty K, Rybicki L, Carey WD. The Child–Pugh classification as a prognostic indicator for survival in primary sclerosing cholangitis. Hepatology. 1997;25:1049–53.
29. Christensen E. Prognostic models in chronic liver disease: validity, usefulness and future role. J Hepatol. 1997;26:1414–24.
30. Liden H, Norrby J, Gabel M, Friman S, Olausson M. Outcome after liver transplantation for primary sclerosing cholangitis. Transplant Proc. 2001;33:2452–3.
31. Wiesner RH. Liver transplantation for primary sclerosing cholangitis: timing, outcome, impact of inflammatory bowel disease and recurrence of disease. Best Pract Res Clin Gastroenterol. 2001;15:667–80.
32. Christensen E. Primary biliary cirrhosis (PBC) and primary sclerosing cholangitis (PSC), which treatments are of value? (IASL-EASL postgraduate course 2002, Madrid, Spain). In: Shouval D, editor. Prevention and Intervention in Liver Disease. Switzerland: Kenes International, 2002:151–60. Website edition: http://www.easl.ch/PGC/Erik%20Christensen.pdf
33. Neuberger J, Gunson B, Komolmit P, Davies MH, Christensen E. Pretransplant prediction of prognosis after liver transplantation in primary sclerosing cholangitis using a Cox regression model. Hepatology. 1999;29:1375–9.
34. Christensen E, Gunson B, Neuberger J. Optimal timing of liver transplantation for patients with primary biliary cirrhosis: use of prognostic modeling. J Hepatol. 1999;30:285–92.
35. Chianciano concensus conference on prognostic studies in hepatology. Ital J Gastroenterol Hepatol. 1998;30:580–3.
36. Orlandi F, Christensen E. A consensus conference on prognostic studies in hepatology. J Hepatol. 1999;30:171–2.
37. Boberg KM, Spurkland A, Rocca G et al. The HLA-DR3, DQ2 heterozygous genotype is associated with an accelerated progression of primary sclerosing cholangitis. Scand J Gastroenterol. 2001;36:886–90.

Section VII
Primary sclerosing cholangitis –
an autoimmune disease?

24
Is primary sclerosing cholangitis an autoimmune disease?

J. M. VIERLING

INTRODUCTION

Neither the aetiology nor the pathogenetic mechanisms of primary sclerosing cholangitis (PSC) have been defined. Both autoimmune and non-autoimmune pathogenetic mechanisms have been postulated to explain the histopathological changes associated with diffuse strictures found in PSC and in the secondary causes of sclerosing cholangitis[1]. The concept of PSC as an autoimmune disease is based on the finding of strong associations with HLA haplotypes, the presence of autoantibodies and the association with inflammatory bowel disease (IBD) in ≥70% of patients. Although the strong association of PSC with IBD, especially ulcerative colitis, provides circumstantial support for an autoimmunopathogenesis in PSC, several features of PSC differ from those of classic autoimmunity (Table 1).

GENDER

Classic autoimmune diseases preferentially afflict females. In contrast, 60–70% of patients with PSC are male.

HLA ASSOCIATIONS

Molecular genotyping has identified three extended haplotypes associated with susceptibility that have a leucine at position 38 of the DRβ polypeptide[2]. Importantly, ulcerative colitis is not associated with these HLA haplotypes. Two additional haplotypes are strongly associated with resistance to developing PSC. In addition, HLA alleles and haplotypes may also be associated with risk of disease progression and clinical features. As observed in other autoimmune

Table 1 Comparison of classic autoimmune diseases and PSC

Feature	Classic autoimmunity	PSC
Autoantibodies or cell-mediated immunity to defined autoantigen(s)	Yes	No
Disease-specific autoantigenic epitopes	Yes	No
Production of disease in animals by adoptive transfer of autoantibody or self-reactive inflammatory cells	Yes	No
Induction of disease in animals by immunization with specific autoantigens	Yes	No
Production of autoreactive T cells or autoantibodies in animals immunized with specific autoantigens	Yes	No
Female predilection of human disease	Yes	No
Affliction of children and adults	Yes	Yes
Strong HLA associations	Yes	Yes
Autoantibodies	Yes	Yes
Associated autoimmune diseases	Yes	Yes*
Response to immunosuppression	Yes	No

* Inflammatory bowel disease and autoimmune hepatitis.

diseases, immunoregulatory genes encoded outside of the MHC may also contribute to susceptibility, severity or progression.

AUTOANTIBODIES

Between 26% and 88% of PSC patients with or without IBD have perinuclear staining of antineutrophil cytoplasmic antibodies (pANCA)[3]. Typical pANCA are not specific for PSC, but are also found with a frequency of 60–87% in ulcerative colitis, 5–25% in Crohn's disease, 50–96% in type I autoimmune hepatitis and 5% in primary biliary cirrhosis. Because atypical pANCA react with antigens localized in the periphery of the nucleus, the term peripheral antineutrophil nuclear antibodies (pANNA) has been proposed. The molecular identity of the antigens recognized by pANNA remains unknown; thus no PSC-specific autoantigen(s) have been detected. Evidence that bacterial antigens are essential for the development of colitis and pANCA in T-cell receptor α 'knockout' mice suggests that bacteria may also induce pANNA in PSC. Crossreactivity of pANCA with bacterial antigens is consistent with evidence that 81% of PSC patients have antibodies against enterobacterial proteins. Indeed, bacterial/permeability-increasing protein (BPI), a LPS-binding neutrophil leucocyte-granular protein with antibacterial and anti-endotoxin activity, has been proposed as the target antigen for ANCA in PSC, IBD, cystic fibrosis and vasculitis. Multiple other non-species- and non-organ-specific autoantibodies are also found in PSC, including antinuclear antibodies (ANA), smooth muscle antibodies (SMA), and antimitochondrial antibodies (AMA), anticardiolipin, antithyroperoxidase, antithyroglobulin, and rheumatoid factor[4]. However, their role in pathogenesis is unknown. Anticolon autoantibodies have been identified in PSC that crossreact with hepatobiliary tissues[5]. These findings suggest that immune responses could be directed against shared antigens and colonic and biliary epithelia.

IMMUNOPATHOLOGY

Portal inflammation in PSC is composed of increased neutrophils, CD4 T cells, macrophages and decreased proportions of natural killer (NK) cells compared to peripheral blood[1]. Peribiliary CD8 cytotoxic T lymphocytes (CTL) are infrequently identified in precirrhotic biopsies. The failure of biliary epithelial cells (BEC) to concomitantly express class II HLA and ICAM-1 suggests that only a minority of BEC might present antigen or be targets for CTL. This is in accord with the observation that direct CTL destruction of the biliary epithelia (non-suppurative destructive cholangitis) is not a feature of PSC. Recent studies of T-cell lines obtained from common bile duct specimens of PSC patients indicated an oligoclonal T-cell antigen receptor (TCR), suggesting reactivity to a limited number of antigens[6]. The fact that MadCAM-1, an adhesion molecule important for the homing of T cells to the gut, is aberrantly expressed by hepatic endothelial cells in IBD and PSC may explain the adhesion of gut-derived $\alpha_4\beta_7$ integrin-positive T cells[7]. Evidence that peribiliary capillary plexi surrounding each bile duct are pushed away from the ducts as concentric fibrosis progresses indicates that fibrogenesis emanates from the ducts and that arterial ischaemia is a secondary event[8].

IMMUNOPATHOGENESIS

Recently we hypothesized that BEC responding to bacterial pathogen-associated molecular patterns (e.g. lipopolysaccharide (LPS), peptidoglycan polysaccharide) and proinflammatory cytokines (interleukin 1β, interferon gamma, tumour necrosis factor alpha), secrete chemokines and cytokines that chemoattract, activate and promote the particular periportal inflammation conducive to periductular fibrogenesis[9]. This hypothesis is supported by a rat model of small bowel bacterial overgrowth, and is also consistent with immunogenetic studies showing that the class III HLA TNFA2 allele predisposes to PSC and evidence of LPS accumulation in the BEC of patients with PSC. An instigating role for bacterial components in the pathogenesis of PSC fits well with the data, indicating that antigens recognized by pANCA may be crossreactive with bacteria. Of interest, the chemokines expressed by BEC in PSC include interleukin 8, which may promote a peribiliary cytokine milieu conducive to generation of concentric fibrosis.

CONCLUSIONS

Available evidence supports the concept that immunogenetically susceptible males with ulcerative colitis are at highest risk of developing PSC. The absence of key features of classical autoimmunity in PSC argues against it being an autoimmune disease. An alternative explanation involves the interaction between the innate immune response of macrophages and BEC and its influence on the magnitude and polarity of the adaptive immune response.

References

1. Vierling JM. Hepatobiliary complications of ulcerative colitis and Crohn's disease. In: Zakim D, Boyer TD, editors. Hepatology. Philadelphia: Saunders, 2002:1221–72.
2. Donaldson PT, Norris S. Immunogenetics in PSC. Best Pract Res Clin Gastroenterol. 2001;15: 611–27.
3. Terjung B, Worman HJ. Anti-neutrophil antibodies in primary sclerosing cholangitis. Best Pract Res Clin Gastroenterol. 2001;15:629–42.
4. Angulo P, Peter JB, Gershwin ME et al. Serum autoantibodies in patients with primary sclerosing cholangitis. J Hepatol. 2000;32:182–7.
5. Mandal A, Dasgupta A, Jeffers L et al. Autoantibodies in sclerosing cholangitis against a shared peptide in biliary and colon epithelium. Gastroenterology. 1994;106:185–92.
6. Probert CS, Christ AD, Saubermann LJ et al. Analysis of human common bile duct-associated T cells: evidence for oligoclonality, T cell clonal persistence, and epithelial cell recognition. J Immunol. 1997;158:1941–8.
7. Grant AJ, Lalor PF, Hubscher SG, Briskin M, Adams DH. MAdCAM-1 expressed in chronic inflammatory liver disease supports mucosal lymphocyte adhesion to hepatic endothelium (MAdCAM-1 in chronic inflammatory liver disease). Hepatology. 2001;33:1065–72.
8. Washington K, Clavien PA, Killenberg P. Peribiliary vascular plexus in primary sclerosing cholangitis and primary biliary cirrhosis. Hum Pathol. 1997;28:791–5.
9. Vierling JM, Braun M, Wang H. Immunopathogenesis of vanishing bile duct syndromes. In: Alpini G, Alvaro D, LeSage G, LaRusso N, editors. Pathophysiology of the Biliary Epithelia. Georgetown, Texas: Landes Bioscience/Eurekah.com, 2003:349–75.

25
Autoimmune markers and their role in the pathogenesis of primary sclerosing cholangitis

I. G. McFARLANE

INTRODUCTION

Primary sclerosing cholangitis (PSC) is a chronic cholestatic disease manifest by progressive inflammation and fibrosis of the intrahepatic and/or extrahepatic bile ducts, resulting in characteristic beading and stricturing of the biliary tree which can usually be visualized by cholangiography[1,2]. The pathogenesis of PSC remains unknown but it is thought to be autoimmune. Part of the evidence for an autoimmune diathesis comes from the observation that the condition is strongly associated with ulcerative colitis and other extrahepatic disorders which are thought to have an immunological basis[3]. In common with several autoimmune diseases it is also associated with inheritance of the HLA B8 and DR3 allotypes, and a number of extended HLA haplotypes have been identified which appear to define susceptibility or resistance to the condition[4]. Additionally, PSC shares some serological and morphological features with autoimmune hepatitis (AIH)[5], especially in children[6], to an extent that an overlapping syndrome of AIH with PSC is well recognized[7–11]. In particular, hypergamma-globulinaemia due mainly to elevations in serum IgM and IgG concentrations, as well as a high frequency of a wide range of tissue autoantibodies (Table 1), are frequent findings[12–14]. Other abnormalities include high levels of circulating immune complexes and complement activation[15]. The hypergammaglobulin-aemia, immune complexes and complement activation are relatively non-specific markers of an inflammatory process and the HLA associations are discussed elsewhere in this volume. The present discussion will therefore focus on the question of whether any of the various autoantibodies plays a patho-genetic role.

Table 1 Autoantibodies in primary sclerosing cholangitis

Frequent*	Rare or absent
Antinuclear (ANA)	Anti-liver–kidney type 1 (anti-LKM1)
Anti-smooth muscle (SMA)	Anti-liver cytosolic antigen 1 (anti-LC1)
Antineutrophil cytoplasmic antibodies (ANCA)	Anti-SLA/LP†
Anti-cardiolipin	Antimitochondrial (AMA)
Anti-endothelial cell	
Anti-colon	
Anti-thyroid	
Rheumatoid factor	

* Frequencies vary widely between different studies, from about 20% to greater than 90%.
† Anti-SLA/LP (anti-soluble liver antigen/liver–pancreas antigen) has not been reported in uncomplicated PSC but has been found in up to 40% of patients with PSC/AIH overlap syndrome (see text).

ANTINUCLEAR, CYTOSKELETAL, MICROSOMAL, LIVER CYTOSOLIC, AND MITOCHONDRIAL AUTOANTIBODIES

Antinuclear (ANA) and anti-smooth muscle (SMA) autoantibodies occur, mainly at modest titres (1:40–1:80), in between 20% and 70% of patients with PSC[13,14,16]. The reasons for the wide variability between different studies are not clear. In many patients the ANA give the 'homogeneous' immunofluorescent pattern of staining of nuclei which is typical of ANA in systemic lupus erythematosus and in AIH, and which reflects reactivities with double-stranded DNA or histones, or both. However, as in AIH, other staining patterns (nuclear dot, centromeric, nucleolar, peripheral) reflecting reactivities with other nuclear antigens are also frequently observed, although the different patterns appear not to have any clinical significance in either disease[17,18]. It is presumed that the SMA in PSC, as in AIH and other conditions[19], react with a variety of cytoskeletal components including intermediate filaments[16] but no detailed studies of their specificities appear to have been undertaken.

Autoantibodies against liver microsomal and cytosolic components seem to be very rare in PSC. In particular, type 1 liver–kidney microsomal antibodies (anti-LKM1) which react with the cytochrome P4502D6 isoform and which characterize so-called type 2 AIH[20,21] have not been found, apart from very occasionally in children with the PSC/AIH overlap syndrome termed 'autoimmune sclerosing cholangitis'[22]. Similarly, an autoantibody reacting with a liver cytosolic antigen (LC1), which has been identified as formiminotransferase cyclodeaminase and which is also associated with type 2 AIH, has not been reported in PSC[23–25]. The recently described anti-SLA/LP autoantibody, which reacts with a UGA suppressor serine tRNA–protein complex and has a high degree of specificity for AIH[26–29], seems not to occur in uncomplicated PSC but has been reported in up to 40% of patients with PSC/AIH overlap syndrome[26,29,30,31]. Antimitochondrial antibodies, particularly the M2 subtype that targets epitopes on the pyruvate dehydrogenase complex and which is characteristic of primary biliary cirrhosis

(PBC), also seem to be rare in PSC. Indeed, their presence should raise doubts about the diagnosis.

ANTINEUTROPHIL AUTOANTIBODIES

Antineutrophil cytoplasmic antibodies (ANCA) are the autoantibodies that are most frequently associated with PSC. These are a heterogeneous group of autoantibodies reacting with proteins in neutrophils (and less frequently in monocytes) which were first described in patients with various vasculitic disorders such as Wegener's granulomatosis, segmental necrotizing glomerulonephritis and microscopic polyangiitis. Two staining patterns obtained by immunofluorescence on ethanol-fixed neutrophils provide the basis for the classification of ANCA: diffuse cytoplasmic staining characterizing cANCA, and a rim-like staining of the perinuclear cytoplasm defining pANCA[32-34]. The ANCA staining patterns can usually be distinguished from those given by other autoantibodies (such as antimitochondrial or antinuclear antibodies) by the absence of staining on other cell types. The cANCA pattern is due to reactivities with proteins in azurophilic granules, particularly with proteinase 3 which is a prominent enzyme in the granules. Myeloperoxidase appears to be a major target of classical pANCA but reactivities with a wide range of other proteins, including azurocidin, catalase, cathepsin G, elastase, enolase, and lactoferrin have also been identified[33-35] (Table 2). However, some investigators have failed to find reactivities with myeloperoxidase or elastase[36] and the identification of some of these targets may be complicated by the simultaneous presence of cANCA in pANCA-positive sera. Other reported ANCA targets include the smooth muscle protein actin[37], bactericidal/permeability-increasing protein (BPI)[38], and human lysosomal-associated protein 2 (h-lamp-2)[14,39].

The classical pANCA pattern is an artefact of the ethanol fixation, caused by migration of strongly cationic cytoplasmic proteins (such as myeloperoxidase) to the negatively charged nuclear membrane, and the staining reverts to a cytoplasmic pattern when pANCA-positive sera are tested on neutrophils fixed with crosslinking agents such as formaldehyde[33]. A third type of ANCA, so-called 'atypical pANCA' or 'xANCA', has recently been identified. In contrast to classical

---

Table 2 Some of the reported antigenic targets* of antineutrophil cytoplasmic antibodies (ANCA)

Actin	Elastase
Alpha-enolase	h-lamp-2‡
Azurocidin	Lactoferrin
BPI†	Lysozyme
Beta-glucuronidase	Myeloperoxidase
Catalase	Nuclear membrane proteins
Cathepsin G	Proteinase 3

* The frequencies of reactivities of ANCA with the various antigens vary widely between different studies (see text).
† Bactericidal/permeability-increasing protein.
‡ Human lysosomal-associated protein 2.

pANCA, the perinuclear staining shown by these atypical pANCA is retained on formalin-fixed neutrophils. They appear to react with nuclear lamina components[40,41], and it has been suggested that they should be more correctly described as perinuclear neutrophil antibodies (pANNA) – not to be confused with antineuronal antibodies (ANNA)[41,42].

pANCA occur in 50–90% of patients with PSC[33,34,43]. Indeed, in the context of liver disease it was previously thought that these antibodies were highly specific for PSC. However, they have since been reported in up to 96% of patients with type 1 AIH[36,44–48]. Due to differences in methodology and lack of clarity as to whether investigators are studying classical pANCA, pANNA, or total ANCA, there is some confusion around the antigenic specificities and disease associations of these antibodies[41,49]. Orth et al.[50] have studied antibodies against two presumed pANCA target antigens, enolase and catalase. Anti-enolase antibodies were found at varying frequencies in patients with PSC (27%), type 1 AIH (60%), PBC (36%), and chronic viral hepatitis (15%), but not in pANCA-positive ulcerative colitis patients who did not have PSC, and anti-enolase did not correlate with pANCA positivity. Anti-catalase was found in 60% of PSC patients and in 25% of patients with type 1 AIH, and seemed to be specific to these disorders since they were not found in the other disease groups. However, as with anti-enolase, anti-catalase did not correlate with pANCA positivity in PSC or AIH. Furthermore, in two PSC cases the sera showed a cANCA staining pattern on ethanol-fixed granulocytes[50] and the presence of cANCA in pANCA-positive PSC sera has also been observed by other investigators[43]. Two other groups of investigators have reported the finding of antibodies against another pANCA target, lactoferrin, in 25–100% of patients with PSC, AIH, PBC or 'autoimmune cholangitis' (AIH/PBC overlap syndrome) but only very rarely in patients with chronic viral hepatitis[51,52]. As with anti-enolase and anti-catalase, anti-lactoferrin antibodies did not correlate with pANCA positivity in these studies. Despite the persisting uncertainties, most investigators seem to agree that pANCA generally do not occur in type 2 AIH and are relatively rare in other liver disorders including PBC and viral hepatitis[47,48,53].

OTHER AUTOANTIBODIES

In addition to the above 'conventional' autoantibodies, a number of other autoantibodies have been described in PSC. Chapman et al.[54] reported that 62.5% of patients with PSC with ulcerative colitis had antibodies reacting with colonic epithelium. This was a significantly higher frequency than in patients with ulcerative colitis (17%) or Crohn's colitis (16%) without PSC. Anticolon antibodies were not detected in PSC patients who did not have concurrent ulcerative colitis, or in healthy subjects or in patients with PBC or extrahepatic biliary obstruction. They also noted that there was no correlation between the presence of anticolon antibodies and inheritance of the HLA-B8 allotype. Gur et al.[12] have documented the finding of anti-endothelial cell antibodies in 35% of PSC patients, while Angulo et al.[14] have recently reported finding anti-cardiolipin antibodies in 66% of a large cohort of PSC patients. In the latter study the titres of anti-cardiolipin were shown to correlate with disease severity as measured by Mayo risk scores and histological staging. This correlation was more marked for PSC patients with, than for those without, inflammatory bowel disease.

ROLE OF AUTOANTIBODIES IN THE PATHOGENESIS OF PSC

The question of whether the autoantibodies that have been described in PSC are epiphenomena secondary to tissue damage, or whether any of them play a causative role in the disease, is still unresolved. In part this is due to the very wide variability in frequencies of the various autoantibodies and of their target antigen specificities reported in different patient populations. Additionally, some studies have observed relationships between ANCA and severity of disease in PSC[36,43,50,55], while others have failed to find correlations with any disease-related parameters[46,49,56,57].

For an autoantibody to directly cause tissue damage in an organ-specific autoimmune disease it is presumed that its target antigen must fulfil the following criteria:

1. It should, by definition, be a normal component of the tissue concerned (i.e. not altered by an exogenous agent, although it is recognized that an autoimmune reaction may be triggered by an immune response to an altered antigen).
2. It should be accessible to the immune system *in vivo*, i.e. expressed on the surfaces of the cells in the target tissue.
3. It should be specific to the target tissue (or at least expressed on the surfaces of cells only in that tissue).

Whether the autoantibody should also be specific to the disease is debatable because there are examples of tissue-specific autoantibodies occurring in the absence of disease and, conversely, of some autoantibodies which do not fulfil the above criteria and which have not been shown to be directly involved in tissue damage but which are relatively disease-specific.

None of the autoantibodies discussed above fulfils all of these criteria. It is, however, possible that autoantibodies may be involved in the pathogenesis of PSC in other ways. For example, in the course of their studies on catalase as a target of ANCA, Orth et al.[50] found that PSC sera showed granular cytoplasmic immunofluorescent staining of human gall bladder epithelial cells, which partially co-localized with staining by anti-catalase antibodies and which could be partially abrogated by absorption of the sera with purified catalase. They suggested that, since catalase prevents free radical cell damage, anti-catalase autoantibodies might contribute to the pathogenesis of PSC by diminishing the protective effect of the enzyme, and that this might result in increased oxidative stress leading to ischaemic injury to bile ducts. On the other hand, Angulo et al.[14] noted that many of their PSC patients with anti-cardiolipin antibodies (see above) also had antibodies reacting with two ANCA target antigens, proteinase-3 (in 44%) and BPI (in 29%), although (in contrast to anti-cardiolipin) these did not correlate with severity of disease. The investigators suggested that, since anti-proteinase-3 and anti-BPI are also frequently found in patients with vasculitis, these findings may implicate vascular damage in the pathogenesis of PSC – a view supported by the previous observation (see above) that there is a high prevalence of anti-endothelial cell antibodies in patients with PSC[12].

IMMUNE REACTIONS TO BILIARY TRACT ANTIGENS

Logically, it might be expected that the most important targets of autoreactions that could damage the biliary system would be antigens expressed on cells of the biliary tract, but evidence of such autoreactions is very limited. In the 1960s there were reports of antibodies detected in the sera of patients with various chronic liver diseases that reacted with bile canaliculi or with bile ducts[58,59], but these were generally thought to be artefacts[60] and were not subjected to detailed investigation until the late 1970s, when studies were undertaken in our institute to attempt to identify putative targets of autoimmune reactions in patients with biliary diseases[61]. On the presumption that biliary tract antigens might be shed in bile, proteins were purified from pooled normal human bile. Two components were found which were distinct from plasma proteins and, by immunofluorescent staining of sections of normal human liver with monospecific animal antisera raised against these proteins, it was determined that one appeared to be derived from the bile canalicular portions of hepatocellular membranes and the other from bile duct epithelial cells[61]. Using the leucocyte migration inhibition test it was found that 80% of patients with PSC had circulating T lymphocytes that appeared to recognize these two antigens (Figure 1). A similar proportion of PBC patients showed responses to the antigens, and preliminary evidence was obtained that PBC patients also had serum autoantibodies reacting with the antigens, but PSC sera were not tested in that study[62]. Unfortunately, the technology did not exist at that time to pursue these investigations further. The studies were abandoned and the identities of the antigens remain unknown.

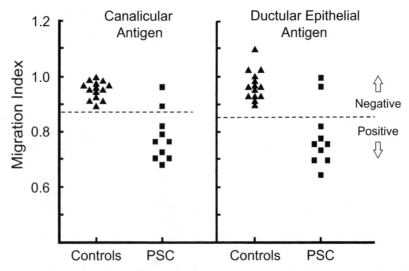

Figure 1 Results of leucocyte migration inhibition tests with peripheral blood mononuclear cells from healthy control subjects and patients with primary sclerosing cholangitis (PSC) against bile canalicular and ductular epithelial antigens. Broken lines indicate the lower normal limits for the test (2 SD below the mean migration indices observed in the control subjects). Values below these lines indicate positive T-cell responses to the antigens

Subsequently, in the course of investigating antibodies reacting with colonic epithelium in ulcerative colitis and PSC, Chapman and colleagues[54] observed that 38% of PSC sera showed immunofluorescent staining of structures in the portal tracts of liver sections from patients with extrahepatic biliary obstruction. These 'portal tract' antibodies were shown to be distinct from anticolon antibodies. Although the investigators could not be certain, the stained structures appeared to be proliferating bile ducts, but the target antigen was not identified. In contrast to the findings of Orth et al.[50] discussed above, no staining of gall bladder epithelium was observed.

Recently, investigators at the Karolinska Institute in Sweden have reported finding autoantibodies against isolated normal human biliary epithelial cells (BEC) in the sera of 63% of PSC patients[63]. Anti-BEC antibodies were also found in 37% of PBC and 16% of AIH patients studied but not in patients with rheumatic disorders. The antibodies in PSC sera were found to react with a 40 kDa component of BEC membranes which was not recognized by anti-BEC in PBC or AIH sera, but the identity of this component has not yet been determined. An intriguing observation was that binding of anti-BEC to the cells induced expression of the cell adhesion molecule CD44, which is the lymphocyte homing receptor that promotes T cell activation and migration of memory and effector cells to sites of inflammation[64]. Binding of the antibodies to BEC also induced production of high levels of the proinflammatory cytokine IL-6. Since IL-6 reportedly has profibrogenic effects, the investigators have suggested that persistent induction of this cytokine by anti-BEC antibodies might contribute to uncontrolled proliferation and fibrosis, leading to the fibro-obliterative inflammation of the biliary tract in PSC.

CONCLUSIONS

The existence and high prevalence of a wide range of markers of inflammation and autoimmunity in PSC strongly support the concept that the disease has a basis in loss of self-tolerance. However, the available evidence does not suggest that any of the 'conventional' markers of autoimmunity is directly involved in bile duct damage in the condition, although some might contribute to this indirectly. The continuing, but very sporadic, reports of autoreactions that are more particularly directed at antigens related to the biliary tract which have appeared over many years would seem to be more relevant to understanding the pathogenesis of PSC, and this should be a fruitful area for further research.

References

1. Talwalker JA, Lindor KD. Sclerosing cholangitis. Curr Opin Gastroenterol. 2002;18:372–7.
2. Björnsson E, Chapman RW. Sclerosing cholangitis. Curr Opin Gastroenterol. 2003;19:270–5.
3. Saarinen S, Olerup O, Broome U. Increased frequency of autoimmune diseases in patients with primary sclerosing cholangitis. Am J Gastroenterol. 2000;95:3195–9.
4. Donaldson PT, Norris S. Evaluation of the role of MHC class II alleles, haplotypes and selected amino acid sequences in primary sclerosing cholangitis. Autoimmunity. 2002;35:555–64.
5. International Autoimmune Hepatitis Group report: Review of criteria for diagnosis of autoimmune hepatitis. J Hepatol. 1999;31:929–38.
6. Mieli-Vergani G, Vergani D. Autoimmune hepatitis in children. Clin Liver Dis. 2002;6:335–46.

7. McNair ANB, Moloney M, Portmann BC, Williams R, McFarlane IG. Autoimmune hepatitis overlapping with primary sclerosing cholangitis in five cases. Am J Gastroenterol. 1998;93:777–84.
8. Van Buuren HR, van Hoogstraten HJF, Terkivatan T, Schalm SW, Veggaar FP. High prevalence of autoimmune hepatitis among patients with primary sclerosing cholangitis. J Hepatol. 2000;33:543–8.
9. Dienes HP, Erberich H, Dries V, Schirmacher P, Lohse A. Autoimmune hepatitis and overlap syndromes. Clin Liver Dis. 2002;6:349–62.
10. Muratori L, Cassani F, Guidi M et al. The hepatitic/cholestatic 'overlap' syndrome: an Italian experience. Autoimmunity. 2002;35:565–8.
11. Heathcote J. Variant syndromes of autoimmune hepatitis. Clin Liver Dis. 2002;6:381–96.
12. Gur H, Shen G, Sutjita M et al. Autoantibody profile of primary sclerosing cholangitis. Pathobiology. 1995;63:76–82.
13. Boberg KM, Fausa O, Haaland T et al. Features of autoimmune hepatitis in primary sclerosing cholangitis: an evaluation of 114 primary sclerosing cholangitis patients according to a scoring system for the diagnosis of autoimmune hepatitis. Hepatology. 1996;23:1369–76.
14. Angulo P, Peter JB, Gershwin ME et al. Serum autoantibodies in patients with primary sclerosing cholangitis. J Hepatol. 2000;32:182–7.
15. Senaldi G, Donaldson PT, Magrin S et al. Activation of the complement system in primary sclerosing cholangitis. Gastroenterology. 1989;97:1430–4.
16. Zauli D, Schrumpf E, Crespi C, Cassani F, Fausa O, Aadland E. An autoantibody profile in primary sclerosing cholangitis. J Hepatol. 1987;5:14–18.
17. Czaja AJ, Cassani F, Cataleta M, Valentini P, Bianchi FB. Antinuclear antibodies and patterns of nuclear immunofluorescence in type 1 autoimmune hepatitis. Dig Dis Sci. 1997;42:1688–96.
18. Nishioka M, Morshed SA, Parveen S, Ming C. Heterogeneity of antinuclear antibodies in autoimmune liver diseases. In: Krawitt EL, Wiesner RH, Nishioka M, editors. Autoimmune Liver Diseases, 2nd edn. Amsterdam: Elsevier, 1998:179–216.
19. Dighiero G, Lymberi P, Monot C, Abuaf N. Sera with high levels of anti-smooth muscle and anti-mitochondrial antibodies frequently bind to cytoskeletal proteins. Clin Exp Immunol. 1990;82:52–6.
20. Geuguen M, Boniface O, Bernard O et al. Identification of the main epitope on human cytochrome P450 IID6 recognized by anti-liver kidney microsome antibody. J Autoimmun. 1991;4:607–15.
21. Vergani D. LKM antibody: getting in some target practice. Gut. 2000;46:449–50.
22. Gregorio GV, Portmann B, Karani J et al. Autoimmune hepatitis/sclerosing cholangitis overlap syndrome in childhood: a 16-year prospective study. Hepatology. 2001;33:544–53.
23. Han S, Tredger M, Gregorio GV et al. Anti-liver cytosolic antigen type 1 (LC1) antibodies in childhood autoimmune liver disease. Hepatology. 1995;21:58–62.
24. Muratori L, Cataleta M, Muratori P et al. Liver/kidney microsomal antibody type 1 and liver cytosol antibody type 1 concentration in type 2 autoimmune hepatitis. Gut. 1998;42:721–6.
25. Lapierre P, Hajoui O, Homberg J-C, Alvarez F. Formiminotransferase cyclodeaminase is an organ-specific autoantigen recognized by sera of patients with autoimmune hepatitis. Gastroenterology. 1999;116:643–9.
26. Wies I, Brunner S, Henninger J et al. Identification of target antigen for SLA/LP autoantibodies in autoimmune hepatitis. Lancet. 2000;355:1510–15.
27. Costa M, Rodriguez-Sanchez JL, Czaja AJ, Gelpi C. Isolation and characterization of cDNA encoding the antigenic protein of the human tRNP[(Ser)Sec] complex recognized by autoantibodies from patients with type-1 autoimmune hepatitis. Clin Exp Immunol. 2000;121:364–74.
28. Volkmann M, Martin L, Baurle A et al. Soluble liver antigen: isolation of a 35-kd recombinant protein (SLA-p35) specifically recognizing sera from patients with autoimmune hepatitis. Hepatology. 2001;33:591–6.
29. Ma Y, Okamoto M, Thomas MG et al. Antibodies to conformational epitopes of soluble liver antigen define a severe form of autoimmune liver disease. Hepatology. 2002;35:658–64.
30. Ballot E, Homberg JC, Johanet C. Antibodies to soluble liver antigen: an additional marker in type 1 autoimmune hepatitis. J Hepatol. 2000;33:208–15.
31. Baeres M, Herkel J, Czaja AJ et al. Establishment of standardised SLA/LP immunoassays: specificity for autoimmune hepatitis, worldwide occurrence, and clinical characteristics. Gut. 2002;51:259–64.

32. Kallenberg CGM, Brouwer E, Weening JJ, Cohen Tervaert JW. Anti-neutrophil cytoplasmic antibodies: current diagnostic and pathophysiological potential. Kidney Int. 1994;46:1–15.
33. Semrad CE, Terjung B, Worman HJ. Antineutrophil cytoplasmic and other autoantibodies in primary sclerosing cholangitis. In: Krawitt EL, Wiesner RH, Nishioka M, editors. Autoimmune Liver Diseases, 2nd edn. Amsterdam: Elsevier, 1998:305–20.
34. Terjung B, Worman HJ. 'ANCA' in liver diseases. In: Manns MP, Paumgartner G, Leuschner U, editors. Immunology and Liver. London: Kluwer, 2000:137–51.
35. Lindgren S, Nilsson S, Nassberger L et al. Anti-neutrophil cytoplasmic antibodies in patients with chronic liver diseases: prevalence, antigen specificity and predictive value for diagnosis of autoimmune liver disease. J Gastroenterol Hepatol. 2000;15:437–42.
36. Mulder AHL, Horst G, Haagsma EB, Limburg PC, Kleibeuker JH, Kallenberg CGM. Prevalence and characterization of neutrophil cytoplasmic antibodies in autoimmune liver disease. Hepatology. 1993;17:411–17.
37. Orth T, Gerken G, Kellner R, Meyer zum Buschenfelde KH, Mayet WJ. Actin is a target antigen of anti-neutrophil cytoplasmic antibodies (ANCA) in autoimmune hepatitis type-1. J Hepatol. 1997;26:37–47.
38. Schultz H, Weiss J, Carroll SF, Gross WL. The endotoxin-binding bactericidal/permeability-increasing protein (BPI): a target of autoantibodies. J Leukocyte Biol. 2001;69:505–12.
39. Kain R, Matsui K, Exner M et al. A novel class of antigens of anti-neutrophil cytoplasmic antibodies in necrotizing and crescentric glomerulonephritis: the lysosomal membrane glycoprotein h-lamp-2 in neutrophil granulocytes and a related membrane protein in glomerular endothelial cells. J Exp Med. 1995;181:585–97.
40. Terjung B, Herzog V, Worman HJ et al. Atypical antineutrophil cytoplasmic antibodies with perinuclear fluorescence in chronic inflammatory bowel diseases and hepatobiliary disorders colocalize with nuclear lamina proteins. Hepatology. 1998;28:332–240.
41. Terjung B, Worman HJ, Herzog V et al. Differentiation of antineutrophil nuclear antibodies in inflammatory bowel and autoimmune liver diseases from antineutrophil cytoplasmic antibodies (p-ANCA) using immunofluorescence microscopy. Clin Exp Immunol. 2001;126:37–46.
42. Terjung B, Worman HJ. Anti-neutrophil antibodies in primary sclerosing cholangitis. Best Pract Res Clin Gastroenterol. 2001;15:629–42.
43. Roozendaal C, de Jong MA, van den Berg AP et al. Clinical significance of anti-neutrophil cytoplasmic antibodies (ANCA) in autoimmune liver diseases. J Hepatol. 2000;32:734–41.
44. Hardarson S, La Brecque DR, Mitros FA, Neil GA, Goeken JA. Antineutrophil cytoplasmic antibody in inflammatory bowel and hepatobiliary diseases: high prevalence in ulcerative colitis, primary sclerosing cholangitis, and autoimmune hepatitis. Clin Microbiol Immunol. 1993;99:277–81.
45. Vidrich A, Lee J, James E, Cobb L, Targan S. Segregation of pANCA antigenic recognition by Dnase treatment of neutrophils: ulcerative colitis, type 1 autoimmune hepatitis and primary sclerosing cholangitis. J Clin Immunol. 1995;15:293–9.
46. Targan SR, Landers C, Vidrich A, Czaja AJ. High-titer antineutrophil cytoplasmic antibodies in type-1 autoimmune hepatitis. Gastroenterology. 1995;108:1159–66.
47. Bansi D, Chapman R, Fleming K. Antineutrophil cytoplasmic antibodies in chronic liver diseases: prevalence, titre, specificity and IgG subclass. J Hepatol. 1996;24:581–6.
48. Zauli D, Ghetti S, Grassi A et al. Anti-neutrophil cytoplasmic antibodies in type 1 and 2 autoimmune hepatitis. Hepatology. 1997;25:1105–7.
49. Lo SK, Fleming K. Investigation of the specific autoantigen of primary sclerosing cholangitis by Western blot and immunoprecipitation. Hepatology. 1993;18:469–70.
50. Orth T, Kellner R, Diekmann O et al. Identification and characterization of autoantibodies against catalase and α-enolase in patients with primary sclerosing cholangitis. Clin Exp Immunol. 1998;112:507–15.
51. Ohana M, Okazaki K, Hajiro K, Uchida K. Antilactoferrin antibodies in autoimmune liver diseases. Am J Gastroenterol. 1998;93:1334–9.
52. Muratori L, Muratori P, Zauli D et al. Antilactoferrin antibodies in autoimmune liver disease. Clin Exp Immunol. 2001;124:470–3.
53. Duerr RH, Targan SR, Landers CJ et al. Neutrophil cytoplasmic antibodies: a link between primary sclerosing cholangitis and ulcerative colitis. Gastroenterology. 1991;100:1385–91.
54. Chapman RW, Cottone M, Selby WS, Shepherd HA, Sherlock S, Jewell DP. Serum autoantibodies, ulcerative colitis and primary sclerosing cholangitis. Gut. 1986;27:86–91.

55. Pokorny CS, Norton ID, McCaughan GW, Selby WS. Anti-neutrophil cytoplasmic antibody: a prognostic indicator in primary sclerosing cholangitis. J Gastroenterol Hepatol. 1994;9:40–4.

56. Seibold F, Weber P, Klein R, Berg PA, Wiedmann KH. Clinical significance of antibodies against neutrophils in patients with inflammatory bowel disease and primary sclerosing cholangitis. Gut. 1992;33:657–62.

57. Schwarze C, Terjung B, Lilienweiss P et al. IgA class antineutrophil cytoplasmic antibodies in primary sclerosing cholangitis and autoimmune hepatitis. Clin Exp Immunol. 2003;133:283–9.

58. Diederichsen H. Hetero-antibody against bile canaliculi in patients with chronic, clinically active hepatitis. Acta Med Scand. 1969;186:299–302.

59. Paronetto F, Schaffner F, Popper H. Immunocytochemical and serologic observations in primary biliary cirrhosis. N Engl J Med. 1964;271:1123–8.

60. Storch WB. Autoantibodies in autoimmune hepatitis. In: Hadziselimovic F, editor. Autoimmune Diseases in Paediatric Gastroenterology. Dordrecht: Kluwer, 2002:13–21.

61. McFarlane IG, Wojcicka BM, Tsantoulas DC, Portmann BS, Eddleston ALWF, Williams R. Leukocyte migration inhibition in response to biliary antigens in primary biliary cirrhosis, sclerosing cholangitis and other chronic liver diseases. Gastroenterology. 1979;76:1333–40.

62. Amoroso P, Vergani D, Wojcicka BM et al. Identification of biliary antigens in circulating immune complexes in primary biliary cirrhosis. Clin Exp Immunol. 1980;42:95–8.

63. Xu B, Broome U, Ericzon B-G, Sumitran-Holgersson S. High frequency of autoantibodies in patients with primary sclerosing cholangitis that bind biliary epithelial cells and induce expression of CD44 and production of interleukin 6. Gut. 2002;51:120–7.

64. Cruickshank SM, Southgate J, Wyatt JI, Selby PJ, Trejdosiewicz LK. Expression of CD44 on bile ducts in primary sclerosing cholangitis and primary biliary cirrhosis. J Clin Pathol. 1999;52:730–4.

26
The HLA system and other genetic markers in primary sclerosing cholangitis

P. T. DONALDSON

INTRODUCTION

Primary sclerosing cholangitis (PSC) is a disease of unknown aetiology. However, a number of factors point to abnormal immune regulation suggesting that the disease may have an autoimmune component. Autoimmunity, an immune response to 'auto' antigen, is thought to occur in genetically susceptible individuals either *sui generis* or following infectious or toxic injury. Most common diseases have a heritable component; however, the pattern of inheritance does not fit into a classical Mendelian or sex-linked (simple) model that we would associate with single-gene disease, but is more complex.

PSC is a 'complex trait', i.e. a disease in which 'one or more genes acting alone or in concert increase or reduce the risk of disease'[1]. The disease alleles in complex traits do not by themselves cause disease, but simply increase the likelihood that under the appropriate circumstances disease will occur. The alleles may also influence the clinical phenotype (severity or progression) of the disease following onset. These two effects are not exclusive and one susceptibility allele may modify the effect of another.

Complex traits have previously been called polygenic (involving several genes) or multifactorial (involving both genes and exogenic/environmental factors). Polygenic and multifactorial diseases rarely aggregate in families and have relatively low heritability compared to single-gene diseases. Complex traits are also characterized by incomplete penetrance, whereby the presence of the disease allele does not always result in disease expression. Hence, many of the susceptibility alleles identified in complex disease are common in the unaffected 'healthy' population.

Identifying the genetic components in complex disease has been heralded as one of the major challenges of the post-genome era[2] with three objectives: (1) to improve diagnosis, (2) to provide useful prognostic indices for disease management (including the development of individualized treatment regimens based on the findings of both immunogenetic and pharmacogenetic studies), and (3) to provide insight into the pathogenesis of these (mostly) idiopathic diseases.

In this chapter I will first discuss the evidence for a genetic component in PSC, briefly update the relevant background on MHC and non-MHC genes, present an overview of the current state of knowledge of the role of HLA and non-HLA genes in PSC and discuss the implications for our understanding of the pathogenesis of PSC and for future genetic studies.

The publication of the human genome project and the accompanying technological revolution in genetics have changed for ever our understanding and approach to the genetics of human diseases. Throughout this chapter I will highlight the potential changes that we expect to see as we apply this knowledge and technology to the search for genes in PSC.

EVIDENCE FOR A GENETIC COMPONENT IN PSC

Before embarking on genetic studies in disease it is useful to gather basic data on the potential genetic risk in order to assess how heritable the disease is. The key facts that concern us are: disease prevalence and incidence, the frequency of familial clusters (though this may result from exposure to environmental risk factors in the family home), concordance rates for monozygotic and dizygotic twins and risk measurements such as the sibling relative risk (λ_s). Geographical clustering is also a useful indicator of genetic risk, but as with familial clustering it too can be an indicator of environmental exposure rather than inherited risk.

In PSC familial clusters are rare and twin data are not available; therefore it is not possible to assess the size of the heritable component in this disease. The main evidence for a genetic component in PSC comes from three observations: (1) the marked male preponderance, (2) the apparent rarity of the disease outside northern Europe and North America, and (3) the common overlap with inflammatory bowel disease.

INVESTIGATING PSC GENETICS

The genetic contribution to any disease may be assessed either through linkage or association studies. Both approaches have advantages and limitations. Linkage analysis is always the preferred first choice, being comprehensive, but may have low sensitivity in terms of statistical power.

In diseases with low heritability and/or late onset (caveats which are particularly applicable to PSC), finding sufficient numbers of such families for linkage analysis may be difficult, if not impossible. Consequently, studies of PSC have been restricted to association analysis and to case–control studies in particular.

The advantages of case–control studies are simplicity and sensitivity. Much larger numbers may be included in this type of study, permitting the identification of disease alleles with relatively small effects (odds ratios less than 1.5). This is particularly important, because current studies of other autoimmune diseases suggest that the genetic risk attributable to many disease alleles (especially non-MHC genes) may be very small[3].

The disadvantages of association studies have been widely aired in the genetics press[4]. The critical factor in any study is statistical power and this is directly proportional to: the number of patients and controls studied, the number of different candidate alleles assessed, and the frequency of the candidate allele in the healthy population. Apart from small sample size, other common errors in association studies include: use of poorly matched controls, analysis of multiple subgroups, over-interpretation of the data, and failure to consider race and linkage disequilibrium[4,5].

All of these problems can be addressed: appropriate controls can be recruited, power calculations to determine the necessary sample size can be performed before studies are started, and the issue of multiple testing, which is common to all analyses (not just genetic studies), can be resolved by confirming the significant associations in a second patient (and control) set[6].

CANDIDATE SELECTION OR WHERE TO LOOK IN THE GENOME

Association analysis is 'hypothesis-driven' and success depends heavily on candidate selection. Candidate genes for genetic studies are selected on the basis of: their location in the genome (if linkage data are available), prior knowledge of similar (related) diseases, knowledge of the disease pathogenesis or of the gene and its function. However, it is also important to remember that candidate genes should be both biologically and functionally relevant[5].

Aside from linkage-based candidates (which are not available in PSC) all of the above involve a degree of speculation. One means of increasing the chance of success is to consider findings from other similar diseases or syndromes. All diseases share common pathways (for example fibrosis is common to most liver diseases) and therefore we would expect only a proportion of disease alleles to be disease-specific. The remainder are non-specific promoters of disease aligned to common pathways.

To date studies in PSC have concentrated on the major histocompatibility complex (MHC) and a few isolated single-nucleotide polymorphisms (SNPs) in other immunoregulatory genes. However, with the human genome project completed, we now realize that almost all immune active proteins are encoded by polymorphic genes and the majority of this genetic variation involves SNPs. These SNPs are found throughout the human genome at frequencies of up to 1 per 1000 base pairs of DNA with a total number[7] in excess of 1.42 million. SNPs are found in the upstream promoter regions, in both coding (exons) and the non-coding regions between exons (introns). These SNPs may have a profound influence on gene transcription and protein function, but also because each amino acid can be encoded by more than one deoxyribose nucleotide triplet, and because many non-coding region SNPs are found outside the regulatory sequences, both the coding and non-coding region SNPs are frequently neutral. Future analyses will not be restricted to single polymorphisms and single genes, but will increasingly involve high-throughput technologies that are capable of screening multiple SNPs in whole pathways or encoded on specific chromosomal regions. This approach, which is more sensible in terms of our understanding of biological pathways, will also be more successful; provided of course that the numbers tested are sufficient.

LINKAGE DISEQUILIBRIUM AND HAPLOTYPES

Susceptibility attributed to a particular allele at a locus may be due to the effect of the identified allele itself, or may simply be due to linkage, and the true susceptibility allele may map elsewhere, but in close proximity to the locus in question. A confounding factor in fine-mapping susceptibility is linkage disequilibrium. Linkage disequilibrium is said to occur when two or more alleles at different loci occur together more frequently than predicted from the simple sum of their individual frequencies (i.e. they are not independently assorted according to Mendel's laws). Alleles at several loci inherited en-bloc are referred to as haplotypes. Where there is extreme linkage disequilibrium, haplotypes may span several mega-bases (Mb) of DNA. This can be problematic for geneticists trying to map disease susceptibility to a single locus, as we will see in PSC with the HLA 8.1 haplotype.

IMMUNOGENETIC STUDIES IN PSC

Immunogenetic studies in PSC have focused mostly on the genes of the MHC and particularly on the role of the human leucocyte antigen (HLA) genes (Tables 1 and 2). More recently there has been growing interest in non-MHC immunogenes in liver disease.

The human MHC

The human MHC occupies a 4 Mb segment of chromosome 6p21.3. The region contains 200-plus different genes; not all are relevant here. The biology of the MHC is frequently reviewed[8]: therefore, I will confine comments here to necessary background only. Up-to-date gene maps for the MHC and other genes

Table 1   Summary of associations with HLA haplotypes in autoimmune liver disease

Haplotype number	Haplotype	Risk ratio
1	*B8-**MICA*008**-TNF*2-DRB3*0101-**DRB1*0301**-DQB1*0201*	2.69[22]
2	*DRB3*0101-DRB1*1301-DQA1*0103-**DQB1*0603***	3.8[22]
3	*MICA*008-DRB5*0101-DRB1*1501-DQA1*0102-**DQB1*0602***	1.52[22]
4	*DRB1*0103-DRB4*0401-DQA1*03-**DQB1*0302***	0.26[22]
5	*DRB4*0103-DRB1*0701-DQA1*0201-**DQB1*0303***	0.15[22]
6	***MICA*002**	0.0–0.15[25]

All studies are based on adult cases unless otherwise marked. Protective haplotypes are tinted, and have risk values <1. Most likely primary susceptibility/resistance alleles are shown in **bold** on each haplotype. In PSC the finding of multiple susceptibility and resistance haplotypes indicates a complex relationship with the MHC. The evidence indicates at least two potential MHC-encoded susceptibility alleles, one of which resides in the class II DR–DQ region and the other closer to the *HLA* B, but not the A locus, for which *MICA* is the current primary candidate.

Table 2 Summary of individual HLA associations in PSC

Allele/genotype	Frequency in PSC	Frequency in controls	Risk ratio	Key references
A1	84/174 (48%)	51/134 (38%)	1.52	Unpublished data
Cw7 (Cw*0701)	48/93 (52%)	34/100 (34%)	2.07	47
B8	86/174 (49%)	33/134 (25%)	3.0	Unpublished data
TNFA2 (−308G allele)	58/110 (58%)	37/126 (29%)	3.35	34
DRB1*0301	70/148 (47%)	35/134 (26%)	2.54	22
DRB1*04	23/148 (16%)	54/134 (40%)	0.27	22
DRB1*0401	14/148 (9%)	31/134 (23%)	0.35	22
DRB1*0701	21/148 (14%)	37/134 (27%)	0.43	22
DRB1*1301	31/148 (22%)	17/134 (13%)	1.82	22
DRB1*1501	42/148 (28%)	27/134 (20%)	1.57	22
MICA*008/MICA*008	65/112 (58%)	26/121 (22%)	4.51–5.51	25
MICA*002	2/112 (2%)	41/121 (34%)	0.00–0.15	25
DRB1*0301/DRB1*0301	23/148 (16%)	4/134 (3%)	5.98	22
DRB1*0301/DRB1*1501	13/148 (9%)	3/134 (2%)	4.2	22

All studies are based on adult cases unless otherwise marked. Protective alleles/genotypes are tinted, and have risk values <1.

referred to herein can be found at www.ensembl.org or at: www.gdb.org, and updates on nomenclature can be found at www.anthonynolan.org.uk.

The human MHC (Figure 1) is divided into three subregions; the MHC class I and class II regions encode the 'transplantation antigens' of the HLA A, B, Cw and DR, DQ and DP families, respectively, whilst the MHC class III encodes a collection of genes, some (but not all) of which are involved in immune regulation. Most of the MHC molecules exhibit a high degree of genetic polymorphism; for example, there are currently more than 1000 different internationally recognized human leucocyte antigen (HLA) sequences.

The human leucocyte antigens

HLA class I and class II antigens are critical for T-cell immunity. HLA molecules present short antigenic peptides that are 8–9 (class I) and 13–23 (class II) amino acid residues in length for recognition by antigen-specific T cells.

MHC class I

HLA class I molecules are found on all nucleated cells and present peptides derived from endogenous antigens (i.e. those found within the cell cytoplasm) to the T-cell receptor (TCR). HLA class I, A, B and Cw genes each encode a single polypeptide; the α-chain, which forms a heterodimer by interaction with β_2-microglobulin (encoded on chromosome 15). The class I molecule has a CD8-binding site which acts as a co-recognition element in the formation of the immune synapse (MHC-peptide-TCR), and this restricts the type of cells to which HLA class I can present peptide. Because of this class I molecules are principally involved in the stimulation of CD8$^+$ T cells (cytotoxic T cells). These cells are particularly important in the recognition of viral antigens.

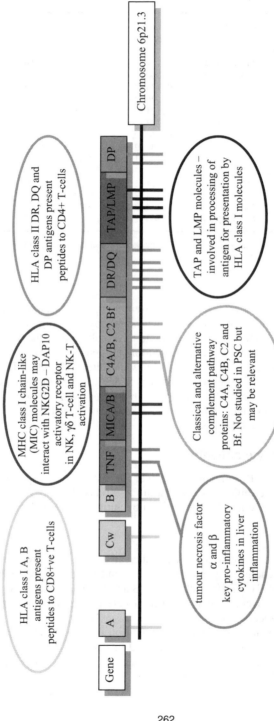

Figure 1 Key genetic components of the MHC and their main functions in immunobiology

Table 3 Arrangement of expressed *DRB* genes by *DRB1* haplotype families

DRB1 *gene family*	DRB *genes on haplotype*
DRB1*01, DRB1*08, DRB1*10	*DRB1 only*
DRB1*03, DRB1*11, DRB1*12, DRB1*13, DRB1*14	*DRB1 and DRB3*
DRB1*04, DRB1*07, DRB1*09	*DRB1 and DRB4*
DRB1*15, DRB1*16	*DRB1 and DRB5*

MHC class II

HLA class II molecules are expressed on a limited number of specialized antigen-presenting cells. Class II molecules present peptide derived from exogenous antigen (i.e. from outside the cell, but captured by endocytosis and processed internally) and are restricted by CD4 co-recognition. Consequently HLA class II molecules are predominantly involved in stimulation of CD4$^+$ helper T cells.

The organization of the HLA class II genes is more complex than that of the HLA class I genes. Firstly, although the expressed HLA class II molecules are also heterodimers, in contrast to HLA class I, both the α and β chains are encoded on chromosome 6p21.3. The α chain is encoded by the A gene and the β chain by the B gene. Second, although, as with HLA class I, there are three families of expressed HLA class II molecules DR, DQ and DP, the DR sub-region may encode more than one B gene depending on the parental haplotype (Table 3). Third, in the case of DQ and DP (but not DR), both the A and B genes exhibit extensive polymorphism.

This added level of complexity in the class II region has a major impact in PSC and complicates the interpretation of the various reported HLA associations (below).

THE RELATIONSHIP BETWEEN HLA CLASS I AND CLASS II GENE POLYMORPHISM AND DISEASE

More than 90% of the inherited variation in the HLA class I and class II genes gives rise to alleles which encode different amino sequences concentrated in the antigen-binding site of the HLA molecule[9]. Thus, different HLA alleles encode structures with different peptide-binding properties. In the competitive environment of the endoplasmic reticulum (ER) and endocytic vesicles (EV), where MHC molecules encounter antigenic peptides, those peptides with higher binding affinities and the preferred structural conformations will be selected over those with lower binding affinities and poor structural conformations. Consequently the structure of the HLA groove dictates which peptides are most likely to be bound. This forms the functional rationale for HLA-encoded disease susceptibility and resistance in complex disease, whereby inheritance of a particular HLA allele may be associated with an increased or reduced risk of disease. Not all individuals with the disease-promoting allele will develop an immune response even if the disease-generating peptide is encountered within the ER or EV. It is important also to remember that a fully heterozygous individual may have 12 or 14 (depending on *DRB1* family of the parental haplotypes, Table 3) different HLA molecules on each cell, each encoding a molecule with different peptide-binding characteristics.

MHC class III

The MHC class III region is particularly interesting in PSC; however, only two of the numerous MHC class III genes have been studied thus far, and therefore I will restrict this discourse to those two immunogenes only.

The first class III region gene to be investigated in PSC was *TNFA*. The *TNFA* gene cluster maps close to *HLA B* telomeric of the *DRB1* locus[10,11] and encodes tumour necrosis factor alpha (TNF-α). There are multiple SNPs in this gene[11], but only two have been investigated thus far. These are both SNPs in the *TNFA* gene promoter at positions −238 and −308 relative to the transcriptional start site. Although there is some evidence to suggest the *TNFA-308*G* allele is associated with higher TNF-α production[12], the functional relevance of these two SNPs remains controversial[13]. However, TNF-α production is one of the earliest events in response to liver injury, and it triggers a cascade of inflammation, cell death, and fibrosis[14]. Therefore, TNF gene polymorphism is an excellent candidate in all types of complex liver disease.

The second MHC class III gene to be investigated in PSC is that encoding the MHC class I chain-like (MIC)-α polypeptide *(MICA)*. MIC molecules are 70 000 M_r single-chain membrane-bound glycoproteins capable of interacting with γδ T cells. The MIC family consists of five members, two of which (*MICA* and *MICB*) have expressed transcripts. The *MICA* gene maps 46.4 kb centromeric of the HLA B locus and has at least 54 different alleles (www.anthonynolan.org.uk).

Although similar to HLA class I molecules, the MIC molecules do not associate with β_2-microglobulin, and they have a restricted tissue distribution, being expressed on gastrointestinal epithelium, keratinocytes, endothelial cells and monocytes. There is extensive polymorphism distributed across all three extracellular domains which is at odds with the diversity in HLA molecules, where the polymorphic sites are concentrated in three so-called 'hypervariable regions'. The *MICA* gene also includes a microsatellite or short tandem repeat (STR) in the transmembrane region. This STR encodes varying numbers of alanine residues (A4, 5, 6 and 9) and one common mutation (A5.1) includes a premature stop codon. The A5.1 STR encodes a glycoprotein with a shortened transmembrane segment and no cytoplasmic tail. This has given rise to speculation that the resulting *MICA* molecule may be unstable or even defective[15].

MIC molecules may be induced by stress and heat shock and appear to activate NK (CD56$^+$) cells and γδ T cells, through the NKG2D activatory receptor and an adaptor protein DAP10A[16]. Engagement of this receptor activates γδ and NK cell effector functions. The 'normal' liver has a large resident population of γδ T cells, NK and natural T cells (NT cells)[17], and increased numbers of γδ and NK cells have been documented in diseased livers[18,19]. Infection may provide a catalyst for heat shock and induce MIC molecules on biliary epithelium. This would lead to the activation of intrahepatic γδ and NK cells. Individuals with aberrant expression of the *MICA* gene may have either persistent immune activation leading to autoimmunity, or failed activation with the consequence of persistent infection.

Increased risk of persistent infection is relevant both in the context of infectious disease and in autoimmunity, where the persistent tissue damage may increase the likelihood of recognition of self (auto) antigens.

The MHC in PSC

There are numerous reviews of the role of MHC genes in PSC[20,21]; therefore I will be brief and concentrate on recent developments only.

All of the major studies of HLA published so far have been based on the European racial group (Tables 1 and 2). Thus far, three different HLA haplotypes have been linked with susceptibility to PSC and three with resistance (Table 1)[21–23]. As with type 1 AIH[24], MHC-encoded susceptibility is strongly linked with *DRB1*, but this alone does not explain all of the MHC associations in this disease, and although there is a general consensus regarding the basic associations, there is some considerable controversy over the interpretation of these observations. There are four possibilities to consider:

1. Susceptibility and resistance to PSC are determined by the *DRB1* locus allele on each haplotype.
2. Susceptibility and resistance are determined by one (or more) shared motifs encoded by the different class II alleles (including both *DRB1* and/or *DQB1*) on each haplotype.
3. Susceptibility and resistance are determined by multiple alleles on each haplotype (including some shared motifs), some of which are shared and some of which are haplotype-specific.
4. Susceptibility and resistance are determined by as-yet-unidentified alleles in linkage disequilibrium on these haplotypes.

I will consider each of these possibilities in turn, and discuss the implications for our understanding of the pathogenesis of PSC.

The first of these three interpretations represents the simplest explanation. The advantages of this hypothesis are that it explains why the different *DRB1* susceptibility alleles on each haplotype may have different effects in terms of disease risk. Thus, the dominant association is with the HLA *B8-DRB1*0301* haplotype which is found in approximately 31% of PSC patients (odds ratio OR = 2.69)[22]. In addition the hypothesis may also explain why we see an increased frequency of *DRB1*0301* homozygotes (OR = 5.98)[22], but not *DRB1*1301* homozygotes or *DRB1*1301/DRB1*0301* heterozygotes in PSC. However, it cannot be used to explain the very strong protective association with *MICA*002*[25].

In most autoimmune diseases reports of inter-population differences in HLA associations have led to development of one or more 'shared motif' hypotheses[24]. By re-analysing these basic HLA associations in terms of amino acids rather than alleles, we can investigate whether the different HLA alleles associated with an increased risk of disease have structural similarities not found on those alleles associated with a reduced risk of disease. This is a more rational approach than comparing alleles by name, which is simply a tag given to specific DNA sequence, for the purposes of developing a standard international nomenclature. Early attempts to do this in PSC led to the publication of a hypothesis predicated on *DRB* alleles (Table 4) encoding leucine (single-letter

Table 4 Shared motif models for PSC: the distribution of key HLA class II encoded amino acids

Residue (no. of copies for maximum effect)	Associated alleles	PSC (n = 148)	Healthy controls (n = 134)	Difference (OR)
Leucine DRβ-38 (two copies)	DRB3*0101 DRB5*0101 DRB1*1201	34%	7%	26% (6.33)
Valine DRβ-86 (two copies)	DRB1*0301 DRB1*1301 DRB1*1501	40%	21%	19% (2.54)
Proline DQβ-55 (one or more)	DQB1*0301 DQB1*0302 DQB1*0303	31%	60%	29% (0.3)
Phenylalanine DQβ-87 (one or more)	DQB1*0601 DQB1*0602 DQB1*0603	43%	26%	17% (2.16)

All studies are based on adult cases unless otherwise marked. Protective amino acids are tinted, and have risk values <1.

code L) at position 38 of the DRβ-polypeptide[26].The leucine-38 hypothesis has been tested and set aside[27]; however, recent analysis of an extended series from the centre where the original report was penned has confirmed the association (Table 4)[22]. Thus, 72% (107/148) PSC patients were found to have one or more leucine-bearing alleles compared with 51% of controls ($p = 0.0003$, OR = 2.46), and 34% of PSC patients had two leucine-38 alleles versus only 7% of controls ($p < 10^{-7}$, OR = 6.33)[22]. In-depth analysis of the same series also suggested a number of other potential models based on: DRβ-86, DQβ-55 and DQβ-87 (Table 4)[22].

Modelling susceptibility on *DQB* alleles as opposed to *DRB* alleles may account for susceptibility and resistance encoded by haplotypes 2, 3, 4 and 5 but does not account for haplotypes 1 or 6 (Table 1). Whereas the leucine-38 model is dependent on the weak association with haplotype 3, this is not found in all populations.

Failure to settle upon a single unified theory to explain the HLA associations in PSC led to the third possible explanation, i.e. that there are multiple susceptibility genes for PSC on these haplotypes. One of these appears to map close to the HLA B locus, perhaps *MICA*[25,28]; the other may be either *DRB1* or *DQB1*[22,26].

In PSC the greatest risk of disease is associated with either homozygosity for *DRB1*0301* (OR = 5.98)[22] or heterozygosity for *DRB1*0301/DRB1*1501* (OR = 4.2)[22] and the greatest protective effect is associated with the *MICA*002* allele (OR$_{(range)}$ = 0.12–0.00)[25]. Since both the *DRB1*0301* and *DRB1*1501* haplotypes (haplotypes 1 and 3) encode *MICA*008* the strong association with *MICA*008* homozygotes (OR value for *008/*008* homozygotes = 4.89)[22], can be accounted for through linkage with HLA 8.1 and the *DRB1*1501-DQB1*0602* haplotype[28]. However, the very strong protective effect of the *MICA*002* allele (pooled OR derived from ref. 25 = 0.069, which is equivalent to 14.45 for a susceptibility effect) cannot be so easily explained. Therefore, *MICA* may have a very important role to play in PSC.

This observation has important implications in terms of disease pathogenesis in PSC. The involvement of the MIC genes may indicate a more prominent role for the innate immune response in PSC. This also dovetails with the current upsurge in interest in the role of the importance of the liver in innate immunity[29,30]. Increased numbers of γδ and NK cells have been documented in PSC livers[18,19]. Thus, if PSC arises as a result of infection, this may provide the catalyst for heat-shock induction of MICα molecules on biliary epithelium, which may in turn lead to the activation of intrahepatic γδ and NK cells.

In individuals homozygous for *MICA*008*, aberrant or unstable expression of the gene may cause either persistent immune activation leading to autoimmunity or failed activation, with the consequence of persistent infection and ultimate recognition of self (auto) antigens. Interestingly the *MICA*008* haplotype encodes the A5.1 STR (above) mutation whilst the *MICA*002* haplotype does not[15,28].

The final possibility is that we have not yet discovered the true susceptibility locus (or loci) for PSC, and that the haplotypes associated with disease so far are simply linkage markers for the undisclosed allele or alleles. This possibility needs to be considered seriously, as there are over 200 genes in the MHC and linkage disequilibrium can span the whole 4 Mb.

The relationship between HLA and disease phenotype in PSC

Early reports suggested that patients with DR3 (the serologically determined equivalent of *DRB1*0301*) and DR4 (which includes most members of the *DRB1*04* subfamily of alleles), may have more severe disease than those without. These observations proved controversial, and were refuted by Olerup et al.[27]. More recently these ideas have resurfaced. There are reports that PSC patients with DR4 alleles may have more rapidly progressing disease[31]; however, it has also been suggested that DR4 encodes resistance to PSC in those with concurrent IBD[22]. Taken together these three observations may seem contradictory, but rapid progression may be more common in the subgroup of PSC patients who do not have IBD.

The total numbers of PSC patients studied so far are very small, and there are many genes in the MHC that have not been investigated; therefore much more work is needed to clarify these associations. Until then we can only speculate about which MHC genes are responsible for these associations.

NON-MHC IMMUNOGENETICS IN PSC

Although antigen presentation and the MHC are crucial there are many other stages in the immune response that may be governed by host genetic variation, and almost any gene that encodes an immune active product can act as an 'immune response gene'. The list of genes that have been investigated in PSC is shown in Table 5; I will consider some of these here.

Table 5 Non-MHC genes that have been investigated in PSC

Gene and SNP	Outcome and study
CTLA4 +49 A/G	Controversial, unpublished
IL1B +3954 G/C	Negative, ref. 35
IL1RN 86bp VNTR	Negative, ref. 35
IL10 −1082 G/C	Negative, ref. 35
IL10 −819 C/T	Negative, ref. 35
IL10 −592 C/T	Negative, ref. 35
TGFB1 +74 G/C	Negative, ref. 43
TGFB1 −509 C/T	Negative, ref. 43
MMP3 −1171 A insertion	Positive, ref. 40
CCR5 32bp deletion	Negative, unpublished
TNFRSF6 (Fas/Apo-1) A/G	Negative, unpublished
MMP2	Negative, unpublished
MMP9	Negative, unpublished
CARD15, C2104T (SNP8), G2722C (SNP12), 3020insC (SNP13)	All negative, ref. 46

CTLA gene polymorphisms in PSC

Critical stages in the immune response include the immediate aftermath of MHC–peptide–TCR interaction in which signalling by accessory molecules determines the characteristics of the resulting immune response. One of these accessory molecules, cytotoxic lymphocyte antigen-4 (ctla-4), is especially interesting. This molecule, expressed on the CD25[+] T cells, competes with CD28 for binding sites on the B7.1 and B7.2 (CD80 and CD86) ligands expressed on the antigen-presenting cell. CTLA-4 binding results in a switch from immune activation to immune memory[3]. There are numerous SNPs in the *CTLA4* gene on chromosome 2q33[32]. Two of these SNPs have been implicated in susceptibility to autoimmune disease; these are: the A+49G[33] and the more recently discovered CT60 SNP[3]. Preliminary studies of the A+49G SNP have failed to identify an association in PSC (Donaldson et al., unpublished data, October 2003); however, this remains controversial as the functional CT60 SNP has not yet been tested.

Cytokine gene polymorphisms in PSC

The immune response is orchestrated, at least in part, by the cytokine network. Cytokines have multiple functions and act through specific cell-surface receptors. The cytokine network is extremely complex and interactive. Genetically determined relative differences in cytokine production may decide whether a cell is activated or not, and (by activating different cells) whether activation leads to a predominantly Th1 or Th2 immune response. The currently identified genetic polymorphisms in the cytokine genes are summarized at www.pam.bris.ac.uk/services/GAI/cytokine4.

The tumour necrosis factor-α gene (*TNFA*), has been implicated in susceptibility to PSC[34], but as it is carried on the HLA 8.1 haplotye this may simply be due to linkage disequilibrium. Other cytokines which have been investigated in PSC include interleukins (IL)-1, and IL-10; both studies were negative[35].

Polymorphism in genes involved in matrix regulation in PSC

Fibrosis is the key processes in PSC; the process is regulated by a series of metalloproteinases (MMPs) and their naturally occurring inhibitors TIMPs (tissue inhibitors of metalloproteinases)[36–39]. These enzymes determine the balance between increased synthesis and collagen deposition versus matrix degradation. In addition cytokines have profound pro- and anti-fibrotic activities. Thus, production of pro-fibrotic cytokines such as TGF-β or TNF-α in tissues will activate periductular fibroblasts, causing them to trans-differentiate into myofibroblasts, whereas high tissue concentrations of IL-10 and IFN-γ will lead to lower levels of fibrosis.

Variation in the genes that regulate collagen metabolism has been investigated in PSC, and preliminary data indicate that a common polymorphism occurring as either a 5A or 6A repeat sequence at position −1171 in the gene encoding *MMP3* (stromelysin chromosome 11q23) may be associated with increased risk of portal hypertension[40]. Stromelysin or MMP-3 degrades type II, IV, IX collagens, laminins, fibronectin, gelatins and elastin, and may activate other metalloproteinases. The 5A variant has been linked with lower levels of gene transcription[41,42]. Though further studies are necessary, confirmation of these data may have important implications for clinical practice.

In addition, two SNPs in the *TGFB1* gene (chromosome 11q23) have been studied in PSC, these are: a G to C at position +74 (resulting in an arginine for proline substitution in codon 25) and a C for T exchange at position −509, though neither polymorphism was positively or negatively associated with disease[43]. This study, however, did not consider the relationship between the degree of fibrosis and these two SNPs, and therefore may be invalid.

CARD15 in PSC

Among the many tempting candidates for PSC is the *CARD15* gene, recently identified as a major susceptibility locus in Crohn's disease[44,45]. The identification of this gene in Crohn's disease has created speculation concerning the role of this and other pattern-recognition receptors in disease. The focus of immunogenetics is increasingly moving away from adaptive to innate immunity, and from early events to late events in immune regulation; such as apoptosis (programmed cell death). The rationale behind this is that apoptosis may be a very effective means of down-regulating the immune response. Therefore, a genetically determined differential in apoptosis could easily 'tip the balance', leading, in some cases, to significant tissue damage and disease genesis. Disease may occur where apoptosis leads to an aberrant expression of otherwise 'cryptic' antigens or where apoptosis of effector cells provides a permissive environment for pathogens to thrive. However, recent studies have failed to link either the *CARD15*[46] mutations or a SNP in the FAS gene (*TNFRSF6*) with susceptibility to PSC (unpublished observations, Donaldson et al., October 2003).

DISCUSSION

Work on non-MHC genes in PSC is not yet complete, and there are many more candidates to examine. Overall the studies published so far suggest that there needs to be a major change in study design. It is simply too naive to base investigations on a single SNP or upon a single cytokine, without considering the other genes that interact with it. The relative success of studies of the MHC by comparison reflects the fact that HLA, and many of the other MHC polymorphisms, are functional, and that most studies test multiple SNPs and/or haplotypes, rather than single SNPs and single genes in isolation. Furthermore it appears MHC genes may have stronger associations with some diseases than many non-MHC genes. Thus it is possible to detect these associations with fewer patients. Recent studies indicate that non-MHC genes may have relatively weak effects in disease. For example, the odds ratio for the CTLA4 CT60 SNP in insulin-dependent diabetes mellitus is 1.14, and for Grave's disease[3] it is 1.51. To confidently detect such weak associations we will need to study thousands rather than hundreds of patients; this observation may cast doubt on the validity of many of the reports above.

Another reason for the lack of success and/or consistency in the majority of investigations of non-MHC genes lies with the complexity of biological networks, the limited scope, as well as the relatively small numbers included in most of these studies. New work on non-MHC genes in PSC needs to be more inclusive, and must be based on larger studies. These new studies need to be based on large collections of well-characterized patients and employ up-to-date high-throughput genotyping to explore whole pathways and networks.

CONCLUSION

Currently we are entering a new era in genetic discovery. The tools we have today would enable us to perform all of the research in PSC of the past 10 years in a few months. What is required is a new focus. We must: (1) assemble DNA banks on large numbers of well-characterized patients with thorough clinical databases; (2) learn the lessons about study design that are apparent in the work to date, especially with regard to non-MHC genes[4]; (3) embrace new technologies and pursue the goal of understanding the genetic basis of PSC, as a primary objective that will inform the pathogenesis of these diseases and ultimately lead to improvements in patient care.

References

1. Haines JL, Pericak-Vance MA. Overview of mapping common and genetically complex disease genes. In: Haines JL, Pericak-Vance MA, editors. Approaches to Gene Mapping in Complex Diseases. New York: Wiley, 1998:1–16.
2. Emery J, Hayflick S. The challenge of integrating genetic medicine into primary care. Br Med Bull. 2001;322:1027–30.
3. Ueda H, Howson JMM, Esposito L et al. Association of the T-cell regulatory gene CTLA4 with susceptibility to autoimmune disease. Nature. 2003;423:506–11.
4. Colhoun H, McKeigue PM, Smith GD. Problems of reporting genetic associations with complex outcomes. Lancet. 2003;361:865–72.
5. Anonymous. Freely associating. Nature Genet. 1999;22:1–2.
6. Rothman KJ. No adjustments are needed for multiple comparisons. Epidemiology. 1990;1:43–6.
7. International SNP Map Working Group. A map of the human genome sequence variation containing 1.42 million single nucleotide polymorphisms. Nature. 2001;409:928–41.

8. Milner CM, Campbell DR, Trowsdale J. Molecular genetics of the human major histocompatibility complex. In: Warrens A, Lechler R, editors. HLA in Health and Disease. London: Academic Press, 2000:35–50.

9. Stern LJ, Brown JH, Jardetsky TS et al. Crystal structure of human class II MHC protein HLA-DR1 complexed with influenza virus peptide. Nature. 1994;368:215–21.

10. Fanning GC, Bunce M, Black CM et al. Polymerase chain reaction haplotyping using 3' mismatches in the forward and reverse primers: application to the biallelic polymorphisms of tumour necrosis factor and lymphotoxin-α. Tissue Ant. 1997;50:23–31.

11. Bidwell J, Keen L, Gallagher G et al. Cytokine gene polymorphism in human disease: on-line databases. Genes Immun. 1999;1:3–19.

12. Wilson AG, Symons JA, McDowell TL et al. Effects of a polymorphism in the human tumour necrosis factor a promoter on transcriptional activation. Proc Natl Acad Sci USA. 1997; 94:3195–9.

13. Wilson AG. Genetics of tumour necrosis factor (TNF) in autoimmune liver diseases: red hot or red herring? J Hepatol. 1999;30:331–3.

14. Simpson KJ, Lukacs NW, Colletti L et al. Cytokines and the liver. J Hepatol. 1997;27: 1120–32.

15. Fodil N, Pellet P, Laloux L et al. MICA haplotypic diversity. Immunogenetics. 1999;49:557–60.

16. Bauer S, Groh V, Wu J et al. Activation of NK cells and T cells by NKG2D, a receptor for stress inducible MICA. Science. 1999;285:727–9.

17. Norris S, Doherty DG, McEntee G et al. Natural T cells in the human liver: cytotoxic lymphocytes with dual T cell and natural killer cell phenotype and function are phenotypically heterogeneous and include Vα24JαQ and γδ T cell receptor bearing cells. Human Immunol. 1999;60:20–31.

18. Martins EBG, Graham AK, Chapman RW, Fleming K. Elevation of γδ T lymphocytes in peripheral blood and livers of patients with primary sclerosing cholangitis and other autoimmune disease. Hepatology. 1996;23:988–99.

19. Hata K, van Thiel DH, Herberman RB, Whiteside TL. Phenotypic and functional characteristics of lymphocytes isolated from liver biopsy specimens from patients with active liver disease. Hepatology. 1992;15:816–23.

20. Donaldson PT. Genetics of autoimmune liver disease. In: Gershwin ME, Vierling JM, Norris S, editors. Liver Immunology. Philadelphia: Hanley Belfus, 2003:291–310.

21. Donaldson PT, Norris S. Immunogenetics in PSC. Best Pract Res Clin Gastroenterol. 2001;15:611–27.

22. Donaldson PT, Norris S. Evaluation of the role of MHC class II alleles, haplotypes and selected amino acid sequences in primary sclerosing cholangitis. Autoimmunity. 2002;35:555–64.

23. Spurkland A, Saarinen S, Boberg KM et al. HLA class II haplotypes in primary sclerosing cholangitis patients from five European populations. Tissue Ant. 1999;53:459–69.

24. Donaldson PT, Czaja AJ. Genetic effects on susceptibility, expression and outcome. Clin Liver Dis. 2002;6:419–37.

25. Norris S, Kondeatis E, Collins R et al. Mapping MHC-encoded susceptibility and resistance in primary sclerosing cholangitis: the role of MICA polymorphism. Gastroenterology. 2001; 120:1475–82.

26. Farrant JM, Doherty DG, Donaldson PT et al. Amino acid substitutions at position 38 of the DRβ polypeptide confer susceptibility and protection from primary sclerosing cholangitis. Hepatology. 1992;16:390–5.

27. Olerup O, Olsson R, Hultcrantz R, Broome U. HLA-DR and HLA-DQ are not markers for rapid disease progression in primary sclerosing cholangitis. Gastroenterology. 1995;108:870–8.

28. Wiencke K, Spurkland A, Schrumpf E, Boberg KM. Primary sclerosing cholangitis is associated to an extended B8-DR3 haplotype including particular MICA and MICB alleles. Hepatology. 2001;34:625–30.

29. Doherty DG, O'Farrelly C. Innate and adaptive lymphoid cells from human liver. Immunol Rev. 2000;174:5–20.

30. Doherty DG, O'Farrelly C. Lymphoid repertoires in healthy liver. In: Gershwin ME, Vierling JM, Manns MP, editors. Liver Immunology Philadelphia: Hanley Belfus, 2003:31–47.

31. Gow PJ, Flemming KA, Chapman RW. Primary sclerosing cholangitis associated with rheumatoid arthritis and DR4: is the association a marker of patients with progressive liver disease? J Hepatol. 2000;34:631–5.

32. Johnson GCL, Esposito L, Barratt BJ et al. Haplotype tagging for the identification of common disease genes. Nature Genet. 2001;29:233–7.

33. Kristiansen OP, Larsen ZM, Pocoit F. *CTLA-4* in autoimmune diseases – a general susceptibility gene to autoimmunity? Genes Immun. 2000;1:170–84.

34. Bernal W, Moloney M, Underhill J, Donaldson PT. Association of tumour necrosis factor polymorphism with primary sclerosing cholangitis. J Hepatol. 1999;30:237–41.

35. Donaldson PT, Norris S, Constantini PK, Harrison P, Williams R. The interleukin-1 and interleukin-10 gene polymorphisms in primary sclerosing cholangitis: no associations with disease susceptibility/resistance. J Hepatol. 2000;32:882–6.

36. Birkedal-Hansen H, Moore GWI, Bodden MK et al. Matrix metalloproteinases: a critical review. Crit Rev Oral Biol Med. 1993;4:197–250.

37. Cawston TE, Billington C. Editorial: metalloproteinases in the rheumatic diseases. J Pathol. 1996;180:115–17.

38. Thomson MP, Arthur MJP. Mechanisms of liver damage and repair. Eur J Gastroenterol Hepatol. 1999;11:949–55.

39. Benyon CR, Iredale JR, Goddard S et al. Expression of tissue inhibitor of metalloproteinase 1 and 2 is increased in human fibrotic liver. Gastroenterology. 1996;110:821–6.

40. Satsangi J, Welsh KI, Bunce M et al. Contribution of the major histocompatibility complex to susceptibility and disease phenotype in inflammatory bowel disease. Lancet. 1996;347:1212–17.

41. Selmi C, Zuin M, Meda F et al. Common variants of the matrix metalloproteinase-3 stromelysin gene promoter in primary biliary cirrhosis. Gastroenterology. 2002;122:247–8.

42. Ye S, Eriksson P, Hamsten A et al. Progression of coronary atherosclerosis is associated with a common genetic variant of the human stromelysin-1 promoter which results in reduced gene expression. J Biol Chem. 1996;271:13055–60.

43. Donaldson PT, Clare MC, Craig W et al. Transforming growth cell factor B-1 (*TGFB1*) gene polymorphisms in primary sclerosing cholangitis and primary biliary cirrhosis. Hepatology. 2000;32:174A (Abstract 45).

44. Hugot J-P, Chamaillard M, Zouali H et al. Association of *NOD2* leucine-rich repeat variants with susceptibility to Crohn's disease. Nature. 2001;411:599–603.

45. Ogura Y, Bonen DK, Inohara N et al. A frameshift mutation in *NOD2* associated with susceptibility to Crohn's disease. Nature. 2001;411:603–6.

46. Cullen SN, Ahmed T, Chapman RW, Jewell DP. No association between NOD2 polymorphism and susceptibility to, or progression of, primary sclerosing cholangitis. Gut 2002;50:A119 [Abstract 439].

47. Moloney MM, Thomson LJ, Strettell MJ et al. HLA-C genes and susceptibility to primary sclerosing cholangitis. Hepatology. 1998;28:660–2.

27
Viruses, protozoans, bacteria and drugs as aetiological factors in primary sclerosing cholangitis

R. W. CHAPMAN

INTRODUCTION

Both the aetiology and pathogenesis of primary sclerosing cholangitis (PSC) remain unknown. It is clear that, since inflammation and cytokines are involved in the generation of both small duct and fibrous ablative cholangitis, all forms of sclerosing cholangitis are associated with an immunopathogenesis. Associations with HLA haplotypes, the presence of autoantibodies such as pANCA, smooth muscle antibodies and antineutrophil antibodies, and the strong association with inflammatory bowel disease, particularly ulcerative colitis, appear to be consistent with a possible autoimmune pathogenesis[1,2]. However, the hypothesis that adult PSC is an autoimmune disease[1,3] remains controversial. It is clear that non-immune factors such as infection with agents such as *Cryptosporidium*, toxic agents, ischaemia and neoplasia can also result in stricturing and dilation of the biliary tree[4]. The bacterial hypothesis was refined by Vierling[5], who has pointed out that biliary epithelia, gut flora and bile all play active roles in both the innate and adaptive immune responses[5] which may be responsible for sclerosing cholangitis lesions[6]. The hypothesis suggests that bacterial constituents in portal blood are the dominant stimuli which initiate the immunopathogenic process of peribiliary inflammation and cytokine-induced circumferential fibrosis in either the presence or absence of inflammatory bowel disease involving the colon.

Hepatic lobules are constantly exposed to bacterial products, gut-derived cytokines and xenobiotics ascending from the gut in portal venous blood. The space between the capillaries and basement membranes of the bile ducts drains lymph, retrogradely from the space of Disse, which contains cytokines and other peptides secreted by Kupffer cells, stellate cells, hepatocytes and fenestrated endothelial cells. Dendritic cells, the most potent professional antigen-presenting cells (APC), are also present in the peribiliary space. Thus, biliary epithelial cells, APC and capillary endothelial cells are in close proximity to non-sterile bile and cytokines in hepatic lymph[6]. In addition, it is established that normal portal tracts contain resident CD4, CD8, and CD4-8-T cells and NK cells.

ANIMAL MODELS IN PSC

Unfortunately there is no single animal model for PSC. There are, however, several models of hepatobiliary disease that are immune-mediated and resemble some but not all aspects of PSC. Surprisingly, only one of the immune-mediated models has had cholangiographic studies performed, and not all the models have related intestinal inflammation to the biliary injury. One of the most interesting models of cholangitis resulted from the injection of formyl peptides administered into the inflamed colons of rats[7]. The colitis was induced by the rectal administration of 15% acetic acid solution. Formyl peptides are proinflammatory agents that are secreted by bacteria and are strongly chemotactic for neutrophils and macrophages. These peptides do not *per se* attract or activate T cells, but they undergo enteropathic circulation and appear in bile within 3 h. When these peptides are injected into inflamed colons, macrophages and granulocytes infiltrate the liver and localize to the portal tracts, and by day 4 CD4-positive and CD8-positive T lymphocytes attach themselves to cholangiocytes. Cholangitis occurs in small ducts with lymphocyte infiltration. However, no cholangiograms were performed, and biliary alkaline phosphatase was not elevated in these animals. Colitis induced with muramycyl dipeptide in rats[7], *Escherichia coli* chemotactic peptide in rats[8] and FMLT in rats[9] were all associated with histological changes similar to PSC, although cholangiography was not performed[7–9].

Another model worthy of further study is that from Kuroe et al., who described a model of granulomatous enterocolitis in rabbits induced by administering muramyl dipeptides (MDP) with Freund's incomplete adjuvant sub-mucosally[10]. Interestingly, this also induced inflammation of the bile ducts with periductal fibrosis. No cholangiograms, however, were performed in this rabbit model, and no T-cell transfer experiments were carried out. The authors suggested that continuous stimulation with bacterial cell wall fragments may be involved in chronic intestinal inflammation and extraintestinal disease such as PSC[10].

Evidence for the role of bacteria in initiating the innate immune response of PSC biliary damage comes from a model of small bowel bacterial overgrowth in susceptible rat strains which induces hepatobiliary injury[11,12]. Following creation of jejunal self-filling blind loops, both male and female Lewis and Wistar rats develop hepatic injury within 4–16 weeks after surgery. Inflammatory lesions were seen in the portal tracts with bile duct proliferation and damage with fibrosis, and cholangiograms demonstrated abnormalities with thickened and tortuous irregular bile ducts. No antibody studies have been performed, and no T-cell transfer experiments have been carried out. It is also relevant that human adults with anaerobic bacterial small bowel overgrowth do not develop hepatic abnormalities.

THE ROLE OF BILIARY EPITHELIAL AND ENDOTHELIAL CELLS AS IMMUNOLOGICAL TARGETS

It remains unclear as to whether biliary epithelial cells (BEC) are the primary targets in PSC. It has been shown that BEC express HLA class 1, and aberrant expression of HLA class 2 and ICAM-1, which are prerequisite for antigen presentation or as target cells for CD4/CD8 BEC-specific cytotoxic lymphocytes[13–15]. Conflicting results have been found regarding the expression of co-stimulatory molecules such as B7 which are also needed for successful antigen presentation. Moreover, in PSC, expression of CD58 (LFA-3), co-stimulatory B7 and Fas (CD95) was modest and intermittent in comparison to PBC BEC[16]. A recent study by Xu et al.[17] demonstrated the presence of autoantibodies to surface antigens expressed on BEC in PSC. In addition the study showed that these autoantibodies induced increased expression of CD44 on the BEC and production of IL-6 by these cells[17].

Several studies, however, have shown that portal tract T cells may be sensitized to epithelial antigens expressed by the gut[18,19], and one hypothesis to explain the association with inflammatory bowel disease is that bile duct injury could be secondary to T-cell crossreactions between enterocytes and BEC which are derived from the embryonic foregut[20]. This could explain the finding that between 20% and 50% of patients with PSC also have stricturing of the pancreatic ducts where, again, T cells are derived from the embryonic foregut, and would suggest common epithelial antigens. Recently Grant et al.[21] have proposed the existence of an enterohepatic circulation of lymphocytes whereby some mucosal lymphocytes produced in the inflamed gut persist as memory cells, capable in certain circumstances of causing hepatobiliary inflammation of recirculation through the liver. This concept of dual homing lymphocytes may help to explain how PSC can develop some years after colectomy[21].

An alternative hypothesis has been suggested by Vierling[5]. He suggested that the pathogenesis of PSC requires an immunogenetically susceptible host and exposure to bacteria or bacterial cell wall products in the portal venous blood. This exposure would naturally be increased in the setting of either acute or chronic colitis. The innate immune response of hepatic macrophages would then promote secretion of IL-1β, TNF-α, IL-12 and IL-18 that would be transported in lymph into the hepatobiliary space of the portal tracts. Increased concentrations of TNF-α endotoxin in this space could stimulate BEC secretion of chemokines and cytokines, and the promotion of the regurgitation of bile into the peribiliary space, and interfere with the cholehepatic circulation. In turn the peribiliary chemokines and cytokines would attract and activate neutrophils, monocytes, macrophages, T cells and fibroblasts, which would promote enzymatic digestion and extracellular matrix, collagen synthesis by activated myofibro-blasts resulting in peribiliary fibrosis. The expanding layers of concentric fibrosis would cause separation of the peribiliary capillary plexi from the bile duct, in turn causing progressive ischaemia and BEC atrophy. This hypothesis, while attractive, does not explain the development of pancreatic stricturing which is present in about 10–50% of PSC patients.

SPECIFIC BACTERIA IMPLICATED IN THE PATHOGENESIS OF PSC

Recently, in an attempt to identify possible infective agents implicated in the pathogenesis of PSC, Ponsioen et al.[22] carried out serological screening for antibodies against 22 common viruses as well as *Chlamydia* spp. and *Mycoplasma pneumoniae* in PSC patients compared with normal and disease controls. No positive results were identified in any of the viruses tested. Interestingly, a marked elevation in the seroprevalence of *Chlamydia*–LPS antibodies was observed compared with the normal and disease controls, which included patients with inflammatory bowel disease[22]. However, the increased seroprevalence was not confirmed in the more specific *C. trachomatis* and *C. pneumoniae* assays. Furthermore the actual prescence of *Chlamydia* bodies could not be demonstrated in liver tissue. While these results are intriguing, clearly further studies are needed to confirm that *Chlamydia* may be involved in the pathogenesis of PSC.

Recent studies have proposed a role for *Helicobacter pylori* in Sjögren's syndrome[23]. Interest in the biliary system was raised by study in Chilean patients, which found that patients with chronic cholangitis were commonly infected by bile-tolerant *Helicobacter* species[24]. In a report from Nilsson et al. bile and liver samples were positive for *Helicobacter* DNA by polymerase chain reaction (PCR) in nearly half of 24 patients with primary biliary cirrhosis and PSC, confirmed by immunoblot analysis[25]. Furthermore a strong correlation was found between bile duct malignancies and the presence of *H. pylori* DNA in bile[26]. Further evidence for a possible role of *Helicobacter* in PSC comes from the isolation of a novel *Helicobacter* species from cottontop tamarins which have a high incidence of an ulcerative colitis-like condition with a high rate of colonic malignancy[27].

VIRUSES, PROTOZOANS AND PSC

Although viruses have been suggested to be important in the pathogenesis of PSC, the common hepatotrophic viruses (hepatitis A, B and C) have been excluded as causative factors. Early studies showed that reovirus type 3 causes cholangitis and biliary atresia in weanling mice and primates[28,29]. However, no differences were found in the titre of antibodies to reovirus type 3 between PSC patients and normal controls[30].

Since 1986, infection of the bile ducts with the protozoan *Cryptosporidium* and cytomegalovirus (CMV) in AIDS patients has been associated with the development of cholangiographic abnormalities similar to PSC[31]. Further evidence of CMV-induced biliary damage is the high incidence of chronic hepatic rejection in patients with orthotopic liver transplantation with hepatic CMV infection, characterized by loss of intralobular and small bile ducts rejection (vanishing bile duct disease, VBD)[32]. In a preliminary study from the USA, CMV-DNA was detected in seven of seven PSC but in only five of 20 controls[33]. However in a later, larger study from Oxford[34], using PCR on liver tissue from 36 PSC patients, CMV-DNA could be detected in only one patient. Current evidence does not suggest that CMV is involved in the pathogenesis of PSC.

Human intracisternal A-type particle (HIAP) has been isolated from the salivary glands of Sjögren's syndrome patients[35]. Other endogenous human retroviruses have been implicated in the pathogenesis of multiple sclerosis and type 1 diabetes[36]. These findings encouraged Mason et al.[37] to investigate, using a Western blotting technique, the possibility that retroviruses could be implicated in PBC, PSC and other idiopathic biliary disorders. HIV-1 p24 gag seropositivity was found in 35% of PBC and 39% of PSC patients compared with only 4% of controls. A positive association was also found with two HIAP proteins. The authors interpreted their findings as either an autoimmune response to antigenically related cellular proteins induced by the retroviral proteins, or an immune response to uncharacterized viral proteins which could share antigenic determinants with these retroviruses. Further confirmatory studies are required to assess the potential role of retroviruses in PSC.

DRUGS AND PSC

Therapy with the cytotoxic agent floxuridine (FUDR) infused intra-arterially has been shown to give cholangiographic appearances similar to PSC. The pathogenesis of the bile duct damage is believed to be ischaemic in type[38]. However, the relevance to the pathogenesis of PSC remains unclear.

References

1. Chapman RW, Jewell DP. Primary sclerosing cholangitis – an immunologically mediated disease? West J Med. 1985;143:193–5.
2. Vierling J, Hu K-Q. Immunologic mechanism of hepatobiliary injury. In: Kaplowitz NE, editor. Liver and Biliary Disease. Baltimore, MD: Williams & Wilkins, 1996:55–87.
3. Chapman RW. Role of immune factors in the pathogenesis of primary sclerosing cholangitis. Semin Liver Dis. 1991;11:1–4.
4. Sherlock S. Pathogenesis of sclerosing cholangitis: the role of nonimmune factors. Semin Liver Dis. 1991;11:5–10.
5. Vierling J. Aetiopathogenesis of primary sclerosing cholangitis. In: Manns M, Stiehl A, Chapman RW, Wiesner RH, editors. Primary Sclerosing Cholangitis. Dordrecht: Kluwer Publishers, 1998:37–45.
6. Reynoso-Paz, Coppel RL, Mackay IR, Bass NM, Ansari AA, Gershwin ME. The immunobiology of bile and bilary epithelium. Hepatology. 1999;30:351–7.
7. Hobson CH, Butt JJ, Ferry DM, Hunter J, Chadwick VS, Broom MF. Enterohepatic circulation of bacterial chemotactic peptide in rats with experimental colitis. Gastroenterology. 1988;94: 1006–13.
8. Kuroe K, Haga Y, Funakoshi O, Mizuki I, Kanazawa K, Yoshida Y. Extra-intestinal manifestations of granulomatous enterocolitis induced in rabbits by long-term submucosal administration of muramyl dipeptide emulsified with Freund's incomplete adjuvant. J Gastroenterol. 1996;31:199–206.
9. Yamada S, Ishii M, Liang LS, Yamamoto T, Toyota T. Small duct cholangitis induced by N-formyl L-methionine L-leucine L-tyrosine in rats. J Gastroenterol. 1994;29:631–6.
10. Yamada S, Ishii M, Kisara N, Nagatomi R, Toyota T. Macrophages are essential for lymphocyte infiltration in formyl peptide-induced cholangitis in rat liver. Liver. 1999;19:253–8.
11. Lichtman SN, Bachmann S, Nunoz SR et al. Bacterial cell wall polymers (peptidoglycan-polysaccharide) cause reactivation of arthritis. Infect Immun. 1993;61:4645–53.
12. Lichtman SN, Okoruwa EE, Kebu J, Schwab JH, Sartor RB. Degradation of endogenous bacterial cell wall polymers by the muralytic enzyme mutanolysin prevents hepatobiliary injury in genetically susceptible rats with experimental intestinal bacterial overgrowth. J Clin Invest. 1992;90:1313–22.

13. Leon MP, Bassendine MF, Gibbs P, Thick M, Kirby JA. Immunogenicity of biliary epithelium: study of the adhesive interaction with lymphocytes. Gastroenterology. 1997;112:968–77.

14. Leon MP, Kirby JA, Gibbs P, Burt AD, Bassendine MF. Immunogenicity of biliary epithelial cells: study of the expression of B7 molecules. J Hepatol. 1995;22:591–5.

15. Tsuneyama K, Harada K, Yasoshima M, Kaji K, Gershwin ME, Nakanuma Y. Expression of co-stimulatory factor B7-2 on the intrahepatic bile ducts in primary biliary cirrhosis and primary sclerosing cholangitis: an immunohistochemical study. (In process citation). J Pathol. 1998;186:126–30.

16. Spengler U, Leifeld L, Braunschweiger I, Dumoulin FL, Lechmann M, Sauerbruch T. Anomalous expression of costimulatory molecules B7-1, B7-2 and CD28 in primary biliary cirrhosis. J Hepatol. 1997;26:31–6.

17. Xu B, Broome U, Ericzon BG. High frequency of autoantibodies in patients with primary sclerosing cholangitis that bind biliary epithelial cells and induce expression of CD44 and production of interleukin 6. Gut. 2002;51:120–7.

18. Dienes HP, Lohse AW, Gerken G et al. Bile duct epithelia as target cells in primary biliary cirrhosis and primary sclerosing cholangitis. Virchows Arch. 1997;431:119–24.

19. Broome U, Hultcrantz R, Scheynius A. Lack of concomitant expression of ICAM-1 and HLA-DR on bile duct cells from patients with primary sclerosing cholangitis and primary biliary cirrhosis. Scand J Gastroenterol. 1993;28:126–30.

20. Chapman RW. Primary sclerosing cholangitis as an autoimmune disease: pros and cons. In: Manns MP, Paumgartner G, Leuscher U, editors. Immunology and Liver. Dordrecht: Kluwer, 2000:279–88.

21. Grant AJ, Lalor PF, Salmi M, Jalkanen S, Adams DH. Homing of mucosal lymphocytes to the liver in the pathogenesis of hepatic complications of inflammatory bowel disease. Lancet. 2002;359:150–7.

22. Ponsioen CY, DeFoer J, Fiebo JW et al. A survey of infectious agents as risk factors for primary sclerosing cholangitis: are *Chlamydia* species involved? Eur J Gastrohepatol. 2002;14:641–8.

23. Figura N, Giordano S, Burroni D. Sjögren's syndrome and *Helicobacter* infection. Eur J Gastroenterol. 1994;6:321–2.

24. Fox JG, Dewhirst FE, Shen Z et al. Hepatic *Helicobacter* species identified in bile and gall bladder tissue from Chileans with chronic cholecystitis. Gastroenterology. 1998;114:755–63.

25. Nilsson I, Lindgren S, Eriksson S et al. Serum antibodies to *Helicobacter hepaticus* and *Helicobacter pylori* in patients with chronic liver disease. Gut. 2000;46:410–14.

26. Bulajic MMM, Jovanovic IRB, Loehr M. *Helicobacter pylori* infection in patients with bile duct malignancies. Gut. 2000;47:A90.

27. Wadstrom T, Ljungh A, Willen R. Primary biliary cirrhosis and primary sclerosing cholangitis are of infectious origin. Gut. 2001;49:454.

28. Phillips PA, Keast D, Papadimitriou JM, Walters MN-I, Stanley NF. Chronic obstructive jaundice induced by reovirus type 3 to weanling mice. Pathology. 1969;1:193–203.

29. Morecki R, Glaser JH, Cho S, Balistreri WF, Horwitz MS. Biliary atresia and reovirus type 3 infection. N Engl J Med. 1982;307:481–4.

30. Minuk GY, Rascannin N, Paul RW, Lee PW, Buchan K, Kelly JK. Reovirus type 3 infection in patients with primary biliary cirrhosis and primary sclerosing cholangitis. J Hepatol. 1987;5:8–13.

31. Jacobson MA, Cello JP, Sande MA. Cholestasis and disseminated cytomegalovirus disease in patients with the acquired immunodeficiency syndrome. Am J Med. 1988;84:218–24.

32. O'Grady JG, Alexander GJM, Sutherland S et al. Cytomegalovirus infection and donor/recipient HLA antigens; interdependent cofactors in the pathogenesis of vanishing bile duct syndrome after liver transplantation. Lancet. 1988;1:302–5.

33. Mason AL, Rosen G, White H, Perrilo RP. Detection of cytomegalovirus (CMV) DNA in the liver of patients with primary sclerosing cholangitis (PSC) by the polymerase chain reaction. Hepatology. 1991;14:91A.

34. Mehal WZ, Hattersley AT, Chapman RW, Fleming K. A survey of cytomegalovirus (CMV) DNA in primary sclerosing cholangitis (PSC) liver tissues using a sensitive polymerase chain reaction (PCR) based assay. J Hepatol. 1992;15:396–9.

35. Garry RF, Firmin CD, Hart DJ, Alexander SS, Donehower LA, Luo-Zhang H. Detection of a human intracisternal protein antigenically related to HIV. Science. 1990;250:1127–9.

36. Conrad B, Weissmahr RN, Boni J, Arcari R, Schupbach J, Mach B. A human endogenous retroviral superantigen as candidate autoimmune gene in type 1 diabetes. Cell. 1997:90:303–13.
37. Mason AL, Xu L, Guo L et al. Detection of retroviral antibodies in primary biliary cirrhosis and other idiopathic biliary disorders. Lancet. 1998;351:1620–4.
38. Ludwig J, Kim CH, Wiesner RH et al. Floxuridine induced sclerosing cholangitis: an ischemic cholangiopathy? Hepatology. 1989;9:215–18.

Section VIII
Primary sclerosing cholangitis and associated diseases

28
Primary sclerosing cholangitis and inflammatory bowel disease: when and how do they relate to each other?

E. SCHRUMPF and K. M. BOBERG

INTRODUCTION

The concomitant occurrence of inflammatory bowel disease (IBD) and liver pathology has been known for a long time[1]. The great variety of hepatic disorders in IBD was previously emphasized and primary sclerosing cholangitis (PSC) was for long considered a rare disease – fewer than 100 cases were reported in the English-language literature before 1980. In that particular year three studies appeared[2-4] indicating that PSC might be far more common than previously recognized. Both the Norwegian study[2] and later studies from Oxford, England[5] and Sweden[6], have all demonstrated that PSC is the most common type of chronic liver disease in patients with IBD; in fact other benign liver disorders are not often seen in IBD[7,8].

PSC IN IBD

PSC in ulcerative colitis (UC)

Our group demonstrated that 4% of all patients with UC had concomitant PSC[2]. A study from England gave a prevalence of 2.4% of PSC among patients with UC[5], whereas the Swedish experience was that 3.7% of all UC patients also suffered from PSC[6]. It has long been known that, in patients with concomitant UC and PSC, the entire colon is usually affected[2-4]. Accordingly, the Swedish study revealed a much higher incidence of PSC among patients with substantial colitis (5.5%) than in patients with distal colitis (0.5%)[6].

PSC in Crohn's disease

PSC also occurs in Crohn's disease, but almost exclusively in Crohn's colitis (and ileocolitis). In a study from Southampton, England, 6.4% out of a group of 125 patients with Crohn's disease were shown to have concomitant PSC[9]. All these patients – apart from one – had extensive colonic involvement; in some cases together with ileal affection. Although the majority of patients with PSC and IBD suffer from UC, a considerable number of patients suffer from Crohn's colitis. Therefore, when considering patients with extensive UC and extensive Crohn's colitis, there may be no difference in the relative risk of having PSC.

IBD in PSC

The prevalence of IBD in PSC varies considerably between different populations. In Western countries between 50% and 100% of PSC cases are associated with IBD[8]. In Japan, where IBD is less prevalent, only around 20% of PSC patients have concomitant IBD[10]. In India, Italy and Spain, where the prevalence of IBD is also low, around 50% of PSC patients suffer from concomitant IBD[11-13]. Many of the patients are asymptomatic, and the absence of IBD should be based on colonoscopy with multiple biopsies. Rectal sparing may be seen in a number of patients; the right side of the colon is usually most severely affected. A correct classification is often difficult; in many series the IBD seen in PSC is unclassified or indeterminate[14]. In one review paper the average percentages in PSC of UC, Crohn's disease and indeterminate colitis respectively were: 60%, 11%, and 9%[8].

UC in PSC

In the majority of PSC–UC patients the colitis is mild and quiescent[14,15]. Thus, colonoscopy should also be performed in PSC patients without bowel symptoms. Endoscopic findings may be most pronounced in the right side of the colon. As many patients have histological evidence of bowel disease, with no or few endoscopic findings, multiple biopsies should be taken[14]. PSC–UC patients receive corticosteroids and are hospitalized for colitis significantly less frequently than UC controls[15]. The colectomy rate, however, is higher in PSC–UC patients due to the development of colonic dysplasia[15].

Crohn's disease in PSC

Patients suffering from concomitant PSC and Crohn's disease have been studied less than patients with PSC and UC[9,16,17]. Nevertheless, there seems to be agreement that extensive colonic involvement is a prerequisite among these patients. The low activity of the bowel disease, and the male dominance as seen in PSC–UC, have not been demonstrated in PSC patients with Crohn's disease.

IS PSC SECONDARY TO IBD?

One hypothesis has been that PSC is secondary to IBD in those suffering from both disorders. The findings of IBD developing after PSC in many patients – and not at all in others – have led to the conclusion that PSC and IBD are independent disorders developing in genetically predisposed individuals. However, if one accepts that PSC is a heterogeneous disorder, it cannot be excluded that the bowel disease may be an important predisposition for the development of PSC in a subgroup of patients. PSC may be linked to IBD due to leakage of intestinal bacteria or toxins through an inflamed bowel mucosa into the portal blood. Genes that code for proteins involved in the intestinal mucosal barrier function are thus candidate genes not only for the development of UC and Crohn's disease[18,19], but could also be associated with the development of PSC. An experimental IBD model in mice that are immunologically normal but deficient for the multidrug resistant 1 (*mdr1a*) gene product P-glycoprotein (Pgp) indicates that adenosine triphosphate-binding cassette transporters have an important barrier function and protect the organism against bacteria and their toxins. The association between the C3435T *MDR1* gene polymorphism and susceptibility for UC is of major interest, and suggests that Pgp plays a major role in the defence against bacteria (or toxins). It remains to be seen if this altered barrier function is also linked to the development of PSC. One hypothesis is that an altered barrier function of any aetiology may give rise to leakage of bacteria (and toxins) through the bowel wall into the portal blood and then to the liver, which in turn may lead to development of PSC. In that case one might say that PSC is secondary to IBD, but only in patients with PSC developing after IBD.

ARE IBD AND PSC INDEPENDENT DISEASES?

The finding of PSC without concomitant IBD in a large number of patients, and the fact that PSC may develop after colectomy, give strong support for these disorders to be independent – at least among a number of patients. Nevertheless, the strong linkage between the two disorders means that, when an association has been found between a gene and one of the disorders, this is also a candidate gene for the development of the other disorder.

There is now evidence for an association with Crohn's disease at the IBD1 locus which has been shown to be attributed to mutations in the NOD2/CARD15 gene[20]. This gene encodes a cytoplasmic protein that is thought to be a pattern-recognition receptor for bacterial lipopolysaccharides and to be responsible for the activation of nuclear factor κB and initiation of immunoinflammatory responses. Three major coding region polymorphisms within NOD2/CARD15 have been highly associated with CD among patients of European descent. All three major variants exhibit a deficit in NFκB activation in response to bacterial components. An altered bacterial defence could theoretically give rise not only to the bowel disease but also to PSC. As these NOD2/CARD15 mutations are linked to Crohn's disease in the distal ileum – which is hardly seen in PSC – these mutations are, however, unlikely to be found in PSC. If demonstrated also in PSC, one interpretation could be that both diseases are secondary to a common genetic aberration.

The IBD locus 3 on chromosome 6 encompassing the major histocompatibility complex has been implicated for both UC and Crohn's disease. One study even demonstrated this linkage to be sex-specific, being observed mostly among males[21]. Strong linkage has been found to the HLA region among patients with PSC[22], which is also linked to the male sex – apart from PSC patients without IBD[23]. Among patients being homozygous for HLA B8,DR3 we found a 20 times increased risk of developing PSC[22]. More recently we have also found that HLA B8,DR3 is linked to this development only in patients with specific MIC (major histocompatibility complex class I chain-related) genes[24]. Such associations have not yet been looked for in IBD, but these genes are candidate genes for the development of concomitant IBD and PSC.

A genome-wide scan in Canadian patients identified a region at chromosome 5 that contributed to Crohn's disease susceptibility[25]. The causative gene(s) and specific risk alleles are not yet identified, but the region contains a number of immunoregulatory genes of possible importance in the pathophysiology of IBD: interleukins 3, 4, 5, and 14. Among Canadian patients other regions (chromosome 19) with linkage to IBD susceptibility have also been found[25]. Candidate genes in this region are genes coding for intercellular adhesion molecule 1, complement component 3, thromboxane A2 receptor, and leukotriene B4 hydroxylase. These are also candidate genes for the development of PSC, but – if a linkage is found – it would be important to decide whether one disease is secondary to the other or whether both disorders are secondary to one common genetic aberration.

These are only a few examples of genes that may be associated to the development of both PSC and IBD. We expect many similar associations to be examined in the near future, and we also expect that PSC – like IBD – will turn out to be a complex genetic disorder with multiple genes influencing the disease expression[19].

Monozygotic twin concordance for IBD is relatively low[19] and the familial occurrence of PSC[26] is very low, so there must definitely be factors other than genes predisposing for and releasing these diseases. Interestingly, cigarette smoking seems to have a protective effect against the development of both UC and PSC[27]. Concomitant UC does not fully explain the association between non-smoking and PSC, suggesting a protective effect in a systemic, rather than colonic, manner; again underlining the independence of these two diseases.

IS PSC A HETEROGENEOUS DISORDER?

Some PSC patients suffer from concomitant IBD, some have extensive disease of both extra- and intrahepatic bile ducts, whereas others have only 'small duct PSC'[28]. Some have a poor prognosis and some even die from cholangiocarcinoma[29]. In other words there is great variation in both presentation and course of the disease. This does not automatically qualify for the designation of a heterogeneous disorder. However, if different phenotypes are linked to different genes as in IBD[19], and possibly also in PSC, this may be helpful to understand the variation in disease pathogenesis, presentation and prognosis (see Figure 1). It is our belief that further identification of genes involved in these processes will lead to a better understanding of both IBD and PSC and their interrelationship, and also to the development of new treatment regimes.

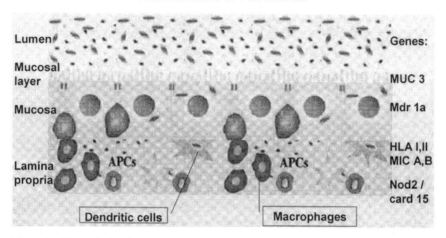

Figure 1 Schematic drawing of mucosa showing some genes of potential importance for development of IBD and PSC

References

1. Thomas HC. Ulceration of the colon with a much enlarged fatty liver. Trans Pathol Soc Phil. 1873;4:87–8.
2. Schrumpf E, Elgjo K, Fausa O et al. Sclerosing cholangitis in ulcerative colitis. Scand J Gastroenterol. 1980;15:689–97.
3. Chapman RW, Arborgh BÅ, Rhodes JM et al. Primary sclerosing cholangitis: a review of its clinical features, cholangiography, and hepatic histology. Gut. 1980;21:870–7.
4. Wiesner RH, La Russo NF. Clinicopathologic features of the syndrome of primary sclerosing cholangitis. Gastroenterology. 1980;79:200–6.
5. Shephard HA, Selby WS, Chapman RWG et al. Ulcerative colitis and persistent liver dysfunction. Q J Med. 1983;52:503–13.
6. Olsson R, Danielsson Å, Järnerot G et al. Prevalence of primary sclerosing cholangitis in patients with ulcerative colitis. Gastroenterology. 1991;100:1319–23.
7. Schrumpf E, Fausa O, Elgjo K, Kolmannskog F. Hepatobiliary complications of inflammatory bowel disease. Semin Liver Dis. 1988;8:201–9.
8. Loftus EV Jr, Sandborn WJ, Lindor KD, LaRusso NF. Interactions between chronic liver disease and inflammatory bowel disease. Inflamm Bowel Dis. 1997;3:288–302.
9. McGarity B, Bansi DS, Robertson AF, Millward-Sadler GH, Shepherd HA. Primary sclerosing cholangitis: an important and prevalent complication of Crohn's disease. Eur J Gastroenterol Hepatol. 1991;3:361–4.
10. Okada H, Mizuno M, Yamamoto K et al. Primary sclerosing cholangitis in Japanese patients: association with inflammatory bowel disease. Acta Med Okayama. 1996;50:227–35.
11. Kochhar R, Goenka MK, Das K et al. Primary sclerosing cholangitis: an experience from India. J Gastroenterol Hepatol. 1996;11:429–33.
12. Okolicsanyi L, Fabris L, Viaggi S et al. Primary sclerosing cholangitis: clinical presentation, natural history and prognostic variables: an Italian multicentre study. The Italian PSC Study Group. Eur J Gastroenterol Hepatol. 1996;8:685–91.
13. Escorsell A, Pares A, Rodes J, Solis-Herruzo JA et al. Epidemiology of primary sclerosing cholangitis in Spain. Spanish Association for the Study of the Liver. J Hepatol. 1994;21:787–91.
14. Fausa O, Schrumpf E, Elgjo K. Relationship of inflammatory bowel disease and primary sclerosing cholangitis. Semin Liver Dis. 1991;11:31–9.

15. Lundqvist K, Broome U. Differences in colonic disease activity in patients with ulcerative colitis with and without primary sclerosing cholangitis: a case control study. Dis Colon Rectum. 1997;40:451–6.

16. Tobias R, Wright JP, Rottler RE et al. Primary sclerosing cholangitis associated with inflammatory bowel disease in Cape Town, 1975–1981. S Afr Med J. 1983;63:229–35.

17. Rasmussen HH, Fallingborg JF, Mortensen PB et al. Hepatobiliary dysfunction and primary sclerosing cholangitis in patients with Crohn's disease. Scand J Gastroenterol. 1997;32:604–10.

18. Schwab M, Schaeffeler E, Marx C et al. Association between the C3435T *MDR1* gene polymorphism and susceptibility for ulcerative colitis. Gastroenterology. 2003;124:26–33.

19. Bonen DK, Cho JH. The genetics of inflammatory bowel disease. Gastroenterology. 2003; 124:521–36.

20. Hugot JP, Laurant-Puig P, Gower-Rousseau C et al. Mapping of a susceptibility locus for Crohn's disease on chromosome 16. Nature. 1996;379:821–3.

21. Fisher SA, Hampe J, Macpherson AJ et al. Sex stratification of an inflammatory bowel disease genome search shows male-specific linkage to the HLA region of chromosome 6. Eur J Hum Genet. 2002;10:259–65.

22. Spurkland A, Saarinen S, Boberg KM et al. HLA class II haplotypes in primary sclerosing cholangitis patients from five European populations. Tissue Ant. 1999;53:459–69.

23. Rabinovitz M, Gavaler JS, Schade RR et al. Does primary sclerosing cholangitis occurring in association with inflammatory bowel disease differ from that occurring in the absence of inflammatory bowel disease? A study of sixty-six subjects. Hepatology. 1990;11:7–11

24. Wiencke K, Spurkland A, Schrumpf E et al. Primary sclerosing cholangitis is associated to an extended B8-DR3 haplotype including particular MICA and MICB alleles. Hepatology. 2001;34:625–30.

25. Rioux JD, Silverberg MS, Daly MJ et al. Genomewide search in Canadian families with inflammatory bowel disease reveals two novel susceptibility loci. Am J Hum Genet. 2000;119: 1483–90.

26. Quigley EMM, LaRusso NF, Ludwig J et al. Familial occurrence of primary sclerosing cholangitis and ulcerative colitis. Gastroenterology. 1983;85:1160–5.

27. Lofthus EV Jr, Sandborn WJ, Tremaine WJ et al. Primary sclerosing cholangitis is associated with nonsmoking: a case–control study. Gastroenterology. 1996;110:1496–502.

28. Wee A, Ludwig J. Pericholangitis in chronic ulcerative colitis: primary sclerosing cholangitis of the small bile ducts? Ann Intern Med. 1985;102:581–7.

29. Boberg KM, Bergquist S, Mitchell S et al. Cholangiocarcinoma in primary sclerosing cholangitis: risk factors and clinical presentation. Scand J Gastroenterol. 2002;37:1205–11.

29
Extrahepatic and extraintestinal manifestations of primary sclerosing cholangitis

A. W. LOHSE, C. SCHRAMM and K. M. BOBERG

INTRODUCTION

About 70–80% of all patients with primary sclerosing cholangitis (PSC) also suffer from inflammatory bowel disease (IBD), the majority of these from ulcerative colitis. In addition to this obvious association, other conditions may also be associated with PSC. Furthermore, PSC may induce secondary changes and complications, which may manifest extrahepatically and extraintestinally. For the purpose of this chapter we would like to distinguish between these two types of manifestation as primary, meaning associated conditions, and secondary, meaning complications of PSC.

ASSOCIATED CONDITIONS

A multitude of case reports on associated conditions can be retrieved from electronic libraries, but there are only very limited systematic data available on associated conditions. The majority of case reports describe an association with other immune-mediated conditions. A list of reported associations is given in Table 1. In view of the close association with ulcerative colitis it is very difficult to distinguish whether other possible associations are characteristic specifically for PSC or only secondary to ulcerative colitis. However, this point is addressed in a very good systematic study of associated autoimmune disease in PSC: Ulrika Broomé and co-workers studied 119 patients with PSC and compared these with matched controls with inflammatory bowel disease[1].

In this study 25% of the PSC patients were found to have an associated autoimmune condition, but only 9% of the IBD controls ($p < 0.005$). Furthermore, nine of the PSC patients had two or more associated autoimmune conditions, but only one of the IBD patients ($p < 0.02$). The associated conditions observed most frequently were insulin-dependent diabetes mellitus (10% vs 2.9% in IBD patients,

Table 1 PSC-associated conditions

Diabetes mellitus	Multiple sclerosis
Thyroid disorders	Vasculitis
Psoriasis	Sarcoidosis
Rheumatoid arthritis	Fibrosing alveolitis
Nephritis	Sacroiliitis
Coeliac disease	Idiopathic thrombocytopenic purpura
Sjögren's syndrome	Pyoderma gangrenosum
Vitiligo	Retroperitoneal fibrosis
Systemic lupus erythematosus	Chronic/autoimmune pancreatitis

$p < 0.04$) and thyroid disease (8.4% vs 2% in IBD patients, $p = 0.05$). The clinical presentation and outcome of PSC with associated autoimmune disorders were similar to those patients without[1].

The European Study Group of PSC has collected data on a total of 394 patients and recorded the associated conditions. These data are rather provisional as data collection for associated conditions was not undertaken prospectively and was not standardized. It is therefore very likely that the recorded data provide an underestimation of these conditions. However, there also appears to be an increased prevalence of autoimmune conditions, with 3.8% of the patients suffering from type 1 diabetes mellitus, 3.3% from rheumatoid arthritis, 3% from thyroid disease and 1.5% from coeliac disease.

Altogether these data suggest a significant association between extrahepatic and extraintestinal autoimmune conditions and PSC, and this in turn supports the interpretation that PSC might itself be an autoimmune disease, despite various atypical features[2]. Our view of PSC being an autoimmune disease has also been supported by the association with autoimmune hepatitis[3,4] and, in our experience, by a frequently good response to immunosuppressive treatment, if given in sufficient doses and as combination therapy[5].

There are various reports of an association between PSC and sarcoidosis, and this was also recorded in 0.8%[1] (in Sweden) to 1.5% of patients (European Study Group of PSC). However, it is arguable whether these cases really represent patients suffering from PSC, as sarcoidosis can cause changes in the liver that may be very difficult, if not impossible, to distinguish from PSC. In sarcoidosis there is occasional massive granuloma formation in the liver, leading to scar formation and bile duct damage or obstruction[6]. Furthermore, hilar lymphadenopathy in sarcoidosis can cause obstructive jaundice, secondary biliary fibrosis and cirrhosis. Therefore it could be that some of these patients were suffering only from sarcoidosis, and others might represent no more than a coincidence.

There is a clinical finding in the majority of PSC patients that is worth mentioning: an enlarged gallbladder. Many patients have a very large gallbladder, and the size seems to increase as the disease progresses[7]. The mechanism of this gallbladder enlargement is not clear, as relative emptying postprandially appears to be normal. The enlarged gallbladder is so common that it can be considered as a diagnostic clue on ultrasound in patients presenting with laboratory features compatible with PSC.

SECONDARY CONDITIONS

In principle, PSC predisposes to complications of chronic liver disease just as any other chronic progressive liver disease. However, there are several features more typical, and others less typical, for PSC. Clinically, patients with PSC nowadays very rarely present primarily with signs of cirrhosis such as finger clubbing, palmar erythema, spider naevi etc., as these signs tend to develop very late in the disease process, and in many PSC patients never develop at all.

Of all the complications of cirrhosis, patients with PSC are most likely to suffer from manifestations of portal hypertension and its specific secondary complications. Splenomegaly is a hallmark of the disease, and in up to one-third of patients can already be found at presentation[8]. Splenomegaly tends to be relatively pronounced. Clinically, the patients may be suffering from left upper quadrant pain, presumably due to stretching of the splenic capsule. Furthermore, as the disease progresses, hypersplenism may be prominent, with pancytopenia developing. Low platelet counts as a result of hypersplenism may be particularly worrisome in a patient with severe portal hypertension and increased risk of upper gastrointestinal bleeding. Furthermore, splenomegaly may result in splenic infarctions manifesting usually with acute attacks of sharp left upper quadrant pain, but rarely also with severe intra-abdominal bleeding due to secondary splenic rupture.

Portal hypertension in PSC often manifests also with upper gastrointestinal bleeding, mostly variceal in origin. Therefore, regular screening for oesophageal or gastric varices is warranted in patients with more advanced PSC. While splenomegaly and varices develop commonly in PSC, development of ascites is rather uncommon and observed only very late in cirrhosis development[8,9]. The reasons why patients with PSC are more likely to develop splenomegaly and varices rather than ascites are unknown.

As PSC advances, and cholestasis progresses, malabsorption of fat and thus fat-soluble vitamins, as well as calcium, may develop, and may lead to osteoporosis. It is not quite clear how important the risk of osteoporosis in PSC really is. As the majority of the patients is male, and the age at manifestation often relatively young, the primary risk of severe osteoporosis is rather low[10,11]. Nonetheless, bone mineral density in the lumbar spine was found to be lower than in an age- and sex-matched population, and correlated with advanced liver disease, the duration of IBD and age[10,11]. In view of liver transplantation as the therapeutic option in late-stage PSC, and in view of the risks of osteoporosis associated with liver transplantation, it thus makes sense to exercise osteoporosis prophylaxis in patients with PSC and progressive cholestasis. The best approach to osteoporosis prophylaxis in PSC is uncertain, and should probably be individualized according to risk co-factors (such as smoking and lack of physical exercise) as well as bone mineral density measurements[12]. For the majority of patients, supplementation of vitamin D and calcium orally will be sufficient, with parenteral vitamin D, as well as bisphosphonates, being reserved for the at-risk population or patients with demonstrable osteoporosis.

Malabsorption may also contribute to weight loss and muscle wasting in late PSC; therefore nutritional advice and support, such as frequent meals, are warranted in patients with progressive cholestasis. In addition, muscle wasting may be observed, and may serve as an indication for liver transplantation. Steatorrhoea may also develop as a result of fat malabsorption.

Cholestasis can result in severe pruritus, which is the presenting feature in 30–40% of patients with PSC[8,9]. The pathogenesis of pruritus in cholestasis is largely unknown, but might involve an activated opioid neurotransmitter system[13]. Dominant strictures should be treated for the maintenance of bile flow. Several symptomatic treatments may be tried, including reduction of the bile salt pool using cholestyramine and histamine antagonists, which are of little clinical value. In addition, rifampin, and in severe cases opiate antagonists such as naltrexone or naloxone, can be given[13], but care should be taken to avoid opioid withdrawal symptoms when using opioid antagonists, by initiating subtherapeutic doses[14].

References

1. Saarinen S, Olerup O, Broomé U. Increased frequency of autoimmune diseases in patients with primary sclerosing cholangitis. Am J Gastroenterol. 2000;95:3195–9.
2. Talwalkar JA, LaRusso NF, Lindor KD. Defining the relationship between autoimmune disease and primary sclerosing cholangitis. Am J Gastroenterol. 2000;95:3024–6.
3. Boberg KM, Fausa O, Haaland T et al. Features of autoimmune hepatitis in primary sclerosing cholangitis: an evaluation of 114 primary sclerosing cholangitis patients according to a scoring system for the diagnosis of autoimmune hepatitis. Hepatology. 1996;23:1369–76.
4. Gohlke F, Lohse AW, Dienes HP et al. Evidence for an overlap syndrome of autoimmune hepatitis and primary sclerosing cholangitis. J Hepatol. 1996;24:699–705.
5. Schramm C, Schirmacher P, Helmreich-Becker I, Gerken G, zum Buschenfelde KH, Lohse AW. Combined therapy with azathioprine, prednisolone, and ursodiol in patients with primary sclerosing cholangitis. A case series. Ann Intern Med. 1999;131:943–6.
6. Ishak KG. Sarcoidosis of the liver and bile ducts. Mayo Clin Proc. 1998;73:467–72.
7. van de Meeberg PC, Portincasa P, Wolfhagen FH, van Erpecum KJ, VanBerge-Henegouwen GP. Increased gall bladder volume in primary sclerosing cholangitis. Gut. 1996;39:594–9.
8. Dickson ER, Murtaugh PA, Wiesner RH et al. Primary sclerosing cholangitis: refinement and validation of survival models. Gastroenterology. 1992;103:1893–901.
9. Broomé U, Olsson R, Loof L et al. Natural history and prognostic factors in 305 Swedish patients with primary sclerosing cholangitis. Gut. 1996;38:610–15.
10. Angulo P, Therneau TM, Jorgensen A et al. Bone disease in patients with primary sclerosing cholangitis: prevalence, severity and prediction of progression. J Hepatol. 1998;29:729–35.
11. Hay JE, Lindor KD, Wiesner RH, Dickson ER, Krom RA, LaRusso NF. The metabolic bone disease of primary sclerosing cholangitis. Hepatology. 1991;14:257–61.
12. Leslie WD, Bernstein CN, Leboff MS. AGA technical review on osteoporosis in hepatic disorders. Gastroenterology. 2003;125:941–66.
13. Jones EA, Bergasa NV. The pruritus of cholestasis. Hepatology. 1999;29:1003–6.
14. Jones EA. Trials of opiate antagonists for the pruritus of cholestasis: primary efficacy endpoints and opioid withdrawal-like reactions. J Hepatol. 2002;37:863–5.

30
Primary sclerosing cholangitis in paediatrics: what is different?

G. MIELI-VERGANI and D. VERGANI

INTRODUCTION

Sclerosing cholangitis in childhood is a heterogeneous condition, with different aetiopathogeneses. Recognized variants are: neonatal sclerosing cholangitis and sclerosing cholangitis associated with primary or secondary immunodeficiencies, with Langerhans cell histiocytosis, or with cystic fibrosis. In contrast to the experience in adults, sclerosing cholangitis occurring as an idiopathic disease (primary sclerosing cholangitis) is rare. The most common type of sclerosing cholangitis in childhood is an overlap syndrome between sclerosing cholangitis and autoimmune hepatitis. We have proposed calling this condition autoimmune sclerosing cholangitis (ASC)[1].

AUTOIMMUNE SCLEROSING CHOLANGITIS

Clinical, laboratory, and histological features

An overlap syndrome between autoimmune hepatitis (AIH) and sclerosing cholangitis has been anecdotally reported in both children[2-4] and adults[5-7]. A retrospective study from our unit showed that 40% of children with sclerosing cholangitis had clinical, biochemical, immunological, and histological features that are indistinguishable from those of AIH[3]. In both AIH and sclerosing cholangitis the serum IgG level was commonly increased and non-organ-specific autoantibodies, antinuclear (ANA) and/or anti-smooth muscle (SMA), were frequently present. Both diseases also commonly showed portal tract inflammation and interface hepatitis. Indeed, most of the reported cases of overlap were originally diagnosed as AIH[5-8]. Typically, the overlap with sclerosing cholangitis was not recognized until years later, when biliary features on follow-up liver biopsy examination led to the performance of a cholangiography. The sequence of diagnoses was then interpreted as an evolution from AIH to sclerosing cholangitis, but the concurrence of these diseases had not been excluded by cholangiographic studies performed at presentation.

Between 1984 and 1997 we performed a prospective study in an attempt to clarify: (a) the relative prevalence of AIH and ASC, (b) whether any feature other than cholangiography can differentiate between the two conditions, (c) whether AIH can progress to ASC, and (d) whether they both respond equally to treatment[1]. All children referred to our unit with clinical and/or biochemical evidence of liver disease and serological features characteristic of AIH (i.e. positive ANA, SMA or anti-liver–kidney microsomal type 1 (LKM1) antibodies), after exclusion of other possible causes of liver disease, underwent cholangiography, sigmoidoscopy, and liver and rectal biopsies at presentation. Follow-up liver biopsies and cholangiograms were also performed in most patients during the study period. We found that 27 of 55 children who presented with clinical and/or laboratory evidence of AIH had radiological evidence of sclerosing cholangitis at presentation. Bile duct abnormalities on cholangiography were both intrahepatic and extrahepatic in two-thirds of patients and intrahepatic in one-third.

Of the 27 patients with ASC, 26 were seropositive for ANA and/or SMA, and one for LKM1[1]. Fifty-five per cent were girls, compared to 80% of those with AIH. The mode of presentation was similar to that of the 28 patients with typical AIH diagnosed during the course of the study, though none of the ASC patients presented with acute liver failure, compared to 14% of those with AIH. Symptoms were those of acute hepatitis in 37% and chronic liver dysfunction in 63%. Inflammatory bowel disease was present in 44% of children with cholangiopathy compared to 18% of those with typical AIH, and, akin to AIH, more than 75% of children with ASC had greatly increased serum IgG levels. Perinuclear antineutrophil cytoplasmic antibodies (pANCA) were present in 74% of patients with ASC compared to 36% of patients with AIH. Compared to healthy controls, frequency of the human leucocyte antigen (HLA) DR3 was increased in ANA/SMA-positive AIH, but not in LKM1-positive AIH and ASC.

There was only a partial concordance between the histological and radiological findings, six patients with ASC (22%) having histological features more compatible with AIH than sclerosing cholangitis. Interestingly, all patients with ASC fulfilled the criteria for the diagnosis of 'definite' or 'probable' AIH established by the International Autoimmune Hepatitis Group (IAIHG)[9]. Indeed, in several patients the diagnosis of sclerosing cholangitis was possible only because of the cholangiographic studies.

Treatment and outcome

Children with ASC responded satisfactorily to the same immunosuppressive treatment used for classical AIH[1]. Prednisolone, 2 mg/kg per day (maximum dose 60 mg/day), was the initial treatment. The dose was gradually decreased over a period of 4–8 weeks if there was a progressive improvement of the serum aminotransferase level. The patient was then maintained on the minimal dose of prednisolone necessary to keep the serum aminotransferase level normal (usual maintenance dose 2.5–5 mg/day, depending on age). During the first 6–8 weeks of treatment, liver function tests were checked weekly, to allow a constant and frequent fine-tuning of the treatment, avoiding severe steroid side-effects. If a progressive normalization of the liver function tests was not obtained over this period of time, or if too high a dose of prednisolone was required to maintain normal transaminases, azathioprine was added at a starting dose of 0.5 mg/kg per day which, in the absence of signs of toxicity, was increased up to a maximum of 2 mg/kg per day until biochemical control was achieved. Although an 80% decrease of the initial transaminase levels was obtained within 6 weeks in most patients, the complete normalization of the liver function took a median of 2 months (range 0.2–107). Since 1992, ursodeoxycholic acid (UDCA, 20 mg/kg per day) was also added to the treatment schedule following the first reports of its value in the treatment of adult PSC[10–11]. After 1 year of normal liver function tests, normal immunoglobulin and negative or low titre ($< 1:20$) autoantibodies, if a follow-up liver biopsy showed minimal or no inflammatory changes, cessation of treatment was attempted. Cessation of treatment was successful in 13% of ASC patients, in comparison to 19% of ANA/SMA-positive AIH and none of the LKM1-positive AIH patients.

Follow-up liver biopsy assessments in this series showed no progression to cirrhosis, although one patient with ASC did develop a vanishing bile duct syndrome and required transplantation 7 years after diagnosis. Follow-up cholangiograms showed static bile duct disease in half of our patients with ASC and progression of the bile duct abnormalities in the other half, two patients with progressive disease requiring transplantation 7 and 10 years after diagnosis. Interestingly, one of the children with AIH who was followed prospectively developed sclerosing cholangitis 8 years after presentation despite effective treatment with corticosteroids (i.e. normal transaminases from the second month of treatment and persistently normal during follow-up) and no biliary changes on several follow-up liver biopsies. This experience suggests that AIH and ASC may be part of the same pathogenetic process and that prednisolone and azathioprine, effective in abating the parenchymal inflammation, may not be as helpful in controlling the bile duct component of the disease.

The medium-term prognosis of ASC is good[1]. All patients in our series were alive after a median follow-up of 7 years. Four patients with ASC, however, required liver transplantation after 2–11 years of observation. In contrast, liver transplantation was not required by any of the 28 children with typical AIH followed for the same period of time.

Primary sclerosing cholangitis

During the 16-year prospective study described above, only nine children were diagnosed with PSC, i.e. chronic liver disease with abnormal cholangiogram, negative ANA, SMA and LKM1, and no identifiable aetiology, in our centre. Six of these patients were male, one presented with a prolonged acute hepatitic illness, the others with signs of chronic liver disease, without history of jaundice. Three had ulcerative colitis, one thyroiditis, three a family history of autoimmune disease and four were positive for pANCA. Liver biopsy showed definite biliary features in seven, chronic hepatitis in one and non-specific portal inflammation in one.

A comparison of the liver function tests at presentation among PSC, ASC, and AIH showed that the alkaline phosphatase/aspartate aminotransferase ratio was significantly higher in PSC and ASC compared to AIH, while bilirubin, aspartate aminotransferase levels, and international normalized prothrombin ratio were significantly higher in AIH than in ASC and PSC. There was no significant difference in levels of gamma-glutamyl transpeptidase, alkaline phosphatase or albumin among the three conditions. Only one of the children with PSC fulfilled the IAIHG criteria for 'probable' AIH at diagnosis[9]. Four patients were treated with UDCA, two with colchicine (in one in combination with penicillamine), one with prednisolone and azathioprine for inflammatory bowel disease, while one received no treatment. One of the four patients receiving UDCA, whose liver biopsy at presentation suggested chronic hepatitis and who scored as 'probable' AIH, became LKM1-positive during follow-up and was then treated with immunosuppression. At a median follow-up of 6 years, six patients were alive and well, one had died of ischaemic hepatitis and two were lost to follow-up.

CONCLUSIONS

Adult-type PSC is rare in paediatric age, where the most common form of sclerosing cholangitis is ASC. The prevalence of ASC and AIH is similar in a tertiary paediatric hepatology referral centre. The differential diagnosis between the two conditions requires visualization of the biliary tree by cholangiogram, no other investigation being able to clearly differentiate between them. Though in our prospective study this was achieved by endoscopic retrograde cholangiography, this procedure should be performed only when the necessary expertise is available. With continuing improvement of the resolution of magnetic resonance cholangiography, this much safer technique will soon be used instead.

Response to immunosuppression is satisfactory in both AIH and ASC, though medium-term transplant-free survival is better in AIH than ASC. AIH can evolve to ASC despite effective immunosuppressive treatment, and in the absence of histological features of sclerosing cholangitis. Whether ASC and AIH are different diseases or different manifestations of the same pathological process remains to be clarified. Equally, the relationship between ASC and adult-type PSC is still unclear, though it is possible that at least some forms of adult PSC represent a 'burnt-out' form of ASC starting in childhood.

References

1. Gregorio GV, Portmann B, Karani J et al. Autoimmune hepatitis/sclerosing cholangitis overlap syndrome in childhood: a 16-year prospective study. Hepatology. 2001;33:544–53.
2. Debray D, Pariente D, Urvoas E, Hadchouel M, Bernard O. Sclerosing cholangitis in children. J Pediatr. 1994;124:49–56.
3. el-Shabrawi M, Wilkinson ML, Portmann B et al. Primary sclerosing cholangitis in childhood. Gastroenterology. 1987;92:1226–35.
4. Wilschanski M, Chait P, Wade JA et al. Primary sclerosing cholangitis in 32 children: clinical, laboratory, and radiographic features, with survival analysis. Hepatology. 1995;22:1415–22.
5. Gohlke F, Lohse AW, Dienes HP et al. Evidence for an overlap syndrome of autoimmune hepatitis and primary sclerosing cholangitis. J Hepatol. 1996;24:699–705.
6. McNair AN, Moloney M, Portmann BC, Williams R, McFarlane IG. Autoimmune hepatitis overlapping with primary sclerosing cholangitis in five cases. Am J Gastroenterol. 1998;93:777–84.

7. Rabinovitz M, Demetris AJ, Bou-Abboud CF, Van Thiel DH. Simultaneous occurrence of primary sclerosing cholangitis and autoimmune chronic active hepatitis in a patient with ulcerative colitis. Dig Dis Sci. 1992;37:1606–11.
8. Sisto A, Feldman P, Garel L et al. Primary sclerosing cholangitis in children: study of five cases and review of the literature. Pediatrics. 1987;80:918–23.
9. International Autoimmune Hepatitis Group report: Review of criteria for diagnosis of autoimmune hepatitis. J Hepatol. 1999;31:929–38.
10. Beuers U, Spengler U, Kruis W et al. Ursodeoxycholic acid for treatment of primary sclerosing cholangitis: a placebo-controlled trial. Hepatology. 1992;16:707–14.
11. Lebovics E, Salama M, Elhosseiny A, Rosenthal WS. Resolution of radiographic abnormalities with ursodeoxycholic acid therapy of primary sclerosing cholangitis. Gastroenterology. 1992;102:2143–7.

Section IX
Treatment options in primary sclerosing cholangitis

31
Ursodeoxycholic acid: high-dose, monotherapy or combination therapy?

H. R. VAN BUUREN

INTRODUCTION

Most patients who are diagnosed with primary sclerosing cholangitis (PSC) are young. After diagnosis they are informed that the expected median time to death or liver transplantation averages 12 years[1–3]. To date there is no evidence that any therapy alters this grave prognosis except liver transplantation for patients with end-stage disease or otherwise untreatable complications. Repeated balloon dilation in combination with ursodeoxycholic acid (UDCA) has been reported to significantly improve prognosis for patients developing dominant bile duct stenoses[4]. However, in this study an indirect comparison of the actual and the predicted course was made, and the intriguing results await confirmation by controlled trials. It is generally accepted that treatment of concomitant inflammatory bowel disease (IBD) does not influence the course of PSC. Although PSC is a disease with autoimmune features there is currently no, or insufficient, proof that immune-modulating or immune-suppressive agents – including corticosteroids, azathioprine, cyclosporin, tacrolimus[5], pentoxifylline[6] or 2-cholodeoxyadenosine[7] – have major therapeutic effects. The same applies to a variety of drugs such as D-penicillamine[8], colchicine[9], pirfenidone[10] and oral[11] or transdermal[12] nicotine. The majority of these drugs has not been evaluated by adequate randomized investigations.

UDCA THERAPY IN PSC: CONTROLLED TRIALS

Among agents potentially effective in PSC, UDCA has aroused most interest, and has been most extensively studied. Nevertheless the number of controlled studies is limited, and only one trial was reported during the past 6 years[13]. This

Table 1 Randomized controlled trials of UDCA versus placebo or no treatment in PSC

Main author and refs	Year	Patients (UDCA/placebo)	UDCA dose (mg/kg per day)	Duration of treatment (months)
Beuers[14]	1992	6/8	13–15	12
Lo[17]	1992	8/10	10	24
Stiehl[18]	1994	10/10	10.7	3
de Maria[15]	1996	20/20*	8.6	24
Lindor[16]	1997	53/52	13–15	Median 26.4
Mitchell[13]	2001	13/13	20	24
Total		110/113	8.6–20	Median 24

* UDCA versus no treatment.

is in sharp contrast to the evaluation of UDCA therapy in primary biliary cirrhosis (PBC): at least 16 randomized trials involving more than 1400 patients have been conducted in this cholestatic liver disease. This suggests that there is major difficulty in studying PSC.

The total number of reported randomized controlled trials comparing UDCA with placebo or no treatment published since 1992 is six[13–18] (Table 1). Most trials were small with an average sample size of 37 (range 14–105) patients. Given the slowly progressive course of PSC all studies have been of short duration. According to a recent Cochrane review[19] none of the trials was of high methodological quality, i.e. was (completely) adequate with respect to generation of the allocation sequence, allocation concealment, double-blinding and report of follow-up data. None of the trials reported data on cost-effectiveness or quality of life. These trial characteristics should be taken into account when assessing the current evidence for UDCA in PSC.

The following effects of UDCA on end-points as reported in the six trials were extracted from the Cochrane Review[19].

Mortality

In the total group of 110 UDCA-treated patients four deaths were reported, compared with five out of 113 placebo-treated patients. Meta-analysis confirmed that UDCA did not reduce the risk of death in patients treated with UDCA (RR 0.86, 95% CI 0.27–2.73).

Treatment failure

Two trials[13,16] reported the number of treatment failures. There was no significant difference between UDCA and placebo treatment with respect to treatment failures (liver transplantation, varices, ascites, encephalopathy) (RR 0.94, 95% CI 0.63–1.42).

Liver histology

Deterioration of liver histology was assessed in four trials[13–16]. Meta-analysis revealed absence of a significant beneficial effect of UDCA treatment (RR 0.89,

95% CI 0.95–1.74). In the trial by Mitchell et al.[13] high-dose UDCA therapy had a statistically significant beneficial effect on progression of the histological stage of the disease (OR 6.5; 95% CI 0.97–43.9; $p = 0.05$). A simultaneous positive trend was noted in inflammatory activity; however, the observed differences were not significant. In the trial by Beuers et al.[14] histopathological features were also found to be improved after 1 year treatment, while in the trials of De Maria et al.[15] and Lindor[16] no differences between the treatment groups were observed.

Cholangiographic deterioration

Three trials[13,15,18] (one with placebo treatment for only 3 months[18]) reported on this rather problematic end-point. Four out of 43 UDCA-treated patients were reported with cholangiographic deterioration compared with 10/43 control patients (RR 0.43, 95% CI 0.18–1.02; n.s.).

Clinical symptoms

No significant effect of UDCA on fatigue or pruritus was apparent in a meta-analysis of data as reported in three trials (RR 0.66, 95% CI 0.2–2.19)[13,16,18].

Liver biochemistry

The Cochrane Review confirmed previous uncontrolled and controlled observations that UDCA has a marked effect on laboratory parameters in PSC. UDCA significantly decreased serum bilirubin concentrations (weighted mean difference −14.6 μmol/L, 95% CI −18.7 to −10.6, reduction ranged from 33% to 60%), serum alkaline phosphatase (weighted mean difference −506 U/L, 95% CI −583 to −430; reduction ranged from 45% to 67%), serum-gamma-glutamyltranspeptidase (weighted mean difference −260 U/L, 95% CI −315 to −205; reduction ranged from 70% to 79%) and serum aspartate aminotransferase activity (mean weighted difference −46 IU/L, 95% CI −77 to −16; reduction ranged from 41% to 48%). No significant effect on serum albumin concentration was found.

Safety

The Cochrane Review confirmed that UDCA is safe and free from serious adverse events.

HIGH-DOSE UDCA IN PSC

The most frequently used dose of UDCA in PSC is 13–15 mg/kg per day. Considering the lack of clear clinical improvements obtained with conventional doses two groups have evaluated higher doses. In a 1-year open-label study[20] 30 PSC patients were treated with UDCA at a dose of 25–30 mg/kg per day. Changes in the Mayo risk score at 1 year of treatment and projected survival at 4 years were compared with that observed in patients who participated in a previous trial evaluating UDCA 13–15 mg/kg per day versus placebo. High-dose UDCA therapy was well tolerated, but three patients developed diarrhoea and/or nausea and withdrew from the study. Significant laboratory improvements occurred, not only in serum alkaline phosphatase and serum transaminases but also in serum bilirubin and albumin. Changes in the Mayo risk score after 1 year were significantly different among the three groups. The expected mortality at 4 years was significantly improved for patients in the high-UDCA group when compared with placebo. In a randomized controlled trial[13] 26 patients were treated with UDCA (20 mg/kg per day) or placebo during 2 years. No significant side-effects were noted. UDCA did not improve symptoms. In this trial high-dose UDCA had no significant effect on serum aspartate aminotransferase, bilirubin or albumin. UDCA treatment was associated with a significant reduction in progression of cholangiographic appearances ($p = 0.015$) and liver fibrosis ($p = 0.05$).

THE PROBLEM OF (NEW) UDCA TRIALS IN PSC

It is a gloomy fact that, 15 years after the first controlled studies with UDCA in PSC were initiated, the true significance of this treatment remains unknown. Reasons why trials evaluating UDCA, or other agents, in PSC have been few, small and of limited duration all seem related to the unique character of the disease. Features contributing to the difficulty of organizing and conducting meaningful (UDCA) trials in PSC include:

1. The highly variable and unpredictable course of PSC. Patients with minor cholestasis may remain stable for a long time, while others may develop disease-specific (cholangitis, dominant bile duct strictures, cholangiocarcinoma) and other complications due to inflammatory bowel disease, portal hypertension or end-stage liver disease.
2. Presence or development of inflammatory bowel disease and, to a lesser extent, autoimmune hepatitis. These conditions may interfere with the course of PSC and may require simultaneous or intercurrent treatments, thereby obscuring effects of UDCA.
3. Failure to recruit sufficient numbers of patients in single-centre studies (and failure to seek or achieve multicentre cooperation).
4. The modest interest or possibilities of pharmaceutical companies and research organizations to support or initiate studies in orphan diseases.
5. Long-term placebo treatment may not be acceptable for patients.
6. The competitive environment in academic centres, with pressure to publish and lack of patience or possibilities to await long-term results.
7. The huge costs of long-term placebo-controlled trials.
8. Recent reports of a protective effect of UDCA on the development of colorectal neoplasia may hamper patient recruitment in future placebo-controlled trials.
9. UDCA treatment is virtually free of side-effects and, without any doubt, improves liver biochemical tests. Nowadays patients are well informed and, being aware that (other) effective drugs are currently not available, are increasingly reluctant to accept placebo treatment and prefer to be treated with UDCA despite uncertainty regarding its true therapeutic significance.

Table 2 Studies evaluating UDCA in combination with other drugs in PSC

Main author and ref.	Year	No. of patients	Type of study	Other drug	Duration of treatment (months)
Lindor[21]	1996	19	Open	Methotrexate	24
Schramm[22]	1999	15	Open	Prednisolone and azathioprine	Median 41
van Hoogstraten[23]	2000	18	RCT	Prednisone or budesonide	2
Vleggaar[12]	2001	12	RCT	Transdermal nicotine	4

UDCA IN COMBINATION WITH OTHER AGENTS

The apparent limited or absent efficacy of UDCA monotherapy has excited interest in combination therapy. Combining UDCA with a drug with a different mechanism of action could result in a more effective treatment regimen through synergistic or additive effects. Thus far the reported results of this approach are not stimulating (Table 2). In an open-label study[21] methotrexate (0.25 mg/kg orally) had no additional effect to UDCA (13–15 mg/kg per day) whatsoever, but was associated with toxicity. In a case series from Mainz 15 patients were treated with UDCA (500–700 mg/day), azathioprine (1–1.5 mg/kg per day) and prednisolone (initially 1 mg/kg per day, maintenance dose of 5–10 mg/day) during a median period of 41 (range 3–81) months[22]. Adverse drug effects led to discontinuation of azathioprine and/or prednisolone in two cases. Liver biochemistry improved significantly. Positive effects were also noted on liver histology and cholangiographic appearances in a subset of patients. The open character of this study, and the small patient number, preclude clear conclusions with respect to the proposed treatment regimen. Two small, randomized double-blind placebo-controlled trials evaluated the short-term effect of combinations of UDCA with prednisone, budesonide and transdermal nicotine on symptoms and liver biochemistry[12,23]. In these trials no beneficial effects were observed.

UDCA AND COLON CANCER

Many patients with PSC also have inflammatory bowel disease and an associated increased risk for colorectal cancer[24,25]. Therefore it is relevant to briefly review recent data concerning a possible important therapeutic effect of UDCA on the colon.

In a number of *in-vitro* and animal studies UDCA has been shown to have colon cancer-chemoprotective effects. In addition, two recent clinical studies found that UDCA seems to significantly decrease the risk of colorectal neoplasia in patients with PSC and ulcerative colitis (UC). In a cross-sectional study by Tung et al. involving 59 patients with PSC and UC participating in an endoscopic surveillance programme, 26 (44%) patients had a diagnosis of colonic dysplasia at some time during surveillance[26]. No patient developed cancer. Of the 26 patients who had dysplasia, 50% had used UDCA compared with 85% of patients without dysplasia (OR 0.18, 95% CI 0.05–0.61; $p = 0.005$). Multivariate analysis of (potential) risk factors for dysplasia (sex, age, age of onset and duration of UC, duration of PSC, Child–Pugh class and use of sulphasalazine) revealed that use of UDCA (OR 0.14, CI 0.03–0.64; $p = 0.01$) remained a negative risk factor for dysplasia. Pardi et al. studied the cumulative incidence of colorectal neoplasia in patients with PSC and UC colitis who had participated in a previously reported controlled trial evaluating UDCA versus placebo for its effect on the hepatobiliary disease[27]. Of the 85 patients with PSC and UC in the original study 33 (39%) were excluded for several reasons. Three out of 29 patients (10%) assigned to UDCA developed dysplasia compared with 8/23 (35%) patients originally assigned to placebo (two colon cancer, six dysplasia). The relative risk for developing colorectal dysplasia was 0.26 (95% CI 0.06–0.92; $p = 0.034$) for patients initially assigned to the UDCA group. Sixteen of 23 (70%) patients initially assigned to placebo were switched to open-label UDCA treatment. Assigning these patients to the UDCA group from the time they began UDCA treatment did not change the magnitude of the protective effect of UDCA. Interestingly, a recent report indicates that in PBC patients UDCA treatment lowers both the prevalence of colorectal adenomas and the risk of recurrent adenomas after adenoma removal[28].

Taken together these reports suggest that UDCA may act as a powerful chemoprotective drug in patients with PSC and UC, who carry a considerable lifetime risk for colorectal carcinoma. Further trials are necessary to confirm the initial promising data. Further studies also seem warranted to assess a protective effect of UDCA in non-colitis patients with adenomas or previous colorectal cancer, and other risk groups such as families with hereditary non-polyposis colorectal cancer or familial adenomatous polyposis.

CONCLUSIONS

UDCA, in conventional and high doses, leads to significant improvements in liver biochemistry, but there is insufficient evidence to either support or refute an important clinical effect. The observation that, after 15 years of clinical research, a major therapeutic effect has not been documented could point to a true absence of such an effect. Another explanation, favoured by many, is that the studies performed to date simply did not allow us to detect a true therapeutic effect due to methodological shortcomings and the many problems associated with therapeutic studies in PSC. There is currently no evidence to suggest that combined therapy with methotrexate, prednisone, budesonide, azathioprine or nicotine is more effective than UDCA monotherapy.

There is probably consensus that treating PSC patients with UDCA is not fully in accordance with the principles of evidence-based medicine. Nevertheless, given the safety of UDCA, the effects on liver biochemistry, the potential benefit on other outcome measures and the complete lack of alternative medical treatment options, in combination with the opinion of patients, it seems likely that doctors will continue to treat patients with UDCA. This choice will probably be reinforced by recent data suggesting a prophylactic effect of UDCA on colorectal cancer.

THE FUTURE

Ideally new trials should be initiated to finally answer the question whether UDCA is cosmetic or effective therapy[19]. These should be large, of long duration and of high methodological quality, and will require multicentre, probably international, collaboration. The costs will be huge but must be balanced against the costs of continuing potentially ineffective therapy. In the Netherlands the annual costs of UDCA treatment (15 mg/kg per day) of a patient with a body weight of 70 kg amount to €1026. While the actual global economic situation may be unfavourable for new large-scale projects the medical community may, in the present era of evidence-based medicine, be increasingly forced to take new initiatives. It is evident that new trials should address the effect of UDCA on both the hepatobiliary tract and the colon. There seems no need to further assess effects of UDCA on symptoms while the pronounced effect of UDCA on liver biochemical tests renders fully blinded studies difficult, if not impossible. A non-placebo-controlled design could possibly diminish some of the noted problems of UDCA trials in PSC, in particular with respect to costs and the willingness of patients to participate. Methodological problems associated with open trials should be solved in a creative way.

References

1. Harnois DM, Lindor KD. Primary sclerosing cholangitis: evolving concepts in diagnosis and treatment. Dig Dis. 1997;15:23–41.
2. Ponsioen CI, Tytgat GN. Primary sclerosing cholangitis: a clinical review. Am J Gastroenterol. 1998;93:515–23.
3. Lee YM, Kaplan MM. Primary sclerosing cholangitis. N Engl J Med. 1995;332:924–33.
4. Stiehl A, Rudolph G, Kloters-Plachky P, Sauer P, Walker S. Development of dominant bile duct stenoses in patients with primary sclerosing cholangitis treated with ursodeoxycholic acid: outcome after endoscopic treatment. J Hepatol. 2002;36:151–6.
5. Van Thiel DH, Carroll P, Abu-Elmagd K et al. Tacrolimus (FK 506), a treatment for primary sclerosing cholangitis: results of an open-label preliminary trial. Am J Gastroenterol. 1995;90:455–9.
6. Bharucha AE, Jorgensen R, Lichtman SN, LaRusso NF, Lindor KD. A pilot study of pentoxifylline for the treatment of primary sclerosing cholangitis. Am J Gastroenterol. 2000;95:2338–42.
7. Duchini A, Younossi ZM, Saven A, Bordin GM, Knowles HJ, Pockros PJ. An open-label pilot trial of cladibrine (2-chlorodeoxyadenosine) in patients with primary sclerosing cholangitis. J Clin Gastroenterol. 2000;31:292–6.
8. LaRusso NF, Wiesner RH, Ludwig J, MacCarty RL, Beaver SJ, Zinsmeister AR. Prospective trial of penicillamine in primary sclerosing cholangitis. Gastroenterology. 1988;95:1036–42.
9. Olsson R, Broome U, Danielsson A et al. Colchicine treatment of primary sclerosing cholangitis. Gastroenterology. 1995;108:1199–203.
10. Angulo P, MacCarty RL, Sylvestre PB et al. Pirfenidone in the treatment of primary sclerosing cholangitis. Dig Dis Sci. 2002;47:157–61.
11. Angulo P, Bharucha AE, Jorgensen RA et al. Oral nicotine in treatment of primary sclerosing cholangitis: a pilot study. Dig Dis Sci. 1999;44:602–7.
12. Vleggaar FP, van Buuren HR, van Berge Henegouwen GP, Hop WC, van Erpecum KJ. No beneficial effects of transdermal nicotine in patients with primary sclerosing cholangitis: results of a randomized double-blind placebo-controlled cross-over study. Eur J Gastroenterol Hepatol. 2001;13:171–5.
13. Mitchell SA, Bansi DS, Hunt N, Von Bergmann K, Fleming KA, Chapman RW. A preliminary trial of high-dose ursodeoxycholic acid in primary sclerosing cholangitis. Gastroenterology. 2001;121:900–7.

14. Beuers U, Spengler U, Kruis W et al. Ursodeoxycholic acid for treatment of primary sclerosing cholangitis: a placebo-controlled trial. Hepatology. 1992;16:707–14.
15. De Maria N, Colantoni A, Rosenbloom E, Van Thiel DH. Ursodeoxycholic acid does not improve the clinical course of primary sclerosing cholangitis over a 2-year period. Hepato-gastroenterology. 1996;43:1472–9.
16. Lindor KD. Ursodiol for primary sclerosing cholangitis. Mayo Primary Sclerosing Cholangitis–Ursodeoxycholic Acid Study Group. N Engl J Med. 1997;336:691–5.
17. Lo SK, Hermann R, Chapman RW et al. Ursodeoxycholic acid in primary sclerosing cholangitis: a double-blind placebo controlled trial. Hepatology. 1992;16:92A (abstract).
18. Stiehl A, Walker S, Stiehl L, Rudolph G, Hofmann WJ, Theilmann L. Effect of ursodeoxycholic acid on liver and bile duct disease in primary sclerosing cholangitis. A 3-year pilot study with a placebo-controlled study period. J Hepatol. 1994;20:57–64.
19. Chen W, Gluud C. Bile acids for primary sclerosing cholangitis. Cochrane Database Syst Rev. 2003(2):CD003626.
20. Harnois DM, Angulo P, Jorgensen RA, Larusso NF, Lindor KD. High-dose ursodeoxycholic acid as a therapy for patients with primary sclerosing cholangitis. Am J Gastroenterol. 2001;96: 1558–62.
21. Lindor KD, Jorgensen RA, Anderson ML, Gores GJ, Hofmann AF, LaRusso NF. Ursodeoxycholic acid and methotrexate for primary sclerosing cholangitis: a pilot study. Am J Gastroenterol. 1996;91:511–15.
22. Schramm C, Schirmacher P, Helmreich-Becker I, Gerken G, zum Buschenfelde KH, Lohse AW. Combined therapy with azathioprine, prednisolone, and ursodiol in patients with primary sclerosing cholangitis. A case series. Ann Intern Med. 1999;131:943–6.
23. van Hoogstraten HJ, Vleggaar FP, Boland GJ et al. Budesonide or prednisone in combination with ursodeoxycholic acid in primary sclerosing cholangitis: a randomized double-blind pilot study. Belgian–Dutch PSC Study Group. Am J Gastroenterol. 2000;95:2015–22.
24. Jayaram H, Satsangi J, Chapman RW. Increased colorectal neoplasia in chronic ulcerative colitis complicated by primary sclerosing cholangitis: fact or fiction? Gut. 2001;48:430–4.
25. Shetty K, Rybicki L, Brzezinski A, Carey WD, Lashner BA. The risk for cancer or dysplasia in ulcerative colitis patients with primary sclerosing cholangitis. Am J Gastroenterol. 1999; 94:1643–9.
26. Tung BY, Emond MJ, Haggitt RC et al. Ursodiol use is associated with lower prevalence of colonic neoplasia in patients with ulcerative colitis and primary sclerosing cholangitis. Ann Intern Med. 2001;134:89–95.
27. Pardi DS, Loftus EV, Jr., Kremers WK, Keach J, Lindor KD. Ursodeoxycholic acid as a chemo-preventive agent in patients with ulcerative colitis and primary sclerosing cholangitis. Gastroenterology. 2003;124:889–93.
28. Serfaty L, De Leusse A, Rosmorduc O et al. Ursodeoxycholic acid therapy and the risk of colorectal adenoma in patients with primary biliary cirrhosis: an observational study. Hepatology. 2003;38:203–9.

32
Endoscopic treatment of dominant stenoses in patients with primary sclerosing cholangitis

A. STIEHL

INTRODUCTION

Primary sclerosing cholangitis (PSC) is characterized by multiple stenoses of intrahepatic and/or extrahepatic bile ducts[1-4]. In a prospective trial on the effect of ursodeoxycholic acid (UDCA) on bile duct disease in which repeat cholangiographies were performed[4], during treatment with UDCA for 8 years, 35% of the patients had or developed a dominant stenosis of major bile ducts. Such patients need endoscopic treatment of their stenoses, which is highly effective[5-11].

ENDOSCOPIC OPTIONS IN MAJOR DUCT STENOSES

When dominant stenoses of the larger bile ducts are detected by endoscopic retrograde cholangiopancreatography (ERCP) early endoscopic intervention is mandatory. Alternatively dilation or stenting may be used to treat the bile duct stenosis (Table 1). There is increasing evidence that dilation is superior to stenting[9-11]. In most cases a single dilation is not sufficient, and repeated dilations are necessary until the duct remains open[11]. Intermittent stenting has also been used[6-11], but the stents tend to occlude early due to the inflammatory material that is shed from the bile ducts. Since occlusion of the stent leads to bacterial infection of the proximal biliary tree stents in general should be removed or replaced early, i.e. within 1–2 weeks. In our hands dilation is by far the more effective form of endoscopic treatment[11].

In the past only stenoses of the common duct have been treated by endoscopic measures. Since after successful opening of the common duct many patients in addition develop dominant stenoses of the hepatic ducts, the treatment of such stenoses represents a great challenge[11]. Attempts to treat such stenoses endoscopically revealed that short segment stenoses within 2 cm of the bifurcation

Table 1 Endoscopic treatment of patients with PSC with dominant stenoses of major bile ducts

Main author and refs.	No. of patients	Stent	Dilation
Johnson, 1987[6]	35	11	24
Lee, 1995[7]	53	22	31
van Milligen, 1996[8]	25	21	0
Petersen, 2001[9]	71	37*	34
Baluyut, 2001[10]	63	32	140†
Stiehl, 2002[11]	52	5	210†

* Patients with dilation and short-time stent.
† Patients with repeated dilations.

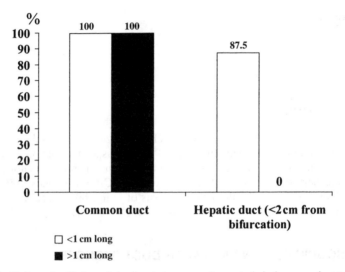

Figure 1 Endoscopic dilation of dominant stenoses: primary technical success in opening the common duct and one of the hepatic ducts

may be treated by endoscopic dilation with good results[11]. In most cases (87.5%) it was possible to open at least one (the right or the left) dominant short segment stenosis of a hepatic duct (Figure 1).

Originally it was thought that only short segment stenoses may be treated by endoscopic means, but there is increasing evidence that long segment stenoses of the common duct of more than 1 cm length may be treated with good success[11]. The situation is different for stenoses of the hepatic ducts situated within 2 cm of the bifurcation, where only short segment stenoses may be treated effectively.

Cholangiography in patients with increasing cholestasis seems essential to detect stenoses of major bile ducts early[5]. Such cholangiographies should be performed under antibiotic prophylaxis[12], since patients with PSC tend to have bacterial cholangitis. This problem appears even more relevant when dominant stenoses, or even complete occlusion of the major ducts, have developed. In such cases endoscopic opening of the duct stenosis is often essential for the successful antibiotic treatment. It is evident that mechanical obstruction of major bile ducts cannot be treated by UDCA effectively, and that endoscopic measures are essential if conservative treatment is to be effective.

SURVIVAL FREE OF LIVER TRANSPLANTATION

PSC is a progressive disease and survival of such patients is reduced. Survival is better in asymptomatic patients than in symptomatic patients. In a recent controlled 2-year study[13], UDCA treatment in conventional doses did not improve survival free of liver transplantation. Treatment with higher doses of UDCA may be more effective[14,15] and studies have been initiated. In a prospective non-randomized study in which patients were treated with UDCA and, whenever necessary, by additional endoscopic dilations the survival after treatment with UDCA and dilation of major duct stenoses was significantly improved[11] compared to the predicted survival with a p value of 0.001.

It is obvious that UDCA will have little or no effect when dominant stenoses are present and are not treated by endoscopic means. Therefore the results of studies in which endoscopic opening of the dominant stenoses did not play a role may be more or less relevant depending on the number of patients with dominant stenoses who were included.

BILE DUCT CARCINOMAS

A problem represents the increased incidence of cholangiocarcinomas and probably also colonic carcinomas in PSC. In a large multicentre study from Sweden[4], in which 305 PSC patients were followed over a median follow-up time of 63 months, a bile duct carcinoma was observed in 8% of patients (Table 2). Very high rates of bile duct carcinomas of over 20% have repeatedly been reported in studies coming from transplantation centres, as it appears that they reflect very selected patient groups[16]. In a controlled study 0/52 of the patients with PSC on UDCA developed a bile duct carcinoma in comparison to 3/53 patients in the control group[13]. In a 13-year prospective study of 106 patients treated with

Table 2 Bile duct carcinomas in PSC

Main author (year), institution and refs.	No. of patients	Observation time (years)	CA (%)
Wiesner (1989), Mayo, Rochester, US[2]	174	6 (mean)	19
Farrant (1991), King's, London, UK[3]	126	5.8 (median)	6
Broome (1996), Multi-centre, Sweden[4]	305	5.2 (median)	8
Stiehl (2002), Dept. Med., Heidelberg, Germany[11]	106	5.0 (median)	2.8*

* All patients treated with UDCA ± endoscopic treatment of dominant stenoses.

UDCA only 3/106 (2.8%) developed a bile duct carcinoma[11]. Of the patients with dominant stenoses a bile duct carcinoma was found in 2/52, indicating that, in this subgroup of patients also, the frequency of such carcinomas is low[11]. It seems possible that the reduced inflammation around the bile ducts observed after UDCA treatment[14,17,18] may reduce the incidence of bile duct carcinomas, but definite proof for this is lacking.

LIVER TRANSPLANTATION

In end-stage disease liver transplantation represents the treatment of choice. The 5-year survival rate after liver transplantation for PSC is approximately 72% (European Transplant Registry). In view of the fact that the incidence of bile duct carcinomas is much lower than the lethality after transplantation it appears unjustified to recommend prophylactic liver transplantation in precirrhotic stages of the disease in order to prevent the development of bile duct carcinomas.

CONCLUSION

We conclude that PSC may be treated conservatively by UDCA with good treatment results and prolongation of survival free of liver transplantation only when patients who develop major duct stenoses are recognized early, and are additionally treated by endoscopic means. In end-stage disease liver transplantation is indicated.

References

1. Chapman RW, Arborgh BA, Rhodes JM et al. Primary sclerosing cholangitis – a review of its clinical features, cholangiography and hepatic histology. Gut. 1980;21:870–7.
2. Wiesner RH, Grambsch PM, Dickson ER et al. Natural history, prognostic factors, and survival analysis. Hepatology. 1989;10:430–6.
3. Farrant MJ, Hayllar KM, Wilkinson ML et al. Natural history and prognostic variables in primary sclerosing cholangitis. Gastroenterology. 1991;100:1710–17.
4. Broome U, Olson R, Lööf L et al. Natural history and prognostic factors in 305 Swedish patients with primary sclerosing cholangitis. Gut. 1996;38:610–15.
5. Stiehl A, Rudolph G, Sauer P et al. Efficacy of ursodeoxycholic acid and endoscopic dilation of major duct stenoses in primary sclerosing cholangitis. An 8-year prospective study. J Hepatol. 1997;26:560–6.
6. Johnson GK, Geenen JE, Venu RP, Hogan WJ. Endoscopic treatment of biliary duct strictures in sclerosing cholangitis: follow up assessment of a new therapeutic approach. Gastrointest Endosc. 1987;33:9–12.
7. Lee JG, Schutz SM, England RE, Leung JW, Cotton PB. Endoscopic therapy of sclerosing cholangitis. Hepatology. 1995;21:661–7.
8. van Milligen AWM, van Bracht J, Rauws EAJ et al. Endoscopic stent therapy for dominant extrahepatic bile duct strictures in primary sclerosing cholangitis. Gastrointest Endosc. 1996;44:293–9.
9. Petersen KM, Angulo P, Baron TH et al. Balloon dilatation compared to stenting of dominant strictures in primary sclerosing cholangitis. Am J Gastroenterol. 2001;96:1059–66.
10. Baluyut AR, Sherman S, Lehman GA, Hoen H, Chalasani N. Impact of endoscopic therapy on the survival of patients with primary sclerosing cholangitis. Gastrointest Endosc. 2001;53:308–12.
11. Stiehl A, Rudolph G, Klöters-Plachky P et al. Development of bile duct stenoses in patients with primary sclerosing cholangitis treated with ursodeoxycholic acid. Outcome after endoscopic treatment. J Hepatol. 2002;36:151–6.

12. Olson R, Björnsson E, Bäckman L et al. Bile duct bacterial isolates in primary sclerosing cholangitis: a study of explanted livers. J Hepatol. 1998;28:426–32.
13. Lindor KD and the Mayo PSC/UDCA Study Group. Ursodiol for the treatment of primary sclerosing cholangitis. N Engl J Med. 1997;336:691–5.
14. Mitchell SA, Bansi D, Hunt N et al. A preliminary trial of high dose ursodeoxycholic acid in primary sclerosing cholangitis. Gastroenterology. 2001;121:900–7.
15. Harnois DM, Angulo P, Jorgensen RA, LaRusso NF, Lindor KD. High-dose ursodeoxycholic acid as therapy for patients with primary sclerosing cholangitis. Am J Gastroenterol. 2001;96:1558–62.
16. Nashan B, Schlitt HJ, Tusch G et al. Biliary malignancies in primary sclerosing cholangitis: timing of liver transplantation. Hepatology. 1996;23:1105–11.
17. Beuers U, Spengler U, Kruis W et al. Ursodeoxycholic acid for treatment of primary sclerosing cholangitis: a placebo controlled trial. Hepatology. 1992;16:707–14.
18. Stiehl A, Walker S, Stiehl L et al. Effects of ursodeoxycholic acid on liver and bile duct disease in primary sclerosing cholangitis. A 3 year pilot study with a placebo-controlled study period. J Hepatol. 1994;20:57–64.

33
How should and how does antifibrotic therapy act in biliary fibrosis?

D. SCHUPPAN, Y. POPOV and E. PATSENKER

INTRODUCTION

Antifibrotic therapies should preferentially be targeted to the activated hepatic mesenchymal cells. Those cells resemble wound-healing myofibroblasts and synthesize an excess of matrix proteins. They derive from quiescent hepatic stellate cells and (myo-)fibroblasts. Several fibrogenic cytokines and other mediators, many of them derived from activated or proliferating bile duct epithelia, trigger their activation. Whereas various agents have been shown to inhibit hepatic stellate cell/myofibroblast proliferation and collagen synthesis *in vitro*, only few of them are effective in suitable animal models *in vivo*, and finally in humans. The best animal model for chronic cholestatic liver diseases is rat secondary biliary cirrhosis. In addition, the speed of reversion of fibrosis after withdrawal of a hepatotoxin such as thioacetamide can be used to test antifibrotic agents *in vivo*.

The interferons (IF-γ > α, β) have proven antiproliferative and fibrosuppressive activity on mesenchymal cells in culture. Retrospective data suggest that IF-α therapy for hepatitis C can halt or even reverse fibrosis. However, this has to be confirmed by randomized prospective studies, and an effect in biliary fibrosis is less probable. Strategies to inhibit the key profibrogenic cytokine transforming growth factor beta (TGF-β), e.g. by soluble decoy receptors, or molecules that are involved in TGF-β signal transduction, are evolving, but results are not yet convincing.

Combination therapy of several potential antifibrotic agents appears most effective, while side-effects of the necessarily long-term or even lifelong treatment are reduced. Such agents are silymarin; a defined mixture of flavonoids; sho-saiko-to which contains related compounds such as baicalein, halofuginone, and other plant-derived drugs; the phosphodiesterase inhibitor pentoxifylline; oral inhibitors of the endothelin-A-receptor or inhibitors of the renin–angiotensin system.

Drug targeting to the fibrogenic liver cells is now possible by use of ligands that bind to receptors which are specifically up-regulated on activated bile duct epithelial or stellate cells, e.g. those for the integrin $\alpha v\beta 6$, platelet-derived growth factor or collagen type VI. Together with the evolving validation of serological markers of fibrogenesis and fibrolysis an effective and individualized treatment of liver fibrosis is anticipated.

MECHANISMS OF HEPATIC FIBROGENESIS

Chronic liver diseases frequently lead to scarring (cirrhosis) which is often accompanied by progressive loss of liver function despite the use of immunosuppressive, antiviral or anti-inflammatory agents.

Fibrosis results from excessive accumulation of extracellular matrix (ECM). The collagens are the most important molecular targets, since (a) they represent the major matrix proteins, (b) they form important mechanical scaffolds and (c) their proteolysis by specific proteases appears to be rate-limiting for ECM removal. The fibril-forming interstitial collagens type I and III, and the sheet-forming basement membrane collagen type IV, are the most abundant ECM components in liver. In cirrhosis their content increases up to tenfold[1]. A variety of adverse stimuli such as toxins, viruses, bile stasis, or hypoxia can trigger *fibrogenesis*, i.e. the excess synthesis and deposition of ECM, usually by activation of cytokine release, or simply by mechanical stress. In the acute phase of liver disease fibrogenesis is balanced by *fibrolysis*, i.e. the removal of excess ECM by proteolytic enzymes, the most important of which are the matrix metalloproteinases (MMP). MMP-1, -2, -3, -8, -9, -12, -13 and -14 are expressed in human liver[2]. With repeated injury of sufficient severity, fibrogenesis prevails over fibrolysis, resulting in excess ECM deposition, i.e. fibrosis. Fibrogenesis is characterized by an up-regulation of ECM synthesis, a down-regulation of MMP secretion and activity, and by an increase of the physiological inhibitors of the MMP, the tissue inhibitors of MMP (TIMP). Among the four known TIMP, the universal MMP-inhibitor TIMP-1 is most important[3]. However, an increase of certain MMP may also be detrimental. Thus activation of MMP at the wrong place and time can lead to removal of the regular, differentiation-inducing ECM, such as basement membranes, with subsequent unfavourable tissue remodelling, architectural distortion and a fibrogenic response. An example is MMP-2 which mainly degrades basement membrane collagen and denatured collagens and which is up-regulated during fibrogenesis. Collagens, MMP and TIMP are mainly produced by myofibroblastic cells (MF) which derive either from activated hepatic stellate cells (HSC) or from activated (portal and perivascular) fibroblasts[4,5] (Figure 1). Activated liver macrophages, i.e. Kupffer cells, or proliferating bile ductular epithelia, but also endothelia, other mononuclear cells and myofibroblasts themselves, are sources of fibrogenic cytokines and growth factors that can stimulate HSC and perivascular fibroblasts to become MF. The prominent profibrogenic cytokine is TGF-β_1, which is released from almost any cell during inflammation, tissue regeneration and fibrogenesis. Apart from

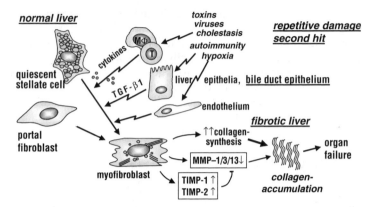

Figure 1 Initiation and maintenance of fibrogenesis. With continuous injury, primarily to hepatocytes or bile duct epithelia, and/or mechanical stress, the normally quiescent hepatic stellate cells and portal fibroblasts undergo activation and transdifferentiation to myofibroblasts. These myofibroblasts produce excessive amounts of collagens, down-regulate release of matrix metalloproteinases (MMP) and show an enhanced expression of the physiological inhibitors of the MMP (TIMP-1 and -2). TIMP-1 can also promote myofibroblast proliferation and inhibit their apoptosis

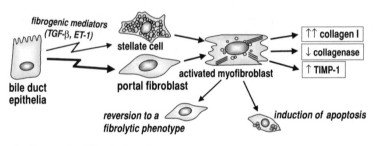

Figure 2 Targets of antifibrotic therapies

immunosuppressive and, in most cell types, antiproliferative effects TGF-β_1 strongly up-regulates production and deposition of the major ECM molecules[5-7]. Therefore, TGF-β_1, as well as activated HSC and MF, are the prime targets for antifibrotic therapies (Figure 2).

ANTIFIBROTIC DRUG DEVELOPMENT

A major obstacle to antifibrotic drug development is the slow evolution of significant fibrosis, which takes years or even decades in humans. Sequential biopsy with semiquantitative and preferably quantitative assessment of fibrous tissue remains the gold standard to monitor fibrosis progression, but sampling error remains a problem since, due to large regenerative nodules that consist mainly of hepatocytes, up to 25% of patients with advanced fibrosis or cirrhosis may be wrongly categorized as only slightly fibrotic[8]. Consequently, prospective studies in patients have to be large, and testing of the large spectrum of potential antifibrotic agents is impossible. First proof of efficacy has to come from cell culture data that show inhibition of proliferation, induction of apoptosis and/or down-regulation of collagen production in the key fibrogenic liver cells, i.e. activated HSC and MF. This has to be followed by suitable animal models of hepatic fibrosis to show the antifibrotic effect *in vivo* in the absence of general toxicity. Rat models are preferable, since significant fibrosis can be produced within 3–10 weeks and, most importantly, total liver collagen, the gold standard for fibrosis, can be determined easily in a representative tissue sample using biochemical methods. However, the *in-vivo* models must include a sizeable number of animals per treatment group ($n = 10$–20) and should be devoid of major hepatocyte necrosis. This is important, since drugs with anti-inflammatory, anti-necrotic or radical scavenging properties can prevent necrosis and collapse, as is the characteristic of the models induced by carbon tetrachloride, dimethylnitrosamine or galactosamine, but are not truly antifibrotic. Thus fibrosis should evolve chronically and reproducibly, with no or little inflammation and necrosis, as in biliary cirrhosis due to bile duct occlusion. In addition, models of fibrosis reversion, e.g. *after* induction by carbon tetrachloride or thioacetamide, are alternatives to predict a 'true' antifibrotic drug effect. Many reports on so-called antifibrotic agents do not fulfil the above-mentioned criteria, and the following examples will refer mainly to those studies that provide sufficient *in-vivo* evidence for an antifibrotic effect. Importantly, in the long term a decrease of fibrosis should be followed by an improvement of portal hypertension and liver function. The targets for antifibrotic therapies are shown in Figure 2.

PHARMACOLOGICAL STRATEGIES TO INHIBIT HEPATIC FIBROSIS

Antifibrotic cytokines

Retrospective analyses and one small prospective study in patients with chronic hepatitis C suggest that IF-α therapy can prevent fibrosis progression, even in non-responders to antiviral therapy[9,10]. The effect was dependent on IF-α dose duration, and most pronounced in sustained responders. However, it remains to be shown if interferon is useful in biliary fibrosis and if its potential antifibrotic effect outweighs high costs and side-effects.

Antagonizing profibrogenic cytokines

TGF-β_1 is considered the most potent fibrogenic cytokine, and its inhibition therefore appears attractive[5-7]. Soluble TGF-β_1 decoy receptors or adenoviral constructs that block TGF-β_1 signalling have been developed that show antifibrotic efficacy *in vitro* and *in vivo*[11-13] (Figure 3). It appears that an approach targeting activated HSC and MF is necessary, since TGF-β receptors are expressed on most cell types, and systemic inhibition that reaches sufficient levels to block hepatic fibrogenesis may trigger autoimmune diseases and cellular de-differentiation.

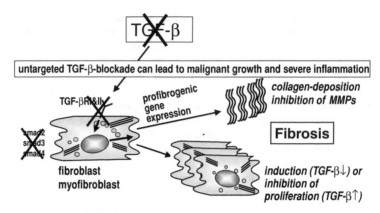

Figure 3 Anti-TGF-β_1 strategies to inhibit fibrogenesis. Strategies have been developed that neutralize TGF-β_1, e.g. by blockage or inactivation of its signalling receptors (TβRI or TβRII), the major signal transducers of the TGF-β pathway, such as smad2, smad3 and smad4

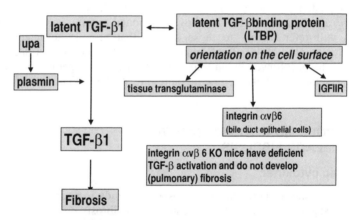

Figure 4 Activation of latent TGF-β and the role of cell surface co-activators. Inhibition of cell surface co-activators that are specifically up-regulated in (biliary) fibrosis, such as integrin $\alpha v\beta 6$, allow a targeted antifibrotic therapy (from refs 15 and 16)

A specific therapy for biliary fibrosis might be possible by inhibiting activation of TGF-β, the precursor of which (latent TGF-β) is highly expressed by proliferating epithelial cells[14]. The epithelial integrin receptor, integrin $\alpha v\beta 6$, is necessary for proteolytic activation of latent TGF-β (Figure 4) and mice lacking this integrin show amazing resistance to induction of pulmonary fibrosis[15,16]. Activation and proliferation of bile duct epithelial cells is a regular finding in biliary fibrosis, and $\alpha v\beta 6$ integrin expression is up-regulated in rat secondary biliary fibrosis (own unpublished data). Our preliminary data indicate that an orally available integrin $\alpha v\beta 6$ antagonist blocks periportal collagen deposition in rat secondary biliary fibrosis.

OTHER ANTIFIBROTIC AGENTS AND COMBINATION THERAPIES

Plant-derived drugs

Several promising drugs derive from plants. *Silymarin*, from the milk thistle, contains three prominent flavonoids, with silibinin representing up to 60% of the dried extract. Silibinin was shown to stimulate hepatocyte RNA synthesis, to act as a radical-scavenger and hepatoprotectant, and to suppress HSC proliferation and collagen synthesis *in vitro*. Importantly, it reduced hepatic collagen accumulation in rat biliary fibrosis secondary to bile duct occlusion, a model which leads to a 10–12-fold hepatic collagen accumulation after 6 weeks, by 30–40%, even when treatment was started in an advanced stage of fibrosis[17]. The major alkaloid baicalein from the traditional Chinese/Japanese plant extract *Sho-saiko-to*, that displays a structure similar to silibinin, has radical-scavenging but also antifibrotic properties in activated HSC *in vitro* and in rat porcine serum-induced fibrosis *in vivo*[18]. *Halofuginone*, a semisynthetic alkaloid derivative from the antimalarial plant *Dichroa febrifuga*, was shown to normalize hepatic collagen content in a fibrosis reversion model *after* induction of hepatic fibrosis by thioacetamide[19]. These drugs appear to mainly act as antioxidants, though probably with different pharmacokinetics, pharmacodynamics and cellular specificities. Intracellular oxidative stress is a relevant contributor to fibrogenesis, and recent studies have shown the induction of profibrogenic TGF-β_1 by peroxide radicals[20,21], providing a rationale for the use of intracellular antioxidants as adjunctive antifibrotic agents (see Figure 6).

Modulators of fibrogenic signal transduction

In vitro the phosphodiesterase inhibitor and cytokine antagonist pentoxifylline suppresses proliferation and collagen production by skin fibroblasts and HSC[22], while in rat biliary fibrosis oral pentoxifylline reduced hepatic collagen accumulation by only 20%. The drug induced a hitherto-unmatched 8-fold down-regulation of hepatic procollagen I mRNA, the product of activated HSC and MF, but this was counterbalanced by a 2-fold increase of hepatic TIMP-1 mRNA expression, with pentoxifylline apparently stimulating bile duct epithelia and hepatocytes to express TIMP-1[23]. Better targeting of pentoxifylline to HSC and MF may prevent up-regulation of the profibrogenic TIMP-1 without compromising the down-regulatory effect on procollagen I expression.

Antagonizing vasoactive mediators

Oral endothelin A receptor (ET$_A$R) antagonists are attractive, since the ET$_A$R mediates HSC/MF contraction, proliferation and possibly also collagen synthesis, whereas the ET$_B$R induces MF relaxation and inhibition of proliferation (Figure 5). In rat biliary fibrosis the oral ET$_A$R antagonist LU135252 reduced hepatic collagen accumulation by up to 60% when given over the full 6 weeks of the experiment, being still effective when treatment was begun after week 3, a time-point with an already 4-fold increased liver collagen[24]. Angiotensin 1

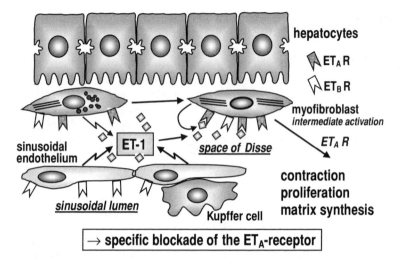

Figure 5 Hepatic endothelin/endothelin receptor system in hepatic stellate cell activation. Upon early activation endothelin A receptors (ET$_A$R) are up-regulated on the perisinusoidal stellate cells (SC). An increased release of endothelin-1 by the injured sinusoidal endothelium and the SC themselves then leads to paracrine and autocrine activation. However, with complete myofibroblastic transformation, SC decrease expression of the profibrogenic ET$_A$R and lower expression of the antifibrogenic ET$_B$R which may be a counterregulatory mechanism. Similar mechnisms are operative in other organs

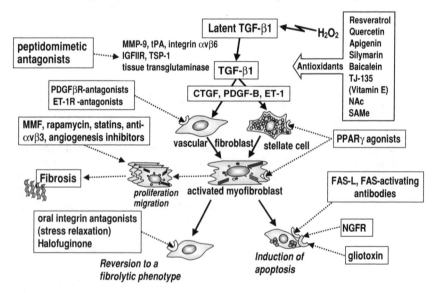

Figure 6 Antifibrotic therapies: specific approaches

receptor antagonists or angiotensin-converting enzyme inhibitors can retard liver fibrosis in suitable rat models[25–27]. However, since the doses applied are up to 100-fold above the doses given in human hypertension, their antifibrotic effect in humans remains controversial.

Table 1 Potential antifibrotic drugs that may be useful in antifibrotic combination therapy. Examples of drugs for which antifibrotic activity has been shown in suitable animal models of liver fibrosis or for which an antifibrotic effect can be anticipated

---

Interferon-$\alpha > \gamma$
Pentoxifylline, PDE-3/4-antagonists (rolipram)
Antioxidants (silymarin, baicalein)
Halofuginone
Prostaglandin E_2
Endothelin A receptor antagonists
Angiotensin system inhibitors
NO-donors (Pyrro-NO)
Mycophenolate, rapamycin, leflunomide
Histone diacetylase inhibitors (trichostatin A, SAHA)
Thioglitazones
Angiogenesis inhibitors (PTK 787, EMD 409915)
Specific integrin antagonists ($\alpha v \beta$)

OTHER DRUGS THAT SHOW AN ANTIFIBROTIC POTENTIAL *IN VITRO*

There is an increasing number of drugs, part of them already in clinical use for other indications, that either block proliferation and migration or induce apoptosis of HSC/MF, while other agents down-regulate matrix production or up-regulate MMP. Some of these drugs have also been shown to inhibit experimental liver fibrosis in more or less reliable rat or mouse fibrosis models (Figure 6).

COMBINATION THERAPY FOR HEPATIC FIBROSIS

It appears that none of the single agents will effectively halt or even reverse liver fibrosis in humans when given in non-toxic concentrations. As in cancer therapy combination of several drugs that show different actions by either blocking fibrogenesis, stimulating fibrolysis, by inducing myofibroblast apoptosis, or reversion to a fibrolytic phenotype, is most promising. This will allow use of lower, non-toxic amounts of single agents for a treatment that will have to be given for years, or even lifelong. Combinations of some of these agents (see Table 1) are currently being tested in suitable *in-vivo* rat fibrosis models.

References

1. Schuppan D, Ruehl M, Somasundaram R, Hahn EG. Matrix as a modulator of hepatic fibrogenesis. Semin Liver Dis. 2001;21:351–72.
2. Benyon RC, Arthur MJ. Extracellular matrix degradation and the role of hepatic stellate cells. Semin Liver Dis. 2001;21:373–84.
3. Iredale JP. Tissue inhibitors of metalloproteinases in liver fibrosis. Int J Biochem Cell Biol. 2001;29:43–54.
4. Knittel T, Kobold D, Saile B et al. Rat liver myofibroblasts and hepatic stellate cells: different cell populations of the fibroblast lineage with fibrogenic potential. Gastroenterology. 1999;117: 1205–21.

5. Friedman SL. Molecular regulation of hepatic fibrosis, an integrated cellular response to tissue injury. J Biol Chem. 2000;275:2247–50.
6. Bissell DM, Roulot D, George J. Transforming growth factor β and the liver. Hepatology. 2001; 34:859–67.
7. Gressner AM, Weiskirchen R, Breitkopf K, Dooley S. Roles of TGF-beta in hepatic fibrosis. Front Biosci. 2002;7:d793–807.
8. Poniachik J, Bernstein DE, Reddy KR et al. The role of laparoscopy in the diagnosis of cirrhosis. Gastrointest Endosc. 1996;43:568–71.
9. Shiffman M, Hoffman CM, Contos MJ et al. A randomised controlled trial of maintenance interferon therapy for patients with chronic hepatitis C virus and persistent viremia. Gastroenterology. 1999;117:1164–72.
10. Poynard T, McHutchison J, Manns M et al. Impact of pegylated interferon alfa-2b and ribavirin on liver fibrosis in patients with chronic hepatitis C. Gastroenterology. 2002;122:1303–13.
11. Qi Z, Atsuchi N, Ooshima A, Takeshita A, Ueno H. Blockade of type beta transforming growth factor signaling prevents liver fibrosis and dysfunction in the rat. Proc Natl Acad Sci USA. 1999;96:2345–9.
12. George J, Roulot D, Koteliansky VE, Bissell DM. *In vivo* inhibition of rat stellate cell activation by soluble transforming growth factor beta type II receptor: a potential new therapy for hepatic fibrosis. Proc Natl Acad Sci USA. 1999;96:12719–24.
13. Yata Y, Gotwals P, Koteliansky V, Rockey DC. Dose-dependent inhibition of hepatic fibrosis in mice by a TGF-beta soluble receptor: implications for antifibrotic therapy. Hepatology. 2002; 35:1022–30.
14. Milani S, Herbst H, Schuppan D, Stein H, Surrenti C. Transforming growth factors β1 and β2 are differentially expressed in fibrotic liver disease. Am J Pathol. 1991;139:1221–9.
15. Munger JS, Huang X, Kawakatsu H et al. The integrin alpha v beta 6 binds and activates latent TGF beta 1: a mechanism for regulating pulmonary inflammation and fibrosis. Cell. 1999;96: 319–28.
16. Morris DG, Huang X, Kaminski N et al. Loss of integrin alpha(v)beta6-mediated TGF-beta activation causes MMP12-dependent emphysema. Nature. 2003;422:169–73.
17. Jia JD, Bauer M, Ruehl M, Milani S, Boigk G, Riecken EO, Schuppan D. Antifibrotic effect of silymarin in rat secondary biliary fibrosis is mediated by downregulation of procollagen I, TIMP-1 and TGF-β1 RNA. J Hepatol. 2001;35:392–8.
18. Shimizu I, Ma YR, Mizobuchi Y et al. Effects of *Sho-saiko-to*, a Japanese herbal medicine, on hepatic fibrosis in rats. Hepatology. 1999;29:282–4.
19. Bruck R, Genina O, Aeed H et al. Halofuginone to prevent and treat thioacetamide-induced liver fibrosis in rats. Hepatology. 2001;33:379–86.
20. De Bleser PJ, Xu G, Rombouts K, Rogiers V, Geerts A. Glutathione levels discriminate between oxidative stress and transforming growth factor-beta signaling in activated rat hepatic stellate cells. J Biol Chem. 1999;274:33881–7.
21. Garcia-Trevijano ER, Iraburu MJ, Fontana L et al. Transforming growth factor beta1 induces the expression of alpha1(I) procollagen mRNA by a hydrogen peroxide-C/EBPbeta-dependent mechanism in rat hepatic stellate cells. Hepatology. 1999;29:960–70.
22. Duncan MR, Hasan A, Berman B. Pentoxifylline, pentifylline, and interferons decrease type I and III procollagen mRNA levels in dermal fibroblasts: evidence for mediation by nuclear factor 1 down-regulation. J Invest Dermatol. 1995;104:282–6.
23. Raetsch C, Boigk G, Herbst H, Riecken EO, Schuppan D. Pentoxifylline retards collagen accumulation in early but not in advanced rat secondary biliary fibrosis. Gut. 2002;50:241–7.
24. Cho JJ, Hocher B, Herbst H et al. An oral endothelin A receptor antagonist blocks collagen synthesis and deposition in advanced rat secondary fibrosis. Gastroenterology. 2000;118:1169–78.
25. Bataller R, Sancho-Bru P, Gines P et al. Activated human hepatic stellate cells express the renin–angiotensin system and synthesize angiotensin II. Gastroenterology. 2003;125:117–25.
26. Jonsson JR, Clouston AD, Ando Y et al. Angiotensin-converting enzyme inhibition attenuates the progression of rat hepatic fibrosis. Gastroenterology. 2001;121:148–55.
27. Paizis G, Gilbert RE, Cooper ME et al. Effect of angiotensin II type 1 receptor blockade on experimental hepatic fibrogenesis. J Hepatol. 2001;35:376–85.

34
Ursodeoxycholic acid to prevent colon cancer in primary sclerosing cholangitis

K. V. KOWDLEY

BACKGROUND

Primary sclerosing cholangitis (PSC) is a relatively uncommon cause of chronic liver disease, but frequently leads to end-stage liver disease and is a major indication for liver transplantation. The worldwide prevalence of PSC has been estimated to be up to 8.5 cases per 100 000. However, PSC is common among patients with inflammatory bowel disease, with an estimated prevalence of 3–5%. It has long been recognized that chronic ulcerative colitis and Crohn's disease of the colon are associated with an increased risk of colon cancer. Recent studies have found that there is a significantly increased risk of colon cancer among patients with PSC. A large study from Sweden found that cumulative risk of developing colorectal dysplasia or cancer was 50% after 25 years of disease, compared to 10% among patients with ulcerative colitis (UC) alone[1]; similar results were found in two other studies[2]. Other risk factors for colorectal neoplasia in chronic UC include age, presence of pancolitis, duration of disease and early age at diagnosis. The pathogenesis of colon cancer in UC has been linked to a 'dysplasia to carcinoma sequence'; it has been postulated that genetic factors, as well as dietary and other environmental influences, contribute to the pathogenesis of colon cancer in UC with and without PSC. Given the high incidence of colon cancer in UC associated with PSC, the difficulty in detecting cancer at an early stage, and the high mortality associated with this disease, there is a need for preventive therapies against colon cancer. There is already a body of work examining the utility and efficacy of multiple such agents for chemoprevention of colon cancer in patients without UC. Such therapies can be classified as nutritional interventions and chemopreventive agents[3].

Both vitamins and other dietary supplements have been used for prevention of colon cancer. These include vitamin C, vitamin E, β-carotene, folate and calcium, as well as dietary fibre. These interventions have been based on observations that colon cancer is much more common in Western countries, where diets rich in fat and red meat are the norm. Vitamin C, vitamin E and vitamin A (β-carotene, retinoids) have all been studied in colon cancer prevention. The possible benefit of vitamin A is controversial because of the many types of vitamin A products used, ranging from β-carotene to retinol, and because vitamin A may actually be carcinogenic in some forms[4]. Other vitamins which have been studied in colon cancer prevention include vitamin C and vitamin E, although human studies have been inconclusive in demonstrating a chemopreventive effect in colon cancer[4]. Folate supplementation is another attractive agent in chemoprevention because folate deficiency may result in DNA hypomethylation and increased risk of malignancy. Two studies have shown that folate repletion at doses >400 μg/day was associated with a reduced risk of colon cancer and colon polyps[5,6]. Furthermore, there may be a genetic basis for the interaction between folate status and DNA hypomethylation[7]. It is hoped that large-scale human studies will confirm the possible benefit of folate supplementation in colon cancer prevention.

Non-steroidal anti-inflammatory drugs (NSAIDs) have been extensively studied in colon cancer prevention. The agents that have been subjected to the most study include aspirin, sulindac, prioxicam, indomethacin and ibuprofen. NSAIDs were shown to prevent colon cancer in animal models[3]. Furthermore, a reduction in colon cancer mortality was reported with aspirin in two studies[8,9]. The mechanism of action of NSAIDs appears to be via inhibition of cyclooxygenase (COX). COX is present in two isoforms, as COX-1, which is expressed constitutively in mammals in almost all tissues, and COX-2, an inducible enzyme that is overexpressed in cancerous and inflamed tissue. COX-2 is present in human colon cancer cells, but has not been found in normal epithelia[10]. Clinical trials are now being conducted to study whether therapy with COX-2 inhibitors such as celecoxib may reduce the incidence of colorectal neoplasia.

Other agents that have been studied in the chemoprevention of colon cancer include difluoromethylornithine, an inhibitor of ornithine decarboxylase, HMG CoA reductase inhibitors[3], histamine 2 receptor antagonists[4], and ursodeoxycholic acid. Ursodeoxycholic acid (UDCA) has been studied extensively as a chemopreventive agent in colon cancer cell lines, murine models of colon cancer and in human studies of high-risk populations. There is a substantial body of data suggesting that hydrophobic bile acids, in particular deoxycholate, may play a role in the development of colon carcinogenesis. These observations, in turn, were based on epidemiological data showing the relatively higher incidence of colon cancer in Western countries, particularly among individuals consuming diets high in fat and red meat. Supporting this hypothesis is the finding that diets high in fat are associated with increased numbers of aberrant crypt foci and other features associated with carcinogenesis in rats[11]. Primary bile acids, namely cholic acid and chenodeoxycholic acid, are synthesized in the liver and subsequently transported via the biliary tree into the intestine; subsequently, these bile acids are metabolized by intestinal bacteria into the secondary bile acids, deoxycholic acid and lithocholic acid. It has been shown that faecal concentrations of secondary bile acids are elevated among high-risk populations for colon cancer[12]. Furthermore, there is a positive relationship between serum faecal concentrations of hydrophobic bile acids and the risk of adenomas in the colon[13,14].

Increased colonic exposure to secondary bile acids may promote carcinogenesis via a number of mechanisms, including direct cytotoxicity, alteration of inflammatory mediators, effects on apoptosis, depletion of mucin and antioxidant defences, and via effects on oncogenes, tumour-suppressor genes and DNA repair mechanisms. Secondary bile acids, most importantly deoxycholic acid, are highly hydrophobic and have been shown to be cytotoxic to colonic cells[15]. Furthermore, recent data suggest that hydrophobic bile acids appear to mediate oxidative stress in the gastric and colonic mucosa. Lechner and colleagues demonstrated up-regulation of thioredoxin reductase after exposure to deoxycholate, suggesting that impairment of antioxidant mechanisms may accelerate tumorigeneses[16]. Several studies have demonstrated that both deoxycholic acid and chenodeoxycholic acid rapidly induce apoptosis in human colon cancer cell lines. The severity of apoptosis is related to the hydrophobicity of the bile acid, with more hydrophobic bile acids promoting apoptosis within a shorter period of time. Other investigators have studied the possible effects of hydrophobic bile acids on intracellular signalling and gene expression as a mechanism for carcinogenesis. Qiao and colleagues showed that deoxycholic acid reduced both intracellular concentrations and transactivation of p53 protein in a colon cancer cell line[17].

Deoxycholate induced expression of p53 mRNA, thus suggesting that the effect of deoxycholate on p53 was post-transcriptionally mediated and via degradation in proteasomes. However, it is of interest that these authors did not demonstrate any alteration of this effect by ursodeoxycholic or cholic acid.

Colonic mucin may have a protective effect in colon cancer, and mucin depletion may be an important mechanism in colon carcinogenesis. Shekels et al. showed that exposure to bile acids is associated with depletion of mucin within enterocytes, via a detergent effect[18]. Co-incubation of Caco-2 and H29 cells with bile acids showed that deoxycholate caused the greatest reduction in enterocyte mucin content; UDCA co-incubation was associated with the least amount of mucin release. Additional pro-carcinogenic effects of hydrophobic bile acids may include mediation of protein kinase C, a member of a family of enzymes involved in cellular differentiation, proliferation and apoptosis. Pongracz and coworkers found lower total protein kinase C activity in cancerous versus non-cancerous tissues[19]. These findings suggest that protein kinase C activity may play a role in the growth and development of cancer, and that modulation of protein kinase C activity may influence tumorigenesis. In summary, there are ample data to suggest that hydrophobic bile acids, if present in increased amounts in the colon, may promote colon cancer by a variety of mechanisms.

By contrast, there are considerable data suggesting that UDCA has cytoprotective and anti-neoplastic properties and may protect against the development of colon neoplasia in colon cancer cell lines, murine models of colon cancer and in humans at increased risk of colonic neoplasia. In colon cancer cell lines, UDCA induced growth arrest in colon cancer cell lines as measured by thymidine incorporation[20]. The effect of UDCA on growth of cell culture models of human colon cancer has been studied. Shekels and colleagues studied the effect of bile acids on growth of a variety of human colonic epithelial cell lines. Co-incubation of taurodeoxycholic acid with tauro-UDCA was associated with reduction of cytotoxicity induced by taurodeoxycholic acid[21].

A recent study examined the effect of UDCA on survivin, a recently discovered inhibitor of apoptosis[22]. Administration of thapsigargin in a hepatoma cell line was associated with decreased survivin levels and resulted in apoptosis. UDCA reduced thapsigargin-induced apoptosis and prevented the reduction in survivin content. Another recent study has examined the effect of butyrate and UDCA on apoptosis in colon adenoma cells[23]. Butyrate, a by-product of the metabolism of fibre in the colon, was associated with apoptosis in the cell culture system. Administration of UDCA was associated with a reduction in butyrate-induced apoptosis. McMillan and co-workers further demonstrated[23] that the mechanism for this UDCA effect was related to activation of PKC-α and MAP kinase.

The anti-neoplastic effect of UDCA has also been studied in murine models of colon cancer. The azoxymethane-treated model is the most commonly used model for colon cancer in rats. Several authors have reported that UDCA may reduce the formation of aberrant crypt foci or overt colon cancer in this model. Chemoprevention with UDCA against colon cancer in the AOM rat model has been studied for almost a decade. Earnest et al. showed in 1994 that UDCA prevented colon cancer in the rats exposed to AOM[24]. Male Fischer 344 rats were fed a diet supplemented with varying concentrations of cholic acid, UDCA, or piroxicam. Animals were sacrificed after 28 weeks and colons were examined for tumours. Cholic acid supplementation was associated with a significant increase in colon tumours. By contrast, UDCA supplementation attenuated the development of tumours in the cholic acid-treated rats and, at higher doses, also prevented the development of colon cancers. UDCA was more effective than piroxicam in preventing the colon tumours. This was the first demonstration that dietary supplementation with UDCA prevented the development of colon cancer in the azoxymethane model of colon cancer. Numerous subsequent studies have demonstrated that UDCA may prevent or decrease the development of colon cancer. Narisawa et al. examined the effect of UDCA and chenodeoxycholic acid on colon cancer development in F344 rats[25]. Treatment with UDCA at doses of 0.4% or 0.08%, respectively, was associated with a 24% and 23% reduction in colonic aberrant crypt foci (ACF); by contrast there was an increase in ACF in the groups treated with chenodeoxycholic acid. Furthermore, UDCA at the two doses reduced the incidence of colon cancers after treatment with N-methyl-nitrosurea (MNU) (36% and 40% vs 68%). The authors suggest that UDCA may suppress MNU-induced telomerase activation. The same group reported that the combination of UDCA and 5-ASA was more effective than UDCA and 5-ASA alone treated groups[26].

Wali et al. showed that UDCA inhibited the initiation and post-initiation phase of colon tumour development in the AOM-treated rat [27]. Ikegami et al. studied group II phospholipase A2 activity in colons of UDCA-treated and untreated rats, as well as the presence of aberrant crypt foci after exposure to azoxymethane[28]. After 12 weeks of exposure, significantly lower numbers of aberrant crypt foci were seen in UDCA-treated versus non-UDCA-treated rats. Furthermore, UDCA-treated rats had lower levels of mucosal PGE_2 and 6-keto $PGF_1\alpha$. In addition, expression of phospholipase A2 was lower in the UDCA-treated rats. Ikegami and colleagues speculated that the chemopreventive effect of UDCA on colon carcinogenesis may be due to its effect on arachidonic acid metabolism in colonic mucosa. Recent work supports this hypothesis. Wali and co-workers showed that

COX-2 expression was increased in AOM-induced tumours and that UDCA blocked this effect[27]. Furthermore, UDCA inhibited formation of aberrant crypt foci and hyperproliferation, by maintaining normal cyclin D1 and E-cathedrin content, which was perturbed by the carcinogen. Finally, K-ras mutations are frequently present in colon cancer and may accelerate tumour growth. Khare and colleagues demonstrated that UDCA inhibited COX-2 induction by both ras-dependent and independent mechanisms[29].

UDCA may also exert effects on nitric oxide synthase, which has been associated with colonic malignancy. Invernizzi and co-workers demonstrated that UDCA reduced inducible nitric oxide synthase activity based on mRNA content, protein and enzymatic activity, but was not associated with toxicity[30]. UDCA may also alter major histocompatibility antigen expression. Rigas and co-workers showed that both UDCA and piroxicam up-regulated the expression of MHC antigens in the colon in F-344 rats treated with azoxymethane along with a simultaneous reduction in the incidence of colon cancer, suggesting that increased immune surveillance may be yet another mechanism whereby UDCA may reduce the risk of colon cancer[31].

It is possible that modification of UDCA may result in improved delivery to the colon, with enhanced efficacy in chemoprevention. Rodrigues and colleagues measured bile acid concentrations in intestine, faeces, urine, plasma and liver tissue of rats following treatment with UDCA and its C-3, C-7 and C-3,7 sulphate derivatives[32]. Use of the sulphated compounds was associated with enhanced delivery of UDCA to the colon, presumably due to decreased bacterial degradation.

The following section reviews the available data with UDCA in the chemoprevention of colon cancer in humans. The effect of UDCA on colonic neoplasia has been studied in primary sclerosing cholangitis and primary biliary cirrhosis. Primary sclerosing cholangitis (PSC) is an attractive model to study the effect of UDCA on the colon. PSC is a disorder of unknown aetiology that is characterized by progressive fibrosis and stricture formation in the medium and large bile ducts within the liver[33]. Progressive damage to the biliary tree leads to cirrhosis and increased risk of cholangiocarcinoma. The majority of patients with PSC also have inflammatory bowel disease (UC and Crohn's disease). The incidence of PSC in UC has been estimated to be between 2% and 5%[33]. Patients with UC have an increased risk of colon cancer; the risk is estimated to be even higher among those with PSC and UC. Therefore, many if not most clinicians routinely perform histological surveillance for dysplasia in their patients with PSC and UC. Many patients with PSC are treated with UDCA, based on the concept that replacement of the bile acid pool with this hydrophilic bile acid may reduce liver damage from retained hydrophobic bile acids, and the empirical observation that serum markers of cholestasis often improve following treatment with UDCA. However, standard doses (10–15 mg/kg per day) of UDCA have not been proven to be effective in improving outcomes of liver disease in PSC. The PSC/UC group therefore represents an attractive model for studying the effect of UDCA on colonic carcinogenesis in a controlled fashion, given the high rate of development of colonic dysplasia and cancer the common practice of colonoscopic surveillance by clinicians.

We studied the effect of UDCA therapy on colonic dysplasia in a group of patients with PSC and UC who were undergoing colonoscopic surveillance at

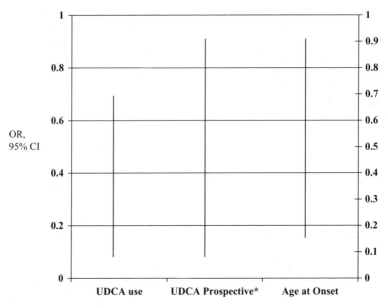

Figure 1 Risk of dysplasia among patients with ulcerative colitis and primary sclerosing cholangitis. UDCA use was associated with lower prevalence of dysplasia both in the overall group, and when patients with dysplasia on the initial colonoscopy were excluded (UDCA Prospective group). * UDCA Prospective = subset of patients who did not have dysplasia on the initial colonoscopy

the University of Washington[34]. The decision to use UDCA was made by the referring or primary physician. The relationship between colonic dysplasia and UDCA therapy was examined after controlling for all other variables associated with development of dysplasia, such as duration of UC, age of onset of colitis, gender, duration of PSC, Child–Pugh classification or use of sulphasalazine. Fifty-nine patients with UC and concomitant PSC were entered into a colon surveillance programme. The majority had been treated with UDCA (69%), and the minority had never been treated with UDCA (31%). The prevalence of dysplasia during the study period was 44%. There was a significant difference in the prevalence of dysplasia in the UDCA-treated group versus those not treated with UDCA (50% vs 85%; $p = 0.005$). UDCA treatment was associated with a significant risk reduction of colon cancer (OR 0.18, 95% CI 0.05–0.61; see Figure 1). UDCA therapy was associated with a reduced prevalence of colonic dysplasia even after controlling for gender, duration of UC, duration of PSC, age at onset of UC, severity of liver disease (as judged by Child–Pugh class), and treatment with sulphasalazine. The protective effect of UDCA was noted regardless of use of other adjuvant therapies such as prednisone, cyclosporin or methotrexate. Duration or total cumulative dose of UDCA therapy did not influence development of dysplasia. There was also no relationship between dose of UDCA and development of dysplasia. UDCA therapy was also inversely related to development of high-grade dysplasia (OR 0.17; 95% CI 0.04–0.68). The protective effect of UDCA against high-grade dysplasia was noted even after adjustment for potential confounding variables such as gender, age of onset of colitis, and duration of UC and PSC. Interestingly, age at onset of colitis but not duration of colitis emerged as an independent variable associated with development of colonic dysplasia. These preliminary findings have now been confirmed by a prospective, randomized trial of UDCA versus placebo in PSC[35]. The patient cohort for this study was derived from the randomized trial of UDCA versus placebo for PSC conducted by Lindor and colleagues. The investigators enrolled 52 patients with PSC and UC who were followed prospectively. The incidence of colon dysplasia or cancer was recorded during surveillance colonoscopy; the authors were able to accumulate 355 person-years of follow-up. The median duration of UDCA therapy was 42 months, compared to a median duration of placebo therapy of 40 months. The median duration of UC was 15 years. There was a similar number of colonoscopies in both groups: 3.96 (UDCA group), versus 3.65 (placebo group). The median interval between colonoscopies was also similar between the UDCA and placebo groups (25.5 months (U), 23.6 months (P)). The average number of biopsies obtained at each colonoscopy was somewhat lower in the Tung study[34] (22 (UDCA group) versus 20 (placebo group)).

Recent data also suggest that UDCA may be protective against development of colon polyps in patients with PBC. Serfaty and colleagues studied the effect of UDCA therapy on development of adenomatous polyps among 114 patients with primary biliary cirrhosis (PBC)[36]. Patients who were already on UDCA at the time of colonoscopic surveillance were compared to those in whom treatment was started after the colonoscopy (mean duration of therapy 46 months). Recurrence of adenoma was compared among treated and untreated patients, and between treated patients and controls who had undergone polypectomy ($n = 205$). Colon epithelial cell proliferation was also studied using anti-Ki67 antibody on colon biopsy tissue in treated and untreated patients. The recurrence rate of adenomas was compared between the treated and untreated groups. Treated patients had a significantly lower rate of adenoma recurrence than controls (7% vs 28%, $p = 0.04$). There appeared to be a trend towards decreased recurrence of adenomas among treated versus untreated PBC patients, although the difference was not statistically significant (13% vs 14%, $p = 0.16$). Markers of colonic epithelial proliferation were significantly lower among the treated group compared to controls ($p = 0.0001$). This interesting observational study suggests that UDCA therapy may reduce the recurrence of colon polyps after primary resection. Additional studies of the effect of UDCA on recurrence of colon polyps appear warranted.

UDCA may have a therapeutic indication in the chemoprevention of other gastrointestinal cancers. A recent preliminary study examined the effect of UDCA on PGE_2 production in Barrett's epithelium and stromal fibroblasts[37]. Primary Barrett's cells were cultivated from endoscopic biopsies. Cell cultures were incubated with varying doses of UDCA for 24 h at concentrations of 0, 1, 5, 10, 50, 100, and 500 mmol/L. PGE_2 levels in the supernatants were assayed using an enzyme-linked immunoassay. Higher concentrations of UDCA were effective in suppressing the production of PGE_2 by Barrett's and fibroblast cells. This effect was prevented by addition of exogenous arachidonic acid. These interesting pilot experiments provide evidence that UDCA may inhibit PGE_2 production via inhibition of arachidonic acid release.

In summary, there are several lines of evidence showing that hydrophobic bile acids are carcinogenic, particularly in colon cancer cell lines and in the AOM rat model for colon cancer. UDCA appears to have chemopreventive properties and may work via several pathways to prevent colon cancer. Data supporting the use of UDCA include epidemiological evidence showing increased faecal and blood levels of hydrophobic bile acids in patients with colon polyps and cancer, prevention against colon cancer in murine models at high risk of colon cancer with UDCA, as well as increased MHC antigen expression in preneoplastic tissues, decreased epithelial cell proliferation, reduction in aberrant crypt foci, modulation of protein kinase C and phospholipase A2 activity, and cytoprotective properties such as increased mucin content in colonocytes and antioxidant functions associated with administration of UDCA. UDCA is safe and well tolerated. It is therefore appropriate that UDCA be studied in prospective, randomized trials designed with the endpoint of reduction in risk of colorectal neoplasia, both in high-risk (patients with pan-ulcerative colitis) and medium-risk (patients with history of adenomatous polyps) populations.

UDCA, when used at doses of 13–15 mg/kg per day, improves transplant-free survival among patients with moderately severe PBC. UDCA treatment is also associated with a reduced incidence of oesophageal varices, and improved histology in PBC. However, UDCA at doses of 13–15 mg/kg per day did not improve outcomes in PSC[38]. Recent studies suggest that much higher doses (20–30 mg/kg per day) of UDCA may be safe, and improve liver disease in PSC[39,40]. The United States National Institutes of Health are currently supporting a multiple, randomized, double-blind controlled trial of high-dose UDCA versus placebo in PSC. Ancillary studies are planned to compare the incidence of colonic neoplasia among the patients with UC in this study, and will provide important information regarding the chemopreventive role of UDCA in high-risk PSC patients. Another study of UDCA versus placebo is being conducted among UC patients with low-grade dysplasia. If UDCA is shown to be an effective chemopreventive agent among patients at high risk of colon cancer, prospective trials of UDCA, and possibly its sulphated form, would be indicated in patients at lower risk, such as those with sporadic colonic adenomas.

References

1. Broome U, Lofberg R, Veress B, Eriksson LS. Primary sclerosing cholangitis and ulcerative colitis: evidence for increased neoplastic potential. Hepatology. 1995;22:1404–8.
2. Leidenius MH, Farkkila MA, Karkkainen P, Taskinen EI, Kellokumpu IH, Hockerstedt KA. Colorectal dysplasia and carcinoma in patients with ulcerative colitis and primary sclerosing cholangitis. Scand J Gastroenterol. 1997;32:706–11.
3. Gwyn K, Sinicrope FA. Chemoprevention of colorectal cancer. Am J Gastroenterol. 2002; 97:13–21.
4. Langman M, Boyle P. Chemoprevention of colorectal cancer. Gut. 1998;43:578–85.
5. Giovannucci E, Stampfer MJ, Colditz GA et al. Multivitamin use, folate, and colon cancer in women in the Nurses' Health Study. Ann Intern Med. 1998;129:517–24.
6. Giovannucci E, Stampfer MJ, Colditz GA et al. Folate, methionine, and alcohol intake and risk of colorectal adenoma. J Natl Cancer Inst. 1993;85:875–84.
7. Friso S, Choi SW, Girelli D et al. A common mutation in the 5,10-methylenetetrahydrofolate reductase gene effects genomic DNA methylation through an interaction with folate status. Proc Natl Acad Sci USA. 2002;99:5606–11.
8. Thun MJ, Namboodiri MM, Heath CW Jr. Aspirin use and reduced risk of fatal colon cancer. N Engl J Med. 1991;325:1593–6.

9. Giovannucci E, Rimm EB, Stampfer MJ, Colditz GA, Ascherio A, Willett WC. Aspirin use and the risk for colorectal cancer and adenoma in male health professionals. Ann Intern Med. 1994;121:241–6.

10. Eberhart CE, Coffey RJ, Radhika A, Giardiello FM, Ferrenbach S, DuBois RN. Up-regulation of cyclooxygenase 2 gene expression in human colorectal adenomas and adenocarcinomas. Gastroenterology. 1994;107:1183–8.

11. Morotomi M, Sakaitani Y, Satou M, Takahashi T, Takagi A, Onoue M. Effects of a high-fat diet on azoxymethane-induced aberrant crypt foci and fecal biochemistry and microbial activity in rats. Nutr Cancer. 1997;27:84–91.

12. McMichael AJ, Jensen OM, Parkin DM, Zaridze DG. Dietary and endogenous cholesterol and human cancer. Epidemiol Rev. 1984;6:192–216.

13. Reddy BS, Wynder EL. Metabolic epidemiology of colon cancer. Fecal bile acids and neutral sterols in colon cancer patients and patients with adenomatous polyps. Cancer. 1977;39:2533–9.

14. Bayerdorffer E, Mannes GA, Richter WO et al. Increased serum deoxycholic acid levels in men with colorectal adenomas. Gastroenterology. 1993;104:145–51.

15. Hori T, Matsumoto K, Sakaitani Y, Sato M, Morotomi M. Effect of dietary deoxycholic acid and cholesterol on fecal steroid concentration and its impact on the colonic crypt cell proliferation in azoxymethane-treated rats. Cancer Lett. 1998;124:79–84.

16. Lechner S, Muller-Ladner U, Neumann E et al. Thioredoxin reductase 1 expression in colon cancer: discrepancy between in vitro and in vivo findings. Lab Invest. 2003 83:1321–31.

17. Qiao D, Gaitonde SV, Qi W, Martinez JD. Deoxycholic acid suppresses p53 by stimulating proteasome-mediated p53 protein degradation. Carcinogenesis. 2001;22:957–64.

18. Shekels LL, Lyftogt CT, Ho SB. Bile acid-induced alterations of mucin production in differentiated human colon cancer cell lines. Int J Biochem Cell Biol. 1996;28:193–201.

19. Pongracz J, Clark P, Neoptelemos JP, Lord JM. Expression of protein kinase C isoenzymes in colorectal cancer tissue and their differential activation by different bile acids. Int J Cancer. 1995;29:35–9.

20. Powell AA, LaRue JM, Batta AK, Martinez JD. Bile acid hydrophobicity is correlated with induction of apoptosis and/or growth arrest in HCT116 cells. Biochem J. 2001;356:481–6.

21. Shekels LL, Beste JE, Ho SB. Tauroursodeoxycholic acid protects in vitro models of human colonic cancer cells from cytotoxic effects of hydrophobic bile acids. J Lab Clin Med. 1996; 127:57–66.

22. Sohn J, Khaustov VI, Xie Q, Chung C Krishnan B, Yoffe B. Survivin expression and the effects of ursodeoxycholic acid on the survivin in thapsigargin-induced apoptosis. Cancer Lett. 2003;191:83–92.

23. McMillan DC, Canna K, McArdle CS. Systemic inflammatory response predicts survival following curative resection of colorectal cancer. Br J Surg. 2003;90:215–19.

24. Earnest DL, Holubec H, Wali RK et al. Chemoprevention of azoxymethane-induced colonic carcinogenesis by supplemental dietary ursodeoxycholic acid. Cancer Res. 1994;54:5071–4.

25. Narisawa T, Fukaura Y, Terada K, Sekiguchi H. Inhibitory effects of ursodeoxycholic acid on N-methylnitrosourea-induced colon carcinogenesis and colonic mucosal telomerase activity in F344 rats. J Exp Clin Cancer Res. 1999;18:259–66.

26. Narisawa T, Fukaura Y, Takeba N, Nakai K. Chemoprevention of N-methylnitrosourea-induced colon carcinogenesis by ursodeoxycholic acid-5-aminosalicylic acid conjugate in F344 rats. Jpn J Cancer Res. 2002;93:143–50.

27. Wali RK, Khare S, Tretiakova M et al. Ursodeoxycholic acid and F(6)-D(3) inhibit aberrant crypt proliferation in the rat azoxymethane model of colon cancer: roles of cyclin D1 and E-cadherin. Cancer Epidemiol Biomarkers Prev. 2002;11:1653–62.

28. Ikegami T, Matsuzaki Y, Shoda J, Kano M, Hirabayashi N, Tanaka N. The chemopreventive role of ursodeoxycholic acid in azoxymethane-treated rats: suppressive effects on enhanced group II phospholipase A2 expression in colonic tissue. Cancer Lett. 1998;134:129–39.

29. Khare S, Cerda S, Wali RK et al. Ursodeoxycholic acid inhibits Ras mutations, wild-type Ras activation, and cyclooxygenase-2 expression in colon cancer. Cancer Res. 2003;63:3517–23.

30. Invernizzi P, Salzman AL, Szabo C, Ueta I, O'Connor M, Setchell KD. Ursodeoxycholate inhibits induction of NOS in human intestinal epithelial cells and in vivo. Am J Physiol. 1997;273:G131–8.

31. Rigas B, Tsiouslias GJ, Allan C, Wali RK, Brasitus TA. The effect of bile acids on MHC antigen expression in rat colonocytes during colon cancer development. Immunology. 1994;83:319–23.

32. Rodrigues CMP, Kren BT, Steer CJ, Setchell KDR. The site-specific delivery of ursodeoxycholic acid to the rat colon by sulfate conjugation. Gastroenterology. 1995;109:1835–44.
33. Lee YM, Kaplan MM. Primary sclerosing cholangitis. N Engl J Med. 1995;332:924.
34. Tung BY, Emond MJ, Haggitt RC et al. Ursodiol use is associated with lower prevalence of colonic neoplasia in patients with ulcerative colitis and primary sclerosing cholangitis. Ann Intern Med. 2001;134:89–95.
35. Pardi DS, Loftus EV Jr, Kremers WK, Keach J, Lindor KD. Ursodeoxycholic acid as a chemopreventive agent in patients with ulcerative colitis and primary sclerosing cholangitis. Gastroenterology. 2003;124:889–93.
36. Serfaty L, Deleusse A, Rosmorduc O et al. Ursodeoxycholic acid decreases recurrence of colorectal adenoma in patients with primary biliary cirrhosis. Gastroenterology. 2002 (abstract A-70).
37. Buttar N, Wang K, Andersen M et al. Ursodeoxycholic acid as a chemopreventive agent in Barrett's esophagus: an *in-vitro* study. Gastroenterology. 2002 (abstract A-292).
38. Lindor KD. Ursodeoxycholic acid for primary sclerosing cholangitis. N Engl J Med. 1997; 336:691.
39. Mitchell SA, Bansi DS, Hunt N, Von Bergmann K, Fleming KA, Chapman RW. A preliminary trial of high-dose ursodeoxycholic acid in primary sclerosing cholangitis. Gastroenterology. 2001;121:900–7.
40. Harnois DM, Angulo P, Jorgensen RA, Larusso NF, Lindor KD. High-dose ursodeoxycholic acid as a therapy for patients with primary sclerosing cholangitis. Am J Gastroenterol. 2001;96:1558–62.

Section X
Malignancies in primary sclerosing cholangitis

35
Hepatocellular carcinoma, cholangiocarcinoma, colon and pancreatic carcinoma in patients with primary sclerosing cholangitis: epidemiology and risk factors

U. BROOMÉ and A. BERGQUIST

EPIDEMIOLOGY OF PRIMARY SCLEROSING CHOLANGITIS AND CHOLANGIOCARCINOMA

Parker and Kendall first described the association between ulcerative colitis (UC) and cholangiocarcinoma in 1954[1]. Later, in 1971, Converse et al. found that bile duct carcinoma in UC most commonly occurs in patients with pre-existing primary sclerosing cholangitis (PSC)[2]. Today we know that PSC can be complicated by cholangiocarcinoma, gall bladder carcinoma and hepatocellular carcinoma. The increased risk for cholangiocarcinoma in PSC is well established but the prevalence of cholangiocarcinoma varies in different studies between 5% and 20%[3,4].

Epidemiological investigations can be performed in order to estimate the frequency or distribution of a disease within a population. The reliability of epidemiological studies is dependent on several factors:

1. the possibility of correct assessment of all patients with the disease being studied;
2. that the disease should be a distinct entity with no overlap to other diseases; and
3. the possibility to accurately define onset of time for the disease.

How do these requirements apply to PSC and cholangiocarcinoma in PSC patients? Today, almost half of all PSC patients are asymptomatic at the time of diagnosis[3,5]. Active screening procedures are therefore needed in order to identify all patients with PSC. There is no single sensitive and specific diagnostic marker for PSC. Diagnosis is made from a combination of clinical, biochemical, radiological and histological features[6,7]. Each diagnostic tool is hampered by overlap with other liver diseases. In a majority of PSC patients the onset is insidious and patients have features of chronic liver disease in general. The insidious onset may lead to problems in defining onset of disease. In several studies it has been shown that the time between first abnormal liver function tests and time to definite diagnosis of PSC is around 5 years[3,8]. In addition, the diagnosis of cholangiocarcinoma in PSC is often difficult to make. It has been recognized in several studies that cholangiocarcinoma in some PSC patients will be found only at autopsy[9]. Thus, there are several major drawbacks concerning epidemiological data regarding PSC, and especially regarding the incidence of cholangiocarcinoma in PSC.

To date only one population-based investigation of PSC epidemiology has been reported using accepted criteria, including cholangiography, for the diagnosis of PSC[10]. In this study from Norway 17 new cases were identified from a defined catchment area over a 10-year period with a point prevalence of 8.5/100 000 persons. The largest study that has evaluated the risk of cholangiocarcinoma in PSC includes 604 Swedish PSC patients identified in 1970–1998[9]. Since Sweden has approximately 8.9 million inhabitants this cohort of PSC patients accounts for a considerable proportion of all Swedish PSC patients. The diagnosis of PSC was based on biochemical, clinical and cholangiographic features. Median time of follow-up was 5.7 years (0–27.8), 79% had concomitant inflammatory bowel disease; 74% of all dead patients without a diagnosis of hepatobiliary carcinoma before death underwent autopsy. Due to an individually unique 10-digit national registration number assigned to all Swedes a follow-up was provided through

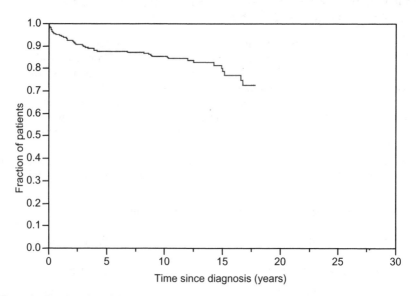

Figure 1 Fraction of surviving patients without hepatobiliary cancer over time in 604 patients with primary sclerosing cholangitis. The event shown is hepatobiliary carcinoma and patients were censored at time for liver transplantation, death without cancer and last date of clinical follow-up

linkages to the Swedish Cancer and Death registries. Cumulative incidence of malignancies and standard incidence ratio (SIR) were calculated with the incidence rates in the Swedish population; 81 patients developed hepatobiliary malignancy (13.3%). The risk for hepatobiliary malignancy was increased 161 times. The prevalence of cholangiocarcinoma in this study was 13%; 37% of the patients with cholangiocarcinoma developed the tumour within 1 year after PSC diagnosis. The incidence rate of cholangiocarcinoma was 1.5% per year in PSC patients with duration of PSC more than 1 year (Figure 1).

PSC AND GALL BLADDER CARCINOMA

The gall bladder epithelium in PSC patients has features of chronic inflammation similar to that found in the liver. Moreover, it has been shown that the frequency of gall bladder polyps in PSC patients is 4%[11]. It therefore seems logical to suppose that patients with PSC are also prone to develop gall bladder carcinoma. In several studies investigating the prevalence of cholangiocarcinoma in PSC, patients with gall bladder carcinomas have been included since there are difficulties in separating these two entities. In a recent study the prevalence of gall bladder cancer was assessed in PSC patients with a gall bladder mass who had undergone cholecystectomy[12]. Among 102 PSC patients who underwent cholecystectomy at the Mayo Clinic between 1977 and 1999, 14 (13.7%) had a gall bladder mass. In eight of the 14 patients the gall bladder mass was caused by adenocarcinoma. In the six patients with benign masses 33% had epithelial cell dysplasia. It is noteworthy that the mass lesions were not recognized preoperatively in five (42%) of the patients at ultrasound. It is important to point out that five of the malignant gall bladder masses were less than 10 mm in size. Thus, gall bladder polyps in patients with PSC should be removed earlier than in other patients, in whom a size more than 10 mm is often required before a cholecystectomy is recommended.

PSC AND HEPATOCELLULAR CARCINOMA (HCC)

There have been several case reports of HCC in PSC[13,14]. In a study from the Mayo Clinic, including 134 PSC patients with cirrhosis undergoing liver transplantation, HCC was found in three (2%) patients[15]. None of the PSC patients with HCC had evidence of hepatitis B or C infection or other risk factors for development of HCC. There were no significant differences in clinical characteristics in PSC patients with and without HCC. Thus, HCC can occur in end-stage PSC, and PSC patients with cirrhosis should be included in surveillance programmes with ultrasonography.

Case reports have also described the association of PSC with fibrolamellar carcinoma.

PSC AND THE RISK OF COLORECTAL CARCINOMA

UC is a well-known risk factor for development of colorectal carcinoma. The two major risk factors for this complication are long duration of the disease and extensive colitis. The cause of neoplastic change in UC remains unexplained; 80–90% of patients with PSC have concomitant inflammatory bowel disease. The majority of the patients with PSC who have an associated inflammatory bowel disease have UC with pancolitis. Lately, the presence of PSC has been shown to increase the risk of colorectal cancer or dysplasia in patients with UC[16–19]. In a study from Sweden the absolute cumulative risk of developing colorectal dysplasia/cancer in the PSC/UC group was 9%, 31% and 50% respectively after 10, 20 and 25 years of disease duration. In the group with UC only the corresponding risk was 2%, 5% and 10%[16]. An almost identical cumulative incidence of colorectal neoplasia was found both in a recent Finnish case–control study including 45 patients with UC and concomitant PSC and 45 pair-matched control patients with UC only, and in a population-based Swedish study including 125 PSC patients[19,20]. However, some studies have shown no increased risk for UC patients with PSC to develop colorectal dysplasia/cancer[21,22]. The discrepancies may be explained by different study designs.

Since published data on the risk of colorectal dysplasia/cancer in patients with PSC are conflicting a meta-analysis was performed[23]. Eleven studies met all eligibility criteria for the meta-analysis. Altogether 16 844 patients with UC were included in the analysis, and 560 had colorectal carcinoma. Of the 564 PSC patients included 60 had colonic carcinoma. It was shown that PSC patients with UC are at an increased risk of colorectal dysplasia/cancer compared with patients with UC alone (OR 4.79; CI 3.58–6.41). This increased risk is still present when the risk of colorectal cancer alone is considered. Due to the well-known risk that studies with null results have not been published, a calculation was made as to how many studies with null results were required to change the conclusion. It was found that 163 studies with null results are necessary in order to change the result of the meta-analysis.

The reason for this increased risk to develop colorectal neoplasia in PSC patients is obscure. Patients with cholestatic liver disease have decreased bile acid excretion and a relatively high proportion of secondary bile acids[24]. It has been speculated that secondary bile acids play a role for carcinogenesis of the colorectal mucosa in PSC. This is supported by the fact that right-sided cancers seem to be more common in patients with PSC compared with patients with UC alone[25]. Moreover, two recent reports have clearly demonstrated that treatment with ursodeoxycholic acid decreased the risk for developing colorectal dysplasia in patients with PSC and UC[26,27]. This further supports the belief that bile acids do play a role in the development of colorectal neoplasia in PSC.

The colitis in PSC often runs a quiescent course compared with UC patients without PSC[28]. This may lead to an underestimation of the presence and duration of UC. Treatment with sulphasalazine/5-ASA has been shown to decrease the risk for colorectal carcinoma in patients with UC. In a study from Sweden this finding could not be confirmed, and the number of patients treated with sulphasalazine/5-aminosalicylic acid (5-ASA) did not differ in UC patients with and without PSC[25]. PSC patients with UC remain at increased risk of developing colon cancer/dysplasia even after they have undergone liver transplantation[29]. In a recent study from Pittsburgh the evolution of inflammatory bowel disease in PSC patients who had been liver transplanted was evaluated. Among 303 PSC patients who underwent liver transplantation 68% had inflammatory bowel disease. The risk of colectomy of intractable disease, but not the risk for colorectal cancer, was increased significantly after orthotopic liver transplant (OLT)[30]. Vera et al. found that the cumulative risk of developing colorectal cancer was 14% and 17%, at 5 and 10 years after liver transplantation[31]. In a multivariate analysis it was shown that duration of colitis more than 10 years and pancolitis were independent risk factors for development of colorectal carcinoma after liver transplantation. Patients developing colorectal cancer have significantly reduced survival. It is therefore of importance to emphasize the necessity that all patients with PSC and UC should be included into colonoscopic surveillance pro- grammes, probably at an earlier time than UC patients without PSC; also, after transplantation, an annual colonoscopy of these patients is suggested. The pre- ferred colectomy procedure in patients with PSC has been to create an ileal pelvic pouch with an ileoanal anastomosis. A recent study investigated whether patients with UC and PSC also have an increased risk of neoplastic transforma- tion or development of atrophy in the ileal pouch mucosa after construction of an ileal pelvic pouch with an ileoanal anastomosis or construction of a continent Kock ileostomy[32]. Flexible video endoscopic examinations of the ileal pouch were performed in 16 patients with UC and PSC and in 16 UC patients without PSC, matched regarding type of reservoir, indication for surgery, pouch duration, age at onset of UC, age at follow-up and UC duration at time of colectomy. Multiple biopsies were sampled from different locations in the pouch for histo- logical assessment of the degree of mucosal atrophy and dysplasia, and for flow cytometric DNA analysis.

The PSC patients developed moderate or severe atrophy in the pouch signifi- cantly more often than UC patients without PSC ($p < 0.01$). Persistent severe mucosal atrophy, a risk factor for neoplastic transformation, was revealed in eight PSC patients and in only two controls. One of the patients with PSC had high-grade dysplasia in multiple locations. Low-grade dysplasia was found in three patients in the PSC group and in two of the controls. UC patients with PSC with an ileal reservoir are more prone to develop mucosal atrophy in the pouch, and seem to have a higher risk of neoplastic transformation in the pouch mucosa than UC patients without PSC.

PANCREATIC CARCINOMA

In the study by Bergquist et al. including 604 PSC patients the risk for developing extrahepatic malignancies was also estimated[9]. For the first time it was found that PSC patients had a 10–14 times increased risk of developing pancreatic car- cinoma compared to the general population. None of these patients had a known history of chronic pancreatitis. There might be a risk for detection bias since it can sometimes be difficult to differentiate pancreatic carcinoma arising from pancreatic caput from cholangiocarcinoma arising from the large bile ducts. Among PSC patients 15–50% have changes at cholangiography indicating chronic pancreatitis[33,34]. Chronic pancreatitis without association to PSC is a known risk factor for development of pancreatic carcinoma[35,36]. In a Swedish study by Isaksson et al. PSC was found to be a risk factor for development of pancreatic carcinoma[37]. In this study the study base comprised all Swedish patients diagnosed with pancreatic carcinoma in 1987–1999. A total of 15 001 patients with pancreatic carcinoma were identified, and all associated diseases among these patients were identified. PSC was shown to be a risk factor for the development of pancreatic carcinoma, the odds ratio for men being 2.7 (CI 1.5–4.6) and for women 3.2 (CI 1.8–5.8). In this study chronic pancreatitis, diabetes and obesity were also identified as risk factors for pancreatic carcinoma.

RISK FACTOR FOR DEVELOPMENT OF CHOLANGIOCARCINOMA IN PATIENTS WITH PSC

Well-performed epidemiological studies can serve as a basis for future investigations of risk factors for cancer development. For a rare disease such as PSC the use of case–control study design is preferable. Control subjects should be PSC patients without cholangiocarcinoma. A bias in case–control studies is the fact that the control is also ill, and harbours the risk of developing cholangiocarcinoma. If the control patient has not been followed long enough there is a risk that the control has an undiagnosed cholangiocarcinoma. Moreover, all studies evaluating risk factors for cholangiocarcinoma development have been retrospective studies, and there is an obvious risk that missing data from medical records can hamper the results. If risk factors for cholangiocarcinoma development in PSC could be identified it might be possible to interfere in the malignant transformation. In addition, knowledge on possible risk factors may be of value to identify PSC patients who should be selected for early liver transplantation. It has been shown in several studies that the prognosis for PSC patients with a diagnosis of cholangiocarcinoma before liver transplantation is poor[14]. The fact that patients with chronic infection with *Clonorchis sinensis* also have an increased risk of developing cholangiocarcinoma may suggest that long-standing inflammation of the bile ducts may enhance the risk for cholangiocarcinoma development. When the cholangiocytes are continuously exposed to chronic inflammation and hydrophobic bile acids it has been suggested that the cholangiocytes may be predisposed to oncogenic mutations, and further progression to malignancies. This may partly be caused by a failure to activate apoptosis and delete cells with genetic damage[38]. Why some PSC patients develop cancer and some do not is, however, still unclear.

In other chronic inflammatory diseases with an increased risk for malignant transformation, e.g. ulcerative colitis, it has been clearly demonstrated that the duration of the inflammatory process is an independent risk factor for cancer development. This is supported by the fact that, in one-third of the PSC patients with cholangiocarcinoma, the cancer is diagnosed within a year after PSC diagnosis. In addition, cholangiocarcinomas in PSC occur both in patients with and without cirrhosis[14]. This is in contrast to the risk of developing hepatocellular carcinoma, which is mostly seen in patients with underlying cirrhosis[15].

PSC can involve the intrahepatic, or the extrahepatic, or most commonly both the intrahepatic and extrahepatic biliary system. In patients with UC it is well known that the colonic distribution of the colitis is an independent risk factor for development of colorectal cancer. UC patients with pancolitis have a significantly higher risk of developing colorectal carcinoma compared to patients with left-sided colitis. In PSC it has not been shown that the distribution of the biliary duct inflammation affects the risk for malignant transformation of the biliary epithelium[14,39]. Small bile duct PSC represent patients with an abnormal liver function test, a characteristic liver histology but a normal cholangiography and no other cholestatic disorder. Three recent studies present data on small bile duct PSC, comprising altogether 83 patients[40–42]. None of these patients was found to acquire cholangiocarcinoma, although one developed hepatocellular carcinoma and 13% progressed to involvement of the large bile ducts. Patients with primary biliary cirrhosis, a biliary disease affecting only the small bile ducts, do not have an increased risk for cholangiocarcinoma development. It therefore seems justified to conclude that only patients having chronic inflammation of the large bile ducts are at an increased risk for cholangiocarcinoma development, regardless of whether only the intrahepatic or extrahepatic biliary tree is affected.

It has been described in a case–control study that PSC patients who are previous or current smokers are at increased risk for development of cholangiocarcinoma[14]. In another recent study investigating risk factors for gall bladder carcinoma in patients without PSC cigarette smoking was found to be an independent risk factor[43]. Moreover, smoking has been considered a risk factor for HCC both in HBsAg chronic carriers and in patients with PBC[44,45]. It is well documented that there is an independent association between non-smoking and PSC in PSC patients without cholangiocarcinoma[46]. However, in another case–control study these findings could not be confirmed, but an association between alcohol consumption and the risk for cholangiocarcinoma development was found[47]. These findings also need confirmation, although it seems wise to recommend PSC patients to abstain from smoking as well as alcohol over-consumption.

The majority of PSC patients have an associated inflammatory bowel disease. In a European multicentre study, including 394 PSC patients from five countries, cholangiocarcinoma was diagnosed in 48 (12.2%) patients[39]. Inflammatory bowel disease was found in 325 (82%) of the patients. It was suggested that a long-standing duration of inflammatory bowel disease was a risk factor for cholangiocarcinoma development. Patients who developed cholangiocarcinoma were diagnosed with inflammatory bowel disease at least 1 year before PSC more often than in the group without cholangiocarcinoma (90% vs 65% respectively; $p = 0.001$). Moreover, the duration of inflammatory bowel disease before diagnosis of PSC was significantly longer in the cancer group, 17.4 years vs 9.0 years in the group without cancer ($p = 0.009$).

The presence of colorectal dysplasia/cancer in patients with concomitant UC seems to be another risk for cholangiocarcinoma development in PSC[16]. In a case–control study comparing 40 PSC patients to 80 age- and sex-matched controls with UC without PSC, 10 PSC patients developed cholangiocarcinoma. Among the 10 PSC patients with cholangiocarcinoma nine also had inflammatory bowel disease. Seven of the patients with cholangiocarcinoma also had colorectal dysplasia/cancer. Thus, cholangiocarcinoma was significantly more common among UC patients with PSC and colorectal neoplasia compared with those patients with UC and PSC without colorectal dysplasia/carcinoma ($p > 0.02$). The finding that colorectal dysplasia/cancer should be a risk factor for the future development of cholangiocarcinoma has, however, not been confirmed in other published studies. The Oxford Group has suggested that biliary duct dysplasia in liver biopsies precedes cholangiocarcinoma in PSC[48]. This is controversial, and Ludwig et al. found only one patient with bile duct dysplasia among 60 cases who underwent liver transplantation[49]. An evaluation of biliary duct dysplasia in PSC has been made, and it seems that, with strict definitions of bile duct dysplasia, an acceptable agreement can be achieved among liver pathologists[50]. The presence of biliary dysplasia in a liver biopsy should therefore increase the suspicion of development of cholangiocarcinoma in another part of the liver.

Patients with PSC are at increased risk of developing cancer at the sites exposed to chronic inflammation: the biliary tree, the gall bladder, the colon and the pancreas. Factors responsible for the malignant development remain unknown, and it is a large challenge for future research to identify this risk factors in order to intervene with these dreadful complications.

Acknowledgements

Financial support from the Knut and Alice Wallenbergs Foundation is greatly appreciated.

References

1. Parker R, Kendall E. The liver in ulcerative colitis. Br Med J. 1954;2:1030–2.
2. Converse C, Reagan J, DeCosse J. Ulcerative colitis and carcinoma of the bile ducts. Am J Surg. 1971;121:39–45.
3. Broomé U, Olsson R, Lööf L et al. Natural history and prognostic factors in 305 Swedish patients with primary sclerosing cholangitis. Gut. 1996;38:610–15.
4. Rosen C, Nagorney D, Wiesner R, Coffey R, LaRusso L. Cholangiocarcinoma complicating primary sclerosing cholangitis. Ann Surg. 1991;213:21–5.
5. Okolicsanyi L, Fabris L, Viaggi S et al. Clinical presentation, natural history and prognostic variables: an Italian multi-center study. Eur J Gastroenterol. 1996;8:685.
6. Chapman R, Arborgh B, Rhodes J et al. Primary sclerosing cholangitis: a review of its clinical features, cholangiography and hepatic histology. Gut. 1980;21:870–7.
7. Wiesner R, La Russo N. Clinicopathologic features of the syndrome of primary sclerosing cholangitis. Gastroenterology. 1980;74:200–6.
8. Boberg K, Rocca G, Egeland T et al. Time-dependent Cox regression model is superior in predicting prognosis in primary sclerosing cholangitis. Hepatology. 2002;35:652–7.
9. Bergquist A, Ekbom A, Olsson R et al. Hepatic and extrahepatic malignancies in primary sclerosing cholangitis. J Hepatol. 2002;36:321–7.
10. Boberg K, Aadland E, Jahnsen J, Raknerud N, Stiris M, Bell H. Incidence and prevalence of primary biliary cirrhosis, primary sclerosing cholangitis, and autoimmune hepatitis in a Norwegian population. Scand J Gastroenterol. 1998;33:99–103.
11. Brandt D, MacCarty R, Charboneau J, LaRusso N, Wiesner R, Ludwig J. Gallbladder disease in patients with primary sclerosing cholangitis. Am J Roentgenol. 1988;150:571–4.
12. Buckles D, Lindor K, Larusso N, Petrovic L, Gores G. In primary sclerosing cholangitis, gallbladder polyps are frequently malignant. Am J Gastroenterol. 2002;97:1138–42.
13. Ismail T, Angrisani L, Hübscher S, McMaster P. Hepatocellular carcinoma complicating primary sclerosing cholangitis. Br J Surg. 1991;78:360–1.
14. Bergquist A, Glaumann H, Persson B, Broomé U. Risk factors and clinical presentation of hepatobiliary carcinoma in patients with primary sclerosing cholangitis – a case control study. Hepatology. 1998;27:311–16.
15. Harnois D, Gores G, Ludwig J, Steers J, LaRusso N, Wiesner R. Are patients with cirrhotic stage primary sclerosing cholangitis at risk for the development of hepatocellular cancer? J Hepatol. 1997;27:512–16.

16. Broomé U, Löfberg R, Veress B, Eriksson S. Primary sclerosing cholangitis and ulcerative colitis: Evidence for increased neoplastic potential. Hepatology. 1995;22:1404–8.

17. Brentnall T, Hagitt R, Rabinovitch P et al. Risk and natural history of colonic neoplasia in patients with primary sclerosing cholangitis and ulcerative colitis. Gastroenterology. 1996; 110:331–8.

18. Marchesa P, Lashner B, Lavery I et al. The risk of cancer and dysplasia among ulcerative colitis patients with primary sclerosing cholangitis. Am J Gastroenterol. 1997;92:1285–8.

19. Kornfelt D, Ekbom A, Ihre T. Is there an excess risk for colorectal cancer in ulcerative colitis patients with primary sclerosing cholangitis? A population-based study. Gut. 1997;41:518–21.

20. Leidenius M, Farkkila M, Karkkainen P et al. Colorectal dysplasia and carcinoma in patients with ulcerative colitis and primary sclerosing cholangitis. Scand J Gastroenterol. 1997;32:706.

21. Loftus E, Sandborn W, Tremaine W et al. Risk of colorectal neoplasia in patients with primary sclerosing cholangitis. Gastroenterology. 1996;110:432.

22. Nuako K, Ahlqvist D, Sandborn W et al. Primary sclerosing cholangitis and colorectal carcinoma in patients with chronic ulcerative colitis: a case control study. Cancer. 1998;82:822.

23. Soetikno R, Lin O, Heidenreich P, Young H, Blackstone M. Increased risk of colorectal neoplasia in patients with primary sclerosing cholangitis and ulcerative colitis: a meta analysis. Gastrointest Endosc. 2002;56:48–54.

24. Nagengast F, Grubben M, vanMunster I. Role of bile acids in colorectal carcinogenesis. Eur J Cancer. 1995;31:1067–70.

25. Lindberg B, Broomé U, Persson B. Proximal colorectal dysplasia or cancer in ulcerative colitis. The impact of primary sclerosing cholangitis and sulfasalazine. Dis Colon Rectum. 2001; 43:77–85.

26. Pardi D, Loftus E, Kremers W, Keach J, Lindor K. Ursodeoxycholic acid as a chemopreventive agent in patients with ulcerative colitis and primary sclerosing cholangitis. Gastroenterology. 2003;124:889–93.

27. Tung B, Emond M, Haggitt R et al. Ursodiol use is associated with lower prevalence of colonic neoplasia in patients with ulcerative colitis and primary sclerosing cholangitis. Ann Intern Med. 2001;134:89–95.

28. Lundqvist K, Broomé U. Differences in colonic disease activity in patients with ulcerative colitis with and without primary sclerosing cholangitis. Dis Colon Rectum. 1997;40:541–6.

29. Bleday R, Lee E, Jessurun J et al. Increased risk of early colorectal neoplasms after hepatic transplant in patients with inflammatory bowel disease. Dis Colon Rectum. 1993;36:908.

30. Dvorchik I, Subotin M, Demetris A et al. Effect of liver transplantation on inflammatory bowel disease in patients with primary sclerosing colangitis. Hepatology. 2002;35:380–4.

31. Vera A, Gunson B, Ussatoff V et al. Colorectal cancer in patients with inflammatory bowel disease after liver transplantation for primary sclerosing cholangitis. Transplantation. 2003;75:1983–8.

32. Ståhlberg D, Veress B, Tribukait B, Broomé U. Atrophy and neoplastic transormation of the ileal pouch mucosa in patients with ulcerative colitis and primary sclerosing cholangitis: a case control study. Dis Colon Rectum. 2003;46:770–8.

33. Epstein O, Chapman R, Lake-Bakaar G, Foo AY, Rosalki S, Sherlock S. The pancreas in primary biliary cirrhosis and primary sclerosing cholangitis. Gastroenterology. 1982;83:1177–82.

34. Lindstrom E, Bodemar G, Ryden B, Ihse I. Pancreatic ductal morphology and exocrine function in primary sclerosing cholangitis. Acta Chir Scand. 1990;156:451–6.

35. Bansal P, Sunnenberg A. Risk factors of colorectal cancer in inflammatory bowel disease. Am J Gastroenterol. 1996;91:44–8.

36. Lowenfels A, Maisonneuve P, Cavallini G et al. Pancreatitis and the risk of pancreatic cancer. N Engl J Med. 1993;328:1433–7.

37. Isaksson B, Jonsson F, Feychting M, Permert J. Pancreatico-biliary inflammation and hyperinsulinemia are risk factors of pancreatic cancer. Pancreatology. 2003;3:209 (abstract).

38. Celli A, Que F. Dysregulation of apoptosis in the cholangiopathies and cholangiocarcinoma. Semin Liver Dis. 1998;18:177–85.

39. Boberg K, Bergquist A, Mitchell S et al. Cholangiocarcinoma in primary sclerosing cholangitis: risk factors and clinical presentation. Scand J Gastroenterol. 2002;37:1205–11.

40. Broomé U, Glaumann H, Lindström E et al. Natural history and outcome in 32 Swedish patients with small duct primary sclerosing cholangitis (PSC). J Hepatol. 2002;36:586–9.

41. Björnsson E, Boberg K, Cullen S et al. Patients with small bile duct primary sclerosing cholangitis have a favourable long term prognosis. Gut. 2002;36:1227–35.

42. Angulo P, Maor-Kendler Y, Lindor K. Small-duct primary sclerosing cholangitis: a long term follow-up study. Hepatology. 2002;35:1494–500.
43. Khan Z, Neugut A, Ahsan H, Chabot M. Risk factors for biliary tract cancers. Am J Gastroenterol. 1999;94:149–52.
44. Floreani A, Baragiotta A, Baldo V, Menegon T, Farinati F, Naccarato R. Hepatic and extrahepatic malignancies in primary biliary cirrhosis. Hepatology. 1999;29:1425–8.
45. Yu M, Hsu F, Sheen I et al. Prospective study of hepatocellular carcinoma and liver cirrhosis in asymptomatic chronic hepatitis B virus carriers. Am J Epidemiol. 1997;145:1039–47.
46. Loftus E, Sandborn W, Tremaine W et al. Primary sclerosing cholangitis is associated with non-smoking; a case control study. Gastroenterology. 1996;110:1496–502.
47. Chalasani N, Baluyut A, Ismail A et al. Cholangiocarcinoma in patients with primary sclerosing cholangitis: a multi-center case–control study. Hepatology. 2000;31:7–11.
48. Martins E, Fleming K, Garrido M, Hine K, Chapman R. Superficial thrombophlebitis, dysplasia, and cholangiocarcinoma in primary sclerosing cholangitis. Gastroenterology. 1994;107:537–42.
49. Ludwig J, Wahlström H, Batts K, Wiesner R. Papillary bile duct dysplasia in primary sclerosing cholangitis. Gastroenterology. 1992;102:2134–8.
50. Fleming K, Boberg K, Glaumann H, Bergquist A, Smith D, Clausen O. Biliary dysplasia as a marker of cholangiocarcinoma in primary sclerosing cholangitis. J Hepatol. 2001;34:360–5.

36
Tumour markers and genetic markers in the diagnosis of bile duct carcinoma

A. BERGQUIST

INTRODUCTION

Cholangiocarcinoma in the setting of primary sclerosing cholangitis (PSC) is difficult to reveal and is often diagnosed at an advanced stage of tumour growth and spread, or accidentally at liver transplantation in end-stage PSC[1–4]. In some patients the cholangiocarcinoma will be revealed only at autopsy[5]. Clinically, biliary malignancy is often suspected when a PSC patient shows rapid, progressive liver disease with increasing bilirubin levels, weight loss and abdominal pain. However, end-stage PSC without cholangiocarcinoma can also present with rapid disease progression, and it is not possible to distinguish clinically between end-stage PSC and PSC complicated by cholangiocarcinoma[6]. The prognosis of PSC patients with cholangiocarcinoma is dismal, with a median survival time of less than 6 months after cancer diagnosis[7], and bile duct carcinoma is a leading cause of mortality in patients with PSC. Not only clinical but also radiological methods have failed to be specific and sensitive diagnostic tools. Therefore other markers are important for the diagnosis of bile duct carcinoma in PSC.

SERUM TUMOUR MARKERS

Serum tumour markers that have been evaluated for detection of bile duct carcinoma in PSC are carbohydrate antigen 19-9 (CA 19-9), carcinoembryonic antigen (CEA), cancer antigen (CA) 50, 125 and 242. CEA is a glycoprotein normally found in the fetal gut, pancreas and liver. CEA was the first tumour marker described to be associated with colorectal carcinoma[8]. CEA has its greatest application in the follow-up of patients with colorectal carcinoma after tumour resection. After curative surgery this marker returns to normal within weeks after resection. CA 19-9 is a mucin-type glycoprotein which has been shown to be increased in serum in malignant pancreatic and biliary tumours[9]. CA 242 is expressed in mucin antigens and is increased in pancreatic and colorectal cancers[10]. Raised levels of serum CA 125 are found in patients with epithelial ovarian cancer, and increased levels in bile are found in gastrointestinal cancers[11]. The best-evaluated, and therefore probably the most commonly used, tumour markers in clinical practice for the detection of bile duct carcinoma in PSC are CEA and CA 19-9.

In 1995 Ramage et al. published a study, including 74 PSC patients, in which a combination of the two tumour markers CA 19-9 and CEA was evaluated in detecting cholangiocarcinoma. Cut-off values of 5 ng/ml for CEA and 200 U/ml for CA 19-9 resulted in a sensitivity of 53% and 60% for CEA and CA 19-9, respectively. The specificity was 86% for CEA and 91% for CA 19-9. Using the formula CA 19-9 + (CEA × 40) with a cut-off level of 400 a sensitivity of 66%, a specificity of 100% and an accuracy of 86% in diagnosing cholangiocarcinoma was achieved[12]. In a study by Björnsson et al. 72 PSC patients were followed with multiple serum measurements of CA 19-9 and CEA[13]. Seven of the 72 PSC patients developed cholangiocarcinoma. Among the PSC patients with cholangiocarcinoma 56% had CA 19-9 values above the upper reference value (37 U/ml), and only 33% had values above 200 U/ml. The sensitivity and specificity of CA 19-9 was 38% and 81% respectively when the cut-off level 200 U/ml was used. In a recent study by Siqueira et al. the sensitivity and specificity of serum levels of CA 19-9 or CEA on diagnosing cholangiocarcinoma in PSC was investigated[14]. Of the 333 PSC retrospectively studied patients the sensitivity and specificity for CEA in 144 patients and CA 19-9 in 55 patients was in line with previous reports, as demonstrated in Table 1. The Ramage formula CA 19-9 + (CEA × 40) < 400 has recently been evaluated by others[13,15]. The sensitivity and specificity has not been shown to be as high as in the original study by Ramage. A summary of sensitivities and specificities of CEA and CA 19-9 in these studies is given in Table 1. However, the use of both markers CA 19-9 and CEA is superior to either of them alone, and it is therefore recommended to use both for the detection of cholangiocarcinoma in PSC.

PSC patients with concomitant cholangitis or an active inflammation in the bile ducts frequently have high levels of serum tumour markers. Björnsson et al. found a correlation between high CA 19-9 values and serum alkaline phosphatase levels[13]. There is, however, no correlation between the levels of the serum tumour markers CEA and CA 19-9 and bilirubin levels, which is a consistent finding in several studies[13,14,16].

Thus, serum tumour markers have a rather good sensitivity and specificity in diagnosing cholangiocarcinoma in PSC. The possibility of *early* detection of tumours or premalignancy by the use of serum CEA and CA 19-9 is very low.

In the study by Ramage et al., eight patients had incidental cholangiocarcinoma diagnosed first at examination of the liver after transplantation[12]. Two of the eight patients had a tumour marker score of less than 400, and they were the only patients in this group with a survival of more than 6 months without tumour recurrence. This indicates that these tumour markers are of limited value for early detection of cholangiocarcinoma in PSC. This is further supported in the

Table 1 Summary of sensitivity and specificity of the tumour markers CA 19-9 and CEA in the diagnosis of cholangiocarcinoma in PSC. King's score is defined as CA 19-9 + (CEA × 40) according to ref. 12

Study	Ramage et al.[12] (n = 74)	Björnsson et al.[13] (n = 72)	Siquera et al.[14] (n = †)	Lindberg et al.[15] (n = 57, 20 PSC)
Sensitivity CA 19-9	60%* (>200 U/ml)	38%* (>200 U/ml); 63%* (>37 U/ml)	67%*(>180 U/ml); 62%* (>37 U/ml)	67%* (>100 U/ml)
Sensitivity CEA	53%* (>5 ng/ml)	33%* (>5 ng/ml)	68% (>5.2 ng/ml)	56%* (>5 ng/ml)
Sensitivity, Ramage's score	66%	33%	Not stated	43%
Specificity CA 19-9	91%* (>200 U/ml)	81%* (>200 U/ml); 50%* (>37 U/ml)	98%* (>180 U/ml); 40%* (>37 U/ml)	89%* (>100 U/ml)
Specificity CEA	86%* (>5 ng/ml)	85%* (>5 ng/ml)	82%* (>5.2 ng/ml)	89%* (>5 ng/ml)
Specificity, Ramage's score	100%	85%	Not stated	89%

* Cut-off level.
† n = 55 for CA 19-9 and n = 144 for CEA.

study by Hultcrantz et al., in which an effort to diagnose cholangiocarcinoma at an early stage was made. Four tumour markers (CA 19-9, CEA, CA 50, and CA 242) were evaluated in 75 PSC patients who were prospectively followed for 3 years[16]. Two patients developed cholangiocarcinoma during the study, one had normal and one increased serum tumour marker levels. Transient, non-cholangiocarcinoma-associated, non-cholangitis-associated elevations of CA 19-9 above 35 U/ml, were seen in five patients. However, none of these patients had CA 19-9 values above 200 U/ml, which was the cut-off level in the study by Ramage et al. In the study by Hultcrantz two additional patients developed cholangiocarcinoma at follow-up (8 years) and none of them had earlier shown elevated tumour markers. It was concluded that these tumour markers were lacking both in sensitivity and specificity, and could not serve as early markers for the detection of cholangiocarcinoma in PSC[16].

Serum CA 242 has shown to be increased in cholangiocarcinoma without PSC with a diagnostic accuracy of 71%[17]. The only study that has investigated CA 242 for the diagnosis of cholangiocarcinoma in PSC is the study by Hultcrantz et al. Only one of the patients in this study with bile duct carcinoma had an increased level of CA 242[16].

The level of CA 125 in serum has recently been evaluated in patients with chronic liver disease with and without ascites. In 50 patients with ascites, and 20 without, it was shown that CA 125 was elevated in all forms of liver disease, especially in those with cirrhotic ascites irrespective of the aetiology of cirrhosis or presence of spontaneous bacterial peritonitis. Five of the patients included in this study had PSC. CA 125 as a possible diagnostic tool for detection of cholangiocarcinoma in PSC can be questioned, although CA 125 has not been separately evaluated for this specific purpose.

In summary, serum tumour markers, especially CEA and CA 19-9, have a role in diagnosing cholangiocarcinoma in patients with PSC. The use of the Ramage formula can improve sensitivity and specificity. A mild rise in CA 19-9 values is unspecific and should be interpreted cautiously. Awareness of the presence of false-negative as well as false-positive results is important. In most transplant centres PSC patients with cholangiocarcinoma will not be accepted for liver transplantation. A rise in the tumour markers CA 19-9 and/or CEA cannot be used for excluding a PSC patient from a potentially life-saving liver transplantation.

TUMOUR MARKERS IN BILE

An early study by Ker et al. evaluated the diagnostic value of CA 19-9 and CA 125 measured in bile for diagnosing cholangiocarcinoma in patients without PSC. This study showed that increased levels of CA 125 in bile had a high specificity for diagnosing cholangiocarcinoma. However, CA 19-9 in bile was not found to be superior to serum analyses in this study. In a recent published study by Chen et al., including 98 patients with biliary obstruction without PSC of whom 28 had cholangiocarcinoma, it was shown that the specificity of CA 125 in bile for the diagnosis of bile duct carcinoma was better than both CA 19-9 and CEA[18]. CA 125 was shown to be less affected by inflammation and hepatolithiasis than CA 19-9 and CEA.

Two recent studies have evaluated CEA and CA 19-9 as diagnostic tools for cholangiocarcinoma in PSC in the bile[13,15]. The results from both of these studies show that measurement of these tumour markers in bile is not clinically useful in diagnosing cholangiocarcinoma in PSC. Therefore, analyses of the tumour markers CEA and CA 19-9 in bile do not seem to have advantages over serum analyses.

Fibronectin is an adhesive glycoprotein involved in a variety of cellular processes including cell-to-substrate adhesion, cell migration, and regulation of cell morphology. Fibronectin has been used as a marker of malignancy, for instance in ascites and urine. The value of biliary fibronectin for the diagnosis of cholangiocarcinoma without PSC has recently been evaluated by Chen et al.[19]. Sixty-two patients with gallstones and cholangitis, five patients with benign biliary stricture and 28 patients with cholangiocarcinoma were included in the study. None of these patients had PSC. The absolute and relative concentrations (concentration of fibronectin divided by the concentration of total bile salts) of fibronectin were measured. The concentration of bile contents may be modified during the various periods of biliary obstruction. Using a relative concentration rather than an absolute concentration can adjust for this. The relative concentration of fibronectin in the study by Chen et al. was higher in the cancer group compared with the gallstone group, 350 vs. 180 592 ng/μmol ($p < 0.05$). The sensitivity and specificity of diagnosing cholangiocarcinoma was 57% and 79%, respectively. This is less than results from a study by Körner et al. investigating 71 patients with biliary strictures, in which a sensitivity of 89% and a specificity of 96% for diagnosing cholangiocarcinoma were found[20]. The difference in results from these two studies can at least partly be explained by the larger number of non-malignant cases with inflammatory activity in the study by Chen et al. in which all non-malignant patients with gallstones had concomitant cholangitis. The value of measuring fibronectin in bile in patients with PSC is not known. Biliary fibronectin increases in response to biliary inflammation, which probably diminishes its use in patients with PSC, although it has to be further evaluated.

Mutations of the *K-ras* oncogene have been described in pancreas and bile duct carcinomas. *K-ras* mutations have also been detected in stools from patients with cholangiocarcinoma and pancreatic cancer[21]. In a study by Saurin et al. bile specimens were obtained from 117 non-PSC patients with biliary strictures to determine if detection of *K-ras* mutations could differentiate between strictures of benign and malignant origin[22]. Detection of *K-ras* gene point mutation was found in bile from 31% (22/90) patients with primary malignancy in the bile ducts and in 4% (1/25) of patients with benign strictures. It was concluded that detection of *K-ras* mutations in bile appears to be specific for differentiating between benign and malignant biliary strictures. However, this does not seem to be the case in patients with an underlying PSC. In PSC, *K-ras* point mutations seem to be present in bile at an early stage of malignancy and are frequent in PSC patients without signs of malignancy. This has recently been demonstrated by Kubicka et al., who studied the occurrence of *K-ras* mutations in the bile fluids obtained by endoscopic retrograde cholangiopancreatography (ERCP) in 56 patients with PSC and 20 patients with other cholestatic liver disease[23]. None of the patients without PSC had *K-ras* mutations in the bile fluid, whereas 17 (30%) of the PSC patients revealed *K-ras* mutations in bile fluid. At follow-up no patient with PSC without *K-ras* mutations developed cholangiocarcinoma. Among the 17 patients with *K-ras* mutations in the bile two developed cholangiocarcinoma at 14 and 34 months after the first detection of *K-ras* gene alteration. Liver transplantation in 19 of the 56 PSC patients revealed two additional patients with incidental cholangiocarcinoma and two with high-grade biliary dysplasia. All four of these patients had previous *K-ras* mutations in the bile.

Thus the presence of *K-ras* mutations in bile from non-PSC patients is specific for biliary malignancy. In patients with PSC, however, *K-ras* mutations in bile might be interpreted as an early sign of malignancy, or even a risk factor for later development of cholangiocarcinoma. The relatively low frequency of *K-ras* mutations (30%) in cholangiocarcinoma tissue from PSC patients may, however, limit the value of such analyses[24].

BRUSH SAMPLES

Brush cytology from strictures obtained at ERCP has a good specificity, but a relatively low sensitivity, in diagnosing cholangiocarcinoma; the method is therefore of limited value in this setting[25–27]. Additional markers for malignancy have been evaluated using brush samples from the biliary tree in PSC patients. In a study by Ponsioen et al. brush cytology samples from 43 PSC patients were investigated. Immunohistochemical analyses of p53 and *K-ras* mutations of bile duct cells from the brush samples were performed and did not supply additional evidence to cytology for the diagnosis of malignancy in PSC[27].

The significance of DNA ploidy determinations in biopsies from cholangiocarcinoma in PSC has been evaluated. A high prevalence of DNA aneuploidy in cholangiocarcinoma (80%) from patients with PSC and a low prevalence of DNA aneuploidy in benign strictures (12%) has been shown[28]. Using DNA measurements from brush samples in the biliary tree might improve the diagnostic yield of malignancy[15,29,30]. In a study by Sears et al. DNA measurements by image cytometry on cytology specimens from biliary strictures (13 PSC) was shown to increase the sensitivity of detection of pancreatic–biliary malignancy compared to cytology analysis only[29]. In the prospective study by Lindberg et al.[15] of biliary strictures (20 PSC), DNA analysis with flow cytometry of brush samples showed alone a sensitivity and specificity of 52% and 96%.

In ulcerative colitis (UC) DNA aneuploidy is presumed to be an early sign of malignant transformation of the colonic mucosa and is sometimes seen prior to the development of colorectal dysplasia in patients with UC. The parallel to PSC is obvious, and this makes it tempting to hypothesize that DNA aneuploidy could precede malignant transformation of bile duct cells in PSC. DNA measurement of bile duct cells from brush samples as an early marker for malignancy has to be further evaluated.

LIVER BIOPSIES

The tumours in PSC are often scirrous in nature and, if a change suspected of being malignant is found at computer tomography or ultrasound, it is still difficult to obtain a representative biopsy specimen. Moreover, even if representative material is gathered, it can still sometimes be difficult to differentiate between non-neoplastic and malignant bile duct changes in needle biopsies from patients with PSC. Boberg et al. found *K-ras* mutations in 33% of cholangiocarcinomas from patients with PSC[24]. Similar figures have been reported in cholangiocarcinoma without PSC[31,32]. Mutation of p53 in PSC-related cholangiocarcinoma varies from 30% to 80%[24,33,34]. However, p53 mutation seems to be a late event in tumour development since no p53 accumulation was seen in areas of biliary dysplasia in a study of PSC patients[34]. It has been shown that loss of chromosome 9p21 and inactivation of the p16 tumour-suppressor gene are common events in PSC-associated cholangiocarcinoma[35]. In addition, a recent study by Tanai et al. investigated the presence of point mutations in the p16INK4a gene. It was shown that p16INK4a gene mutations were present only in PSC cholangiocytes and PSC-associated cholangiocarcinoma cells, and not in cholangiocytes from control liver specimens[36]. All these genetic alterations may contribute to improve the diagnostic yield for malignancy in PSC, especially when tumours are histologically highly differentiated and difficult to separate from changes mediated by the inflammatory process in PSC.

The association between PSC-associated HLA class II genes and the risk of cholangiocarcinoma has been evaluated but no significant increase in risk has been found[37], although a tendency that PSC patients with DR4, DQ8 haplotype were more prone to develop cholangiocarcinoma was found.

COMBINATION OF METHODS

Recent studies have investigated the effectiveness of combining different diagnostic methods for the detection of cholangiocarcinoma in PSC. In the study by

Siqueira et al. the combination of a positive brush cytology and increased levels of CA 19-9 or CEA was investigated[14]. Of the 333 patients included in the study a subset of patients with all three analyses available were separately analysed (PSC = 45, cholangiocarcinoma = 8). It was shown that the combination of an abnormal CEA or CA 19-9 had the highest sensitivity of 100%, and a specificity of 78.4%. The combination of positive brush cytology and/or an abnormal CA 19-9 had a sensitivity and specificity of, respectively, 87.5% and 97.3%. In a prospective study by Lindberg et al. 57 patients (20 with PSC) with biliary strictures were included, and evaluation of different diagnostic methods of malignancy in the biliary tract was investigated[15]. The diagnostic methods studied were brush cytology, the tumour markers CA 19-9 and CEA in serum and bile, DNA analysis by flow cytometry, and radiological evaluation of cholangiograms. All these methods were evaluated separately and in combination. It was shown that a combination of brush cytology, DNA analysis and serum tumour markers CA 19-9 and CEA had the best sensitivity and specificity of 88% and 80% respectively. In this study 20 patients had PSC, of whom seven had cholangiocarcinoma. In the subset of 20 PSC patients a combination of cytology, DNA analysis and CA 19-9 and CEA in serum showed a sensitivity and specificity for cholangiocarcinoma of 100% and 85%, respectively[15].

CONCLUSION

In conclusion, CEA and CA 19-9 in serum have a role as diagnostic tools in the revelation of cholangiocarcinoma in patients with PSC. Assessment of *K-ras* mutations in bile as an early marker for the detection of cholangiocarcinoma in PSC seems promising, but needs further evaluation. A combination of different diagnostic tumour markers and methods increases the diagnostic yield for cholangiocarcinoma in PSC.

Acknowledgements

Financial support from the Knut and Alice Wallenbergs Foundation is greatly appreciated.

References

1. Rosen C, Nagorney D, Wiesner R, Coffey R, LaRusso L. Cholangiocarcinoma complicating primary sclerosing cholangitis. Ann Surg. 1991;213:21–5.
2. Miros M, Kerlin P, Walker N, Harper J, Lynch S, Strong R. Predicting cholangiocarcinoma in patients with primary sclerosing cholangitis before transplantation. Gut. 1991;32:1369–73.
3. Nashan B, Schlitt H, Tusch G et al. Biliary malignancies in primary sclerosing cholangitis: timing for liver transplantation. Hepatology. 1996;23:1105–11.
4. Farley D, Weaver A, Nagourney D. 'Natural history' of unresected cholangiocarcinoma: patient outcome after noncurative resection. Mayo Clin Proc. 1995;70:425–9.
5. La Russo N, Wiesner R, Ludwig J. Sclerosing cholangitis. In: Oxford Textbook of Clinical Hepatology. Oxford: Oxford University Press, 1999;2:1121–30.
6. Bergquist A, Glaumann H, Persson B, Broomé U. Risk factors and clinical presentation of hepato-biliary carcinoma in patients with primary sclerosing cholangitis – a case control study. Hepatology. 1998;27:311–16.

7. Bergquist A, Ekbom A, Olsson R et al. Hepatic and extrahepatic malignancies in primary sclerosing cholangitis. J Hepatol. 2002;36:321–7.
8. Gold P, Freedman S. Specific carcinoembryonic antigens of the human digestive system. J Exp Med. 1965;122:467–81.
9. Pagnuzzi M, Onetto M, Marroni P. CA 19-9 and CA 50 in benign and malignant pancreatic and biliary disease. Cancer. 1988;61:2100–8.
10. Nilsson O, Johansson C, Glimelius B, Persson B, Nörgaard-Pedersen B, Andren-Sandberg Å. Sensitivity and specificity of CA 242 in gastrointestinal cancer. A comparison with CEA, CA 50 and CA 19-9. Br J Cancer. 1992;65:215–21.
11. Haga Y, Sakamoto K, Egami H, Yoshimura R, Mori K, Akagi M. Clinical significance of serum CA 125 values in patients with cancers in the digestive system. Am J Med Sci. 1986;292:30–4.
12. Ramage J, Donaghy A, Farrant J, Iorns R, Williams R. Serum tumor markers for the diagnosis of cholangiocarcinoma in primary sclerosing cholangitis. Gastroenterology. 1995;108:865–9.
13. Björnsson E, Kilander A, Olsson R. CA 19-9 and CEA are unreliable markers for cholangiocarcinoma in patients with primary sclerosing cholangitis. Liver. 1999;19:501–8.
14. Siqueira E, Schoen R, Silverman W et al. Detecting cholangiocarcinoma in patients with primary sclerosing cholangitis. Gastrointest Endosc. 2002;56:612.
15. Lindberg B, Arnelo U, Bergquist A et al. Diagnosis of biliary strictures in conjunction with endoscopic retrograde cholangiopancreaticography, with special reference to patients with primary sclerosing cholangitis. Endoscopy. 2002;34:1–8.
16. Hultcrantz R, Olsson R, Danielsson Å et al. A 3-year prospective study on serum tumor markers used for detecting cholangiocarcinoma in patients with primary sclerosing cholangitis. J Hepatol. 1999;30:669–73.
17. Carpelan-Holmström M, Louhimo J, Stenman U, Alfthan H, Haglund C. CEA, CA 19-9 and CA72-4 improve the diagnostic accuracy of gastrointestinal cancers. Anticancer Res. 2002;22:2311–16.
18. Chen C, Shiesh S, Tsao H, Lin X. The assessment of biliary CA 125, CA 19-9 and CEA in diagnosing cholangiocarcinoma – the influence of sampling time and hepatolithiasis. Hepatogastroenterology. 2002;49:616–20.
19. Chen C, Lin X, Tsao H, Shiesh S. The value of biliary fibronectin for diagnosis of cholangiocarcinoma. Hepatogastroenterology. 2003;50:924–7.
20. Körner T, Kropf J, Hackler R, Brenzel A, Gressner A. Fibronectin in human bile fluid for diagnosis of malignant biliary disease. Hepatology. 1996;23:423–8.
21. Caldas C, Hahn S, Hruban R, Redston M, Yoe C, Kern S. Detection of *K-ras* mutation in the stools of patients with pancreatic adenocarcinoma and pancreatic ductal hyperplasia. Cancer Res. 1994;54:3568–73.
22. Saurin J-C, Joly-Pharaboz M-O, Pernas P, Henry L, Ponchon T, Madjar J-J. Detection of Ki-ras gene point mutations in bile specimens for the differential diagnosis of malignant and benign biliary strictures. Gut. 2000;47:357–61.
23. Kubicka S, Kühnel F, Flemming B et al. *K-ras* mutations in the bile of patients with primary sclerosing cholangitis. Gut. 2001;48:403–8.
24. Boberg K, Schrumpf E, Bergquist A et al. Cholangiocarcinoma in primary sclerosing cholangitis: *K-ras* mutations and Tp53 dysfunction are implicated in the neoplastic development. J Hepatol. 2000;32:374–80.
25. Mansfield J, Griffin S, Wadehra V, Matthewson K. A prospective evaluation of cytology from biliary strictures. Gut. 1997;40:671–7.
26. Rabinovitz M, Zajko A, Hassanein T et al. Diagnostic value of brush cytology in the diagnosis of bile duct carcinoma: a study in 65 patients with bile duct strictures. Hepatology. 1990;12:747–52.
27. Ponsioen C, Vrouenraets S, vanMilligen de Wit A et al. Value of brush cytology for dominant strictures in primary sclerosing cholangitis. Endoscopy. 1999;31:305–9.
28. Bergquist A, Tribukait B, Glaumann H, Broomé U. Can DNA cytometry be used for evaluation of malignancy and premalignancy in bile duct strictures in primary sclerosing cholangitis? J Hepatol. 2000;33:873–7.
29. Sears R, Duckworth C, Decaestecker C et al. Image cytometry as a discriminatory tool for cytologic specimens obtained by endoscopic retrograde cholangiopancreatography. Cancer Cytopathol. 1998;84:119–26.
30. Rumalla A, Baron T, Leontovich O et al. Improved diagnostic yield of endoscopic biliary brush cytology by digital image analysis. Mayo Clin Proc. 2001;76:29–33.
31. Kang Y, Kim W, Lee H, Lee H, Kim Y. Mutation of p53 and *K-ras*, and loss of heterozygosity of APC in intrahepatic cholangiocarcinoma. Lab Invest. 1999;79:477–83.

32. Hidaka E, Yanagisawa A, Seki M, Takano K, Setoguchi T, Kato Y. High frequency of *K-ras* mutations in biliary duct carcinomas of cases with a long common channel in the papilla of Vater. Cancer Res. 2000;60:522–4.
33. Rizzi P, Ryder S, Portmann B, Ramage J, Naoumov N, Williams R. p53 Protein overexpression in cholangiocarcinoma arising in primary sclerosing cholangitis. Gut. 1996;38:265–8.
34. Bergquist A, Glaumann H, Stål P, Wang G, Broomé U. Biliary dysplasia, cell proliferation and nuclear DNA fragmentation in primary sclerosing cholangitis with and without cholangiocarcinoma. J Intern Med. 2001;249:69–75.
35. Ahrendt S, Eisenberger C, Yip L et al. Chromosome 9p21 loss and p16 inactivation in primary sclerosing cholangitis-associated cholangiocarcinoma. J Surg Res. 1999;84:88–93.
36. Tanai M, Higuchi H, Burgart L, Gores G. p16INK4a promoter mutations are frequent in primary sclerosing cholangitis (PSC) and PSC-associated cholangiocarcinoma. Gastroenterology. 2002;123:1090–8.
37. Boberg K, Spurkland A, Rocca G et al. The HLA-DR3,DQ2 heterozygous genotype is associated with an accelerated progression of primary sclerosing cholangitis. Scand J Gastroenterol. 2001;36:886–90.

37
Histology and brush cytology for diagnosis of bile duct carcinoma in primary sclerosing cholangitis

K. A. FLEMING

INTRODUCTION

Cholangiocarcinoma (CC) in primary sclerosing cholangitis (PSC) is the most feared complication of this disease. It is associated with rapid progression and death, usually within 12 months of diagnosis[1]. This poor prognosis arises partly, at least, from the difficulty in diagnosis. There are several reasons for this diagnostic difficulty, which will be discussed in greater detail below, but the main problem is that of differentiating between a benign dominant structure in the extrahepatic ducts and a malignancy.

Before discussing the diagnostic problem further, it is worth briefly highlighting three points regarding the association of CC with and without PSC. The first is the difference in age at presentation. Thus, CC occurring in the absence of PSC has an age at presentation around 70[2], whereas the majority of patients with CC in PSC are in their mid-40s[1]. This presumably reflects the early age of onset of PSC and the fact that PSC is clearly a high-risk factor for CC. Indeed, the lifetime risk is 10–20% (1.5% per year)[1]. The second point is the difference in location of the tumours (Table 1). In CC with PSC, nearly half the tumours arise in the intrahepatic ducts (Figure 1A) while tumours solely of the extrahepatic ducts

Table 1 Cholangiocarcinoma in PSC (percentages)

	PSC	Non-PSC
Extrahepatic bile ducts	10	70–75
Extra/intra	35	
Intrahepatic bile ducts	45	25–30
Lifetime risk	10–20 (1.5 per year)	

354

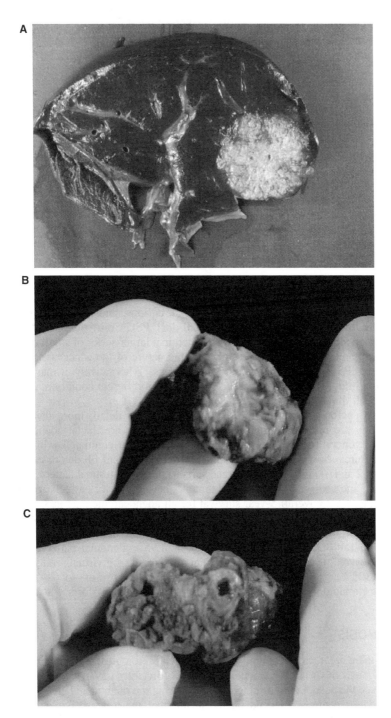

Figure 1 **A**: An example of an intrahepatic cholangiocarcinoma. **B,C**: Cross-section of the extra-hepatic bile duct showing irregularity of the lumen and infiltration of the wall by cholangiocarcinoma

Table 2 Cholangiocarcinoma in PSC: pathology

Adenocarcinoma (95%) (8% 5-year survival)
Mucous, intestinal, clear cell, signet-ring
Papillary (22% 5-year survival)
Squamous
Undifferentiated

Table 3 Cholangiocarcinoma in PSC: pathology grade: percentage of glandular differentiation

> 95%	25% 5-year survival
40–94%	
6–39%	
< 5%	5% 5-year survival

are uncommon (10%) (Figures 1B,C). In contrast, in CC without PSC only 25–30% of tumours arise in the intrahepatic ducts and 70–75% arise in the extrahepatic bile ducts[2]. Thirdly, there is the curious, and recently recognized, apparent low or absent risk of CC in 'small-duct' PSC[3]. Why this should be so is completely obscure, but clearly, if confirmed in a larger series of small-duct PSC cases, this may provide some insight into the nature of the cancer risk in 'conventional' PSC and into the carcinogenic process. Alternatively, it may indicate that small-duct PSC is not a variant of PSC, but a different condition, although, to date, all the data suggest that this is not the case.

Lastly, before discussing the diagnostic issues in detail, more data on the pathology are relevant. Virtually all (> 95%) of CC are ductal adenocarcinomata. In general the tumours are well to moderately differentiated, with glandular structures showing mucus secretion and with abundant fibrous tissue stroma (Figures 2 and 3) (Table 2). Occasional variants have an intestinal pattern of differentiation and less well-differentiated tumours have either a clear-cell or a signet-ring pattern. The overall 5-year survival for all adenocarcinomata is 8%, but the uncommon papillary variant has a 5-year survival of 22%[2]. Similarly, as might be expected, the better differentiated the tumour is, the better the progress is. As shown in Table 3, if the tumour has more than 95% glandular pattern, then the 5-year survival is considerably better than tumours having virtually no glandular pattern (25% vs 6%). The recently recognized alternative form of CC – the intrahepatic cholangiocellular carcinoma[4] – probably does not occur in PSC.

DIAGNOSIS

While there are a variety of clinical, biochemical, serological and imaging criteria for diagnosis of CC in PSC, none of these is sufficiently sensitive and/or specific to replace the need for tissue diagnosis[5]. However, the method and ease of obtaining a tissue diagnosis depend on the location of the tumour. For intrahepatic masses tissue diagnosis is relatively straightforward with a needle biopsy, usually guided by ultrasound, normally being sufficient to obtain appropriate material to

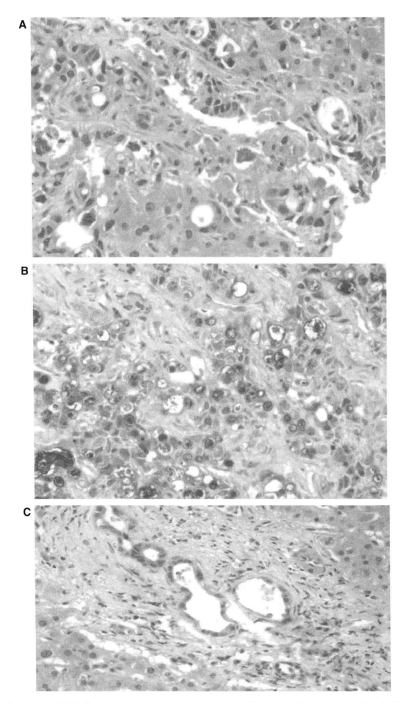

Figure 2 **A,B**: Infiltration of hepatocytes by a poorly differentiated, mucus-secreting (H&E and DPAS) cholangiocarcinoma **C**: A portal tract with dilated, abnormal bile ducts. This may represent infiltrating cholangiocarcinoma or dysplastic interlobular bile ducts (H&E)

allow a diagnosis (Figure 2). The only potential diagnostic difficulty is to differentiate between a primary intrahepatic CC and a secondary mucus-secreting adenocarcinoma, perhaps originating from the gut, ovary, etc. Immunochemistry (for example for cytokeratin 7 and 20) usually resolves this, if there is any doubt.

A much more difficult problem is the diagnosis of an extrahepatic mass. This is the area which gives the diagnosis of CC in PSC its reputation as a diagnostic problem, which then contributes to the poor prognosis. Essentially the crucial differential diagnosis is between a benign, dominant stricture and a malignancy.

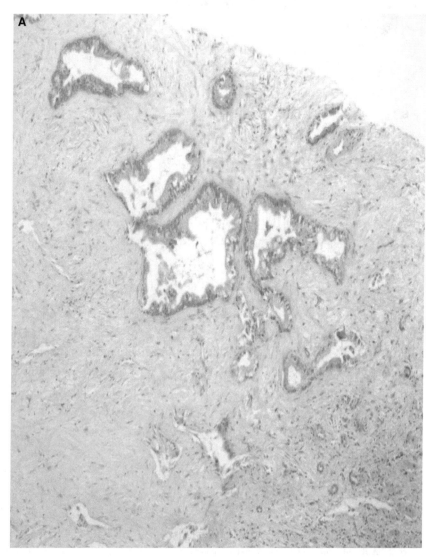

Figure 3 Low- and high-power views of an extrahepatic cholangiocarcinoma showing extensive infiltration, abundant fibrous tissue stroma, and loss of surface epithelium

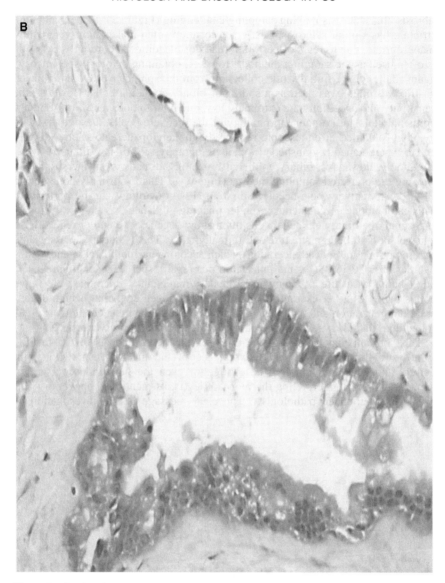

Figure 3 *Continued*

As mentioned above, other diagnostic tests and investigations are insufficiently sensitive or specific to resolve this fundamental problem. However, even tissue diagnosis is difficult. There are three reasons why this is so.

First, sampling is often inadequate[5]. CC of extrahepatic ducts tends to grow submucosally and not in an exophytic manner, diminishing access to tumour cells (Figures 1B,C). In addition, the tumour often has extensive associated fibrosis, this sclerosis making sampling challenging (Figure 3); indeed, a benign stricture has similar sclerosis. Lastly, the location often makes biopsy sampling inappropriate, due to fears of perforation and/or bleeding. Accordingly, cytology is often used as the sampling method. However, obtaining cytology specimens is again challenging[6]. Initially bile collection from the sphincter of Oddi (and even gastric washings) was used as a source of biliary epithelial cells. However, the sensitivity and specificity are extremely low, due both to poor recovery of biliary epithelial cells and to poor morphology of the recovered cells. Despite this, bile cytology obtained at endoscopic retrograde cholangiopancreatography (ERCP) and by percutaneous transhepatic cholangiography (PCT) is still used. Most commonly, nowadays, biliary epithelial brushings, directly from the suspicious site, are the preferred sampling method (Figure 4). This is normally done during ERCP. Alternatively, fine-needle aspiration (FNA) cytology can be performed. This can be done percutaneously (under imaging guidance).

Second, the biliary epithelial cells often show degenerative and/or regenerative changes in both benign stricture and in malignancy. This is due to the associated inflammation (and indeed ulceration) which accompanies both benign and malignant lesions. CC in PSC is not unusual in this regard, such degeneration/regeneration being a feature of many inflammatory/malignancy dilemmas, ulcerative colitis being a further example. Differentiating between epithelial benign degeneration/regeneration and malignant dysplasia is one of the most challenging areas for cellular pathology, and is subject to considerable inter-observer error[7].

This difficulty contributes to the third reason why diagnosis of CC in PSC is not straightforward, namely inexperience of the medical team. Obtaining correct and adequate sampling is testing, for even the best endoscopists and hepatologists, and interpreting the morphology is, as mentioned above, difficult even for experienced pathologists. The clear message is that investigation of

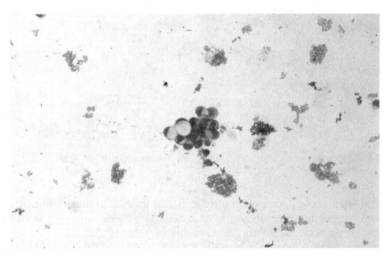

Figure 4 A cytology preparation of a cholangiocarcinoma showing a clump of malignant, signet-ring cells

patients with a differential diagnosis of benign and malignant stricture in PSC should be performed at centres with considerable experience and sufficient workload to maintain that experience.

A variety of methods have been adopted to increase the success rate of tissue sampling[6], including the use of guidewires to obtain samples more accurately and obtaining multiple samples. Greater cytological accuracy can be obtained by rapid processing (with or without storage at 4°C) to decrease degeneration and use of 'block' samples, where all the material present in the sample is centrifuged and the pellet processed and embedded as a tissue biopsy. Recently, a variety of methods have been tried, aimed at the differentiation of benign from malignant cells by analysing the genetic composition. These include image analysis, with measurement of DNA ploidy, and detection of mutant P53, P16, K-ras, c-erB-2, and other oncogenes (by either immunohistochemistry, polymerase chain reaction or *in-situ* hybridization). However, to date none of these methods has demonstrated a superior success rate to conventional morphology, although further trials are awaited[5].

As shown in Table 4, the range of sensitivity of the various cytological methods is exceedingly wide, and although high sensitivities are reported, a sensitivity of around 50% (40–70%) is the normal experience in day-to-day practice[5]. However, as also shown in Table 4, the positive predictive value is high, indicating that if a sample is reported as malignant, it is almost certain to be malignant. The problem is of false negatives when sampling error prevents an accurate diagnosis of malignancy being made.

A key factor, therefore, in investigating a dominant stricture in the extrahepatic biliary system in PSC is correlating all the evidence, including clinical, biochemical, imaging and pathological. This is absolutely necessary since none of the techniques is sufficiently reliable in itself, but the combination of all the factors can lead to a diagnosis. Sometimes, however, it is necessary to wait and repeat the investigations because of the absence of definitive evidence.

An exception to the poor prognosis of CC in PSC is when the tumour is found as an incidental finding at transplantation. If the tumour is less than 1 cm in diameter the evidence is that this has no effect on the success of the transplant – in other words, the surgery is curative[8]. This being so, this suggests that, if one could diagnose CC at this size, then it is possible to cure this otherwise almost universally fatal tumour.

How can this be done, as to date none of the investigative techniques is capable of this? Recent experience from two PSC cases in our own practice suggests one possible approach. In both of these cases the patients presented with deep-vein thrombosis. In one case the investigation revealed a CC in the extrahepatic bile ducts, but importantly a liver biopsy showed dysplasia of the biliary

Table 4 Cholangiocarcinoma in PSC: cytology

Bile	Sensitivity	20–73%
Brushings	Sensitivity	18–82%
Fine-needle aspiration	Sensitivity	40–91%

Positive predictive value 92–100%.

epithelium of the interlobular bile ducts[9]. In the second case the patient, who had long-standing PSC, underwent a liver biopsy, which again showed dysplasia of the intrahepatic biliary epithelium. Extensive investigation failed to reveal a tumour, but 18 months later the patient presented with a CC.

The above suggests that intrahepatic dysplasia exists, and that detection on needle biopsy may be associated with the presence of CC elsewhere in the biliary tract, or that there is a high risk of such a tumour developing in the near future. If this is indeed the case, then two consequences follow. First, discovery of intrahepatic biliary dysplasia should initiate extensive investigation for CC. If a tumour is found, decision regarding surgery or other therapy can then be made on the usual criteria. If no tumour is found, there then arises the issue of whether preventative (or 'curative') transplantation should be performed. This latter approach would clearly be extremely controversial, since liver transplantation is a very major operation, with considerable risk and costs, with shortages of donors, etc. Conversely, and setting aside the very considerable costs and other factors associated with management of patients who develop CC, patients would be cured who would otherwise die. Even if the detection of intrahepatic biliary dysplasia is relatively uncommon, clearly this approach would still be of value.

For such an approach to be worth considering, three things (at least) are necessary. First, it needs to be shown that intrahepatic biliary dysplasia does exist in PSC. In this context there are other occasional case reports in the literature documenting that intrahepatic biliary dysplasia can both predate and coexist with CC[10,11]. Furthermore, a series of cases of PSC from the Mayo Clinic[12] found dysplasia of biliary epithelium in one out of 60 cases. As the incidence is about 1.5% per year this may not be an unexpected frequency. Second, it needs to be shown that this dysplasia can be recognized reliably and reproducibly. Third, it would have to be clearly demonstrated that such dysplasia is indeed a marker of high risk for CC.

As an initial approach to this, in conjunction with pathologists from Sweden and Norway, we investigated retrospectively 26 cases of PSC with coexisting or subsequent CC for presence of interlobular bile duct dysplasia on needle biopsy of the liver[13]. In comparison, 60 cases without CC were also analysed. The pathologists were blinded to the outcome. The objectives were to see if dysplasia was present, whether it could be recognized reliably and whether it was present more frequently in the CC cases, compared to the non-tumour cases. The results are presented in Table 5. This study showed that about 20% of the biopsies from patients with coexisting or subsequent CC had dysplasia compared to none of the non-tumorous biopsies, a highly statistically significant difference. The kappa values (a measure of inter-observer reproducibility) were adequate for the presence of dysplasia, supporting the idea that it is possible to recognize the

Table 5 Interlobular bile duct dysplasia in cholangiocarcinoma (26 cases)

Normal/degenerative/regenerative: 7/26 (27%), kappa 0.4
Indeterminate: 1/26 (4%), kappa 0.2
Dysplasia: 5/26 (19%), kappa 0.4

Absent in 60 cases without cholangiocarcinoma.

lesion reasonably reliably. Accordingly, the results support the hypothesis that bile duct dysplasia exists, can be recognized and is associated with CC. Clearly this was a small, retrospective study and there is a need for further investigations of larger numbers. However, the data are encouraging.

SUMMARY

CC in PSC can be extremely difficult to diagnose, especially extrahepatic tumours. Tissue diagnosis can be problematic because of difficulties in differentiating malignancy from regenerative/degenerative changes and in avoiding false negatives due to sampling error. Because of these problems the need for considerable experience in the team dealing with the patient is paramount, and the results of all diagnostic methods should be correlated, without reliance on one method alone. Interlobular bile duct dysplasia in liver biopsy in PSC should always be looked for and, if detected, investigation for possible CC should be undertaken. Discovery of a tumour less than 1 cm in diameter would warrant transplantation as a curative operation, while absence of a tumour should warrant close follow-up. Indeed, transplantation may be considered, even in the absence of a demonstrable tumour, although further investigations into the significance of intrahepatic dysplasia are needed before this course of management can be unequivocally recommended.

References

1. Berquist A et al. Hepatic and extra-hepatic malignancies in primary sclerosing cholangitis. J Hepatol. 2002;36:321–7.
2. Henson DE, Albores-Saavedra J, Corle D. Carcinoma of the extra-hepatic bile ducts. Cancer. 1992;70:1498–501.
3. Bjornsson E, Boberg KM, Cullen S et al. Patients with small duct primary sclerosing cholangitis have a favourable long-term prognosis. Gut. 2002;51:731–5.
4. Gores GJ. Cholangiocarcinoma: current concepts and insights. Hepatology. 2003;37:961–9.
5. Khan SA et al. Guidelines for the diagnosis and treatment of cholangiocarcinoma: consensus document. Gut. 2002;51(Suppl. 6):vi1–9.
6. Sterrett, Frost Whitaker. Gall bladder and extra-hepatic ducts. In: Gray, McKee, editors. Diagnostic Cytopathology. London: Elsevier, 2003:413–26.
7. Creagh T, Bridger JE, Kupek E, Fish DE, Martin-Bates E, Wilkins MJ. Pathologist variation in reporting cervical borderline epithelial abnormalities and cervical intraepithelial neoplasia. J Clin Pathol. 1995;48:59–60.
8. Goss JA, Shackleton CR, Farmer DG et al. Orthotopic liver transplantation for primary sclerosing cholangitis. A 12-year single center experience. Ann Surg. 1997;225:472–81.
9. Martins EBG, Fleming KA, Garrido MC, Hine KR, Chapman RW. Superficial thrombophlebitis, dysplasia, and cholangiocarcinoma in primary sclerosing cholangitis. Gastroenterology. 1994;107:537–42.
10. Davis RI, Sloan JM, Hood JM, Maxwell P. Carcinoma of the extra-hepatic biliary tree: a clinico-pathological and immunohistochemical study. Histopathology. 1988;12:623–31.
11. Jin SY et al. Microsatellite instability is absent in liver and biliary mucosa of patients with primary sclerosing cholangitis. Dig Dis Sci. 1999;44:595–601.
12. Ludwig J, Wahlstrom HE, Batts KP, Wiesner RH. Papillary bile duct dysplasia in primary sclerosing cholangitis. Gastroenterology. 1992;102:2134–8.
13. Fleming KA, Boberg KM, Glaumann H, Bergquist A, Smith D, Clausen OP. Biliary dysplasia as a marker of cholangiocarcinoma in primary sclerosing cholangitis. J Hepatol. 2001;34;360–5.

38
Primary sclerosing cholangitis: indications for and recurrence after transplantation

O. YE and J. NEUBERGER

INTRODUCTION

Medical management of primary sclerosing cholangitis (PSC) has been disappointing. Immunosuppressive drugs, copper-chelating agents, and antibiotics do not appear to alter progression of the disease. Treatment with ursodeoxycholic acid may slow progression of disease. The judicious use of dilation of strictures can palliate jaundice and may improve survival, but liver transplantation remains the definitive treatment.

INDICATIONS FOR LIVER TRANSPLANTATION

The indications for liver transplantation for patients with PSC are similar to those for patients with other chronic liver diseases: namely a quality of life that, because of the liver disease, is unacceptable to the patient, or end-stage disease. The indications and contraindications are listed in Tables 1 and 2. As with other indications for liver transplantation, increasing serum bilirubin, falling serum albumin, onset of encephalopathy or spontaneous bacterial peritonitis are useful markers of deteriorating liver function. For those with symptomatic but not end-stage disease, features such as progressive osteopenia, intractable pruritus or overwhelming lethargy, clinically significant encephalopathy or progressive hepato-pulmonary syndrome may be good indications for transplantation.

TIMING OF LIVER TRANSPLANTATION IN PSC

Although PSC is a progressive disease its course is associated with fluctuations; thus timing of transplantation is difficult. The optimal timing of transplantation

Table 1   Indications for liver transplantation in PSC

1. Decompensated end-stage chronic liver disease
   Intractable encephalopathy
   Spontaneous bacterial peritonitis
   Recurrent variceal haemorrhage
   Intractable bone disease
   Child–Turcotte–Pugh grade C
   Mayo model score > 4

2. Poor and unacceptable quality of life
   Intractable pruritus
   Severe fatigue and tiredness
   Lethargy

3. Progressive extrahepatic complications
   Hepatopulmonary syndrome
   Osteopenia
   Pulmonary hypertension
   Recurrent bacterial cholangitis

Table 2   Absolute and relative contraindications to liver transplantation

Absolute contraindications
AIDS
Extrahepatic malignancy*
Advanced cardiopulmonary disease
Cholangiocarcinoma†

Relative contraindications
HIV positivity
Age above 70 years
Significant sepsis outside the extrahepatic biliary tree
HBV DNA positivity‡
Active alcohol/substance misuse
Severe psychiatric disorder
Portal venous system thrombosis§
Pulmonary hypertension§

* Haemangioendothelioma and neuroendocrine malignancy are an
exception in some centres.
† Relative contraindication in some centres in conjunction with
experimental approaches.
‡ Most patients can be treated with antiviral therapy.
§ Require assessment at a transplant centre.

is determined by assessing the probability of survival/dying from the disease and the probability of survival/dying after liver transplantation. A Mayo model score of 5 or Child grade C score justify referral for transplantation[1].

Use of prognostic models

Several prognostic models have been developed to help the clinician estimate the chances of survival in patients with PSC; of these age and serum bilirubin are the more important factors. Those factors associated with survival can be incorporated into a prognostic model, and probabilities of survival developed. While such an approach is helpful in that a quantifiable figure is given, confidence intervals are wide so extrapolation to the individual must be done with caution. Most models generated are static models; that is to say that the probability of survival is based on data generated at a set time (usually at referral to a tertiary liver unit) and do not take into account factors such as variceal bleeding which may herald a more rapid progression. Furthermore, the advent of newer techniques which result in improved survival, such as biliary dilation or stenting, may alter the natural history.

Prognosis without transplantation

The Mayo Clinic studied the prognostic factors and survival in 174 patients over a mean follow-up of 6 years. Multivariate analysis (Cox proportional hazards regression modelling) revealed that age, serum bilirubin concentration, blood haemoglobin concentration, presence or absence of inflammatory bowel disease and histological stage on liver biopsy were independent predictors of high risk of dying. This survival model helps in identifying individual PSC patients at low, moderate and high risk of dying[3]. The group then[4] created a survival model based on 405 patients with PSC from five clinical centres using Cox proportional hazards analysis. Based on multivariate analysis of 405 patients a risk score was defined by the following formula:

$$R = 0.03 \text{ (age [years])}$$
$$+ 0.54 \log_e \text{ (bilirubin [mg/dl])}$$
$$+ 0.54 \log_e \text{ (aspartate aminotransferase [U/L])}$$
$$+ 1.24 \text{ (variceal bleeding [0/1])}$$
$$- 0.84 \text{ (albumin [g/dl])}.$$

The risk score was used to obtain survival estimates for up to 4 years.

Other units have established different models: the King's College Hospital Liver Unit analysed 126 patients with PSC to identify prognostic variables and found that on multivariate analysis independent prognostic factors were hepatomegaly, splenomegaly, serum alkaline phosphatase, histological stage, and age[5]. A study from Sweden described the natural outcome of PSC patients in a total of 305 patients followed over a median period of 63 months. The prognostic significance of clinical, biochemical, and histological findings at the time of diagnosis was evaluated using multivariate analysis. The estimated median survival from time of diagnosis to death or liver transplantation was 12 years. Cholangiocarcinoma was found in 8% of the patients and 44% of the patients were asymptomatic at the time of diagnosis. Age, serum bilirubin concentration, and histological stage at the time of diagnosis were independent predictors of a poor prognosis[6].

The Italian PSC Study Group carried out a retrospective multicentre study of unselected patients with PSC in 16 Italian university and regional hospitals to find prognostic variables. A total of 117 PSC patients were studied. At presentation 70% of patients were symptomatic; symptoms did not relate to liver histology. Both intrahepatic and extrahepatic bile duct lesions were detected in 46% of patients at cholangiography. Inflammatory bowel disease was found in 54% of symptomatic patients, ulcerative colitis was found in 36%. Survival at 10 years

Table 3 Univariate Cox proportional hazards models (all patients) (adapted from ref. 8)

Variables	No. of patients	p-Value	Risk ratio	95% confidence interval
Child–Pugh criteria				
Child–Pugh classification				
A	207	–	–	–
B		<0.001	3.6	1.8–7.1
C		<0.001	16.1	6.5–39.9
Encephalopathy (yes vs no)	207	<0.001	15.1	3.9–58.4
Ascites				
None	207	<0.001	–	–
Easily controlled			3.7	2.2–6.5
Poorly controlled			14.1	4.7–42.1
Bilirubin (mg/ml)	207	<0.001		
<2			–	–
2–3			2.0	1.4–2.8
>3			3.9	2.0–7.8
Albumin (g/dl)	207	<0.001		
>3.5			–	–
2.8–3.5			3.4	2.4–5.0
<2.8			11.8	5.6–25.1
Prothrombin time (s prolonged)	207	0.22		
1–4			–	–
4–6			1.9	0.7–5.4
>6			3.7	0.5–29.2
DSM criteria				
Mayo risk score (per 1 unit increase)	139	<0.001	1.9	1.4–2.6
Age (per 10-year increase)	207	<0.001	1.8	1.4–2.3
Splenomegaly (yes vs no)	207	0.53	1.3	0.6–3.2
Bilirubin (per 1 mg% increase)	206	<0.001	1.13	1.1–1.2
Histological stage	140	0.13		
1 or 2			–	–
3			1.2	0.9–1.6
4			1.9	0.8–4.4

was 74%. Features of poor prognosis were cholesterol, aspartate aminotransferase (AST), haemoglobin, and albumin[7].

The Cleveland Clinic explored the value of the Child–Turcotte–Pugh classification (CTP) in the prediction of survival and compared it with a disease-specific model (DSM) (Table 3). A total of 208 PSC patients were studied over a mean follow-up of 70 months. Prognostic variables were measured from the first visit. Kaplan–Meier 7-year survivals for CTP A, B, and C were 90%, 68%, and 25%, respectively. The Cox model identified CTP score and age as the most significant predictors of mortality. Adding the DSM risk score did not significantly improve the fit of the model. It was concluded that CTP is a powerful predictor of survival in PSC; DSM does not enhance the predictive ability of CTP[8].

A time-dependent Cox regression model has the potential to estimate a more precise short-term prognosis in PSC compared with the traditional time-fixed models. In one study consecutive clinical and laboratory follow-up data from the time of diagnosis were collected from the files of 330 PSC patients from five

European centres, followed for a median of 8.4 years. Time-fixed and time-dependent Cox regression analyses, as well as the additive regression model, were applied. Bilirubin, albumin, and age at diagnosis of PSC were identified as independent prognostic factors in multivariate analysis of both the time-fixed and the time-dependent Cox regression models. The importance of bilirubin was more pronounced in the time-dependent model than in the time-fixed analysis. The additive regression model indicated that, once patients survive beyond the first 5 years, the impact on prognosis of albumin at diagnosis ceases. The time-dependent prognostic model was superior to the time-fixed variant in assigning low 1-year survival probabilities to patients who actually survived less than 1 year[9].

Models predicting survival after transplantation

A study from our own unit identified pre-transplant variables associated with survival after transplantation and devised a Cox regression model for prediction of post-transplant survival based on 118 patients transplanted for PSC followed for up to 9 years after the procedure (Table 4). Univariate analyses showed the

Table 4 Pre-transplant variables associated with prognosis after transplantation in 118 transplanted patients with PSC (from ref. 2)

Variable	Direction of association*	p-Value	
		Total observation period	First year
Age (years)	—	0.72	0.94
Males (%)	—	0.97	0.72
Year of transplantation	↓	0.11	0.051
Malignancy (%)	↑	0.0007	0.0002
Ulcerative colitis (%)	↓	0.06	0.004
Crohn's disease (%)	↑	0.005	0.003
Previous upper abdominal surgery (%)	↑	0.01	0.02
Encephalopathy (%)	↑	0.06	0.007
Variceal haemorrhage (%)	↑	0.32	0.18
Ascites (%)	↑	0.006	0.005
Diuretic treatment (%)	—	0.49	0.55
Plasma albumin (g/L)	↓	0.06	0.40
Plasma prothrombin (INR)	↑	0.17	0.06
Plasma bilirubin (μmol/L)	↑	0.02	0.02
Plasma aspartate transaminase (U/L)	—	0.88	0.71
Plasma alkaline phosphatase (U/L)	—	0.51	0.22
Plasma creatinine (μmol/L)	↑	0.02	0.04
Blood group A gene (%)	—	0.30	0.47
Blood group B gene (%)	—	0.07	0.21
Rhesus blood group gene (%)	—	0.20	0.26

Results of univariate analysis using logrank test.
INR, International Normalized Ratio.
*Presence of the characteristic (qualitative variables) or of higher values of the variables (quantitative variables) are associated with a higher risk (↑) (poor prognosis), a lower risk (↓), or not associated with the prognosis (—).

Table 5 Final Cox regression model for pre-transplant prediction of short-term survival (up to 1 year) after transplantation for PSC (from ref. 2)

Variables (p-value)	Scoring	b	SE(b)
Inflammatory bowel disease (0.00004)	No: 0 Ulcerative colitis: 1 Crohn's disease: 4	0.534	0.130
Previous upper abdominal surgery (0.002)	Yes: 1 No: 0	1.393	0.455
Ascites (0.002)	Present: 1 Absent: 0	1.431	0.453
Serum creatinine (0.02)	< 100 μmol/L: 0 = 100 μmol/L: 1	1.111	0.479
Malignancy (0.03)	Present: 1 Absent: 0	1.191	0.547

following variables to be associated with a decreased post-transplant survival: high serum creatinine, high serum bilirubin, biliary tree malignancy, previous upper abdominal surgery, hepatic encephalopathy, ascites, and Crohn's disease. The final multiple Cox regression model included only inflammatory bowel disease (Crohn's disease associated with an increased risk and ulcerative colitis with a decreased risk), ascites, previous upper abdominal surgery, serum creatinine, and biliary tree malignancy (Table 5). The model was validated in a separate group of patients transplanted in Leeds.

These findings can help selection and timing of transplantation. The developed prognostic model for transplantation can be used in parallel with previously published prognostic models for non-transplantation[2].

CHOLANGIOCARCINOMA AND PSC

Cholangiocarcinoma (CC) is a malignant neoplasm deriving from intrahepatic or extrahepatic bile ducts. It affects both sexes, and is most prevalent at the age 50–70 years. CC develop in up to 30% of patients with PSC by 15 years. Diagnosis of CC before transplantation usually contraindicates transplantation, as the post-transplant survival is greatly reduced.

Diagnosis of CC

The diagnosis of CC is often very difficult; several centres have evaluated serological, histological, and imaging techniques to diagnose the condition.

A study from Norway[10] assessed predisposing factors for CC in 394 PSC patients from five European countries. The cohort included 12% of patients with CC. CC was diagnosed within the first year after diagnosis of PSC in 50% and in 27% of the patients at intended liver transplantation. Jaundice, pruritus, abdominal pain, and fatigue were significantly more frequent at diagnosis of PSC in the group who developed CC. The duration of inflammatory bowel disease before diagnosis of PSC was significantly longer in patients who developed CC than in the remaining group. Nashan and his group applied the Mayo survival model to assess optimal timing for transplantation in patients with PSC in 48 patients receiving transplants between 1972 and 1994 (Tables 6 and 7). Of these patients, 10 had a biliary malignancy, which was incidental in nine. According to the Mayo model, low-, moderate-, and high-risk groups of patients could be formed. The actuarial patient survivals at 1 and 7 years were 100% and 100% (low risk), 68.6% and 68.6% (moderate risk), and 54.6% and 46.8% (high risk), respectively. Patients with a biliary malignancy had a 30% survival at 1 year and none survived at 6 years. Analysis of the Mayo model risk scores demonstrated a marked increase in the incidence of biliary malignancies in those with a score above 4.4 and all patients with tumours were found to have a score above 4. Moreover, the prevalence rate rose from 14.3% in the low-risk group to 33.3% in the moderate-risk group. Regular scoring of patients with the Mayo model risk score is suggested, and transplantation should be taken into consideration at scores above 4[11].

The onset of CC is usually insidious, and it is usually difficult to distinguish whether the progression of disease merely reflects end-stage liver failure or malignant development.

In one multicentre case–control study carried out in USA, to determine the risk factors and possible predictors for CC in patients with PSC, the demographic, clinical, and laboratory features of 26 PSC patients with CC diagnosed over a 7-year period at eight academic centres were compared with 87 patients with PSC but no CC (the control group). There was no statistically significant difference in demographics, smoking, signs or symptoms or complications of PSC, indices of disease severity (Mayo risk score or Child–Pugh score), frequency

Table 6 Values for Mayo model variables in 48 patients with PSC classified in risks groups (from ref. 11)

Variables	Low risk (n = 15)	Moderate risk (n = 15)	High risk (n = 26)
Age (years)	32.7 ± 6.2	35.9 ± 11.8	39.4 ± 10.3
Bilirubin (mg/dl)	4.2 ± 6.7	13.2 ± 8.7	22.9 ± 14.3
Splenomegaly	4 (57%)	11 (73%)	26 (100%)
Histological stage	3.6 ± 0.8	3.7 ± 0.5	3.9 ± 0.3
1 and 2	1 (14%)	0	0
3	1 (14%)	4 (27%)	2 (8%)
4	5 (72%)	11 (73%)	24 (92%)
Risk score	3.7 ± 1.0	4.9 ± 0.2	5.8 ± 0.3

Table 7 Distribution and prevalence rate of biliary malignancies in patients with PSC according to risk groups (from ref. 11)

Risk group	Risk score	PSC (n = 38)	PSC + carcinoma (n = 10)	Prevalence rate (%)
Low	= 4.4	6	1	14.3
Moderate	4.4–< 5.3	10	5	33.3
High	> 5.3	22	4	15.4

or duration or complications of inflammatory bowel disease (IBD), frequency of biliary surgery, or therapeutic endoscopy between the two groups. Alcohol consumption was significantly associated with CC in patients with PSC. Serum carbohydrate antigen 19-9 (CA 19-9) was significantly higher in patients with CC than those without. A serum CA 19-9 level greater than 100 U/ml had 75% sensitivity and 80% specificity in identifying PSC patients with CC. Alcohol consumption was a risk factor for having CC in PSC patients. The indices of severity of liver disease were not associated with CC in patients with PSC. Serum CA 19-9 appeared to have good ability to discriminate PSC patients with and without CC[12].

These tumours may be difficult to visualize radiologically (using either ultrasound, CT, MRI, or PET scanning). Recently, FDG positron emission tomography has been suggested to be a sensitive technique in identifying small bile duct cancers. PET scanning can assess metabolism *in vivo*. The glucose analogue [18F]fluoro-2-deoxy-D-glucose (FDG) accumulates in malignant tumours because of high glucose metabolism. PET scanning of the liver was performed after intravenous FDG and hot spots of radioactivity were seen in patients with PSC who had CC.

Bile cytology, brushings at ERCP or direct tumour aspiration may be specific, but are not very sensitive; furthermore, ERCP and biopsy are not without risk to the patient.

Molecular markers of cholangiocarcinogenesis, such as K-ras mutations, may improve the early diagnosis of CC or the timing of liver transplantation. Kubicka analysed K-ras mutations by enriched polymerase chain reaction/restriction fragment length polymorphism in the bile fluid of 56 PSC patients and 20 patients with other cholestatic diseases. To assess the value of K-ras mutations as a risk factor for cholangiocarcinogenesis, patients were prospectively investigated over a mean period of 31.5 months. The result showed that 30% of patients with PSC revealed K-ras mutations in bile fluid. In contrast with the group of PSC patients without K-ras mutations, four instances of CC and two of dysplasia were diagnosed in the group of patients with K-ras mutations during the follow-up investigation, indicating that K-ras mutations in bile fluid of PSC patients represent frequent early events during cholangiocarcinogenesis. However, most of the PSC patients with K-ras mutations remained tumour-free after a long follow-up investigation, which is in agreement with the fact that these mutations are not specific for malignancy but may also occur in normal bile duct mucosa or in dysplasias. Therefore, analysis of K-ras mutations in bile should not be used for diagnosis of CC in PSC patients. However K-ras mutations in bile fluid of PSC patients have to be considered as risk factors for the development of CC, which may have implications for the timing of liver transplantation[13].

Identification of biliary dysplasia in a PSC liver biopsy may indicate developing CC. The strong association of biliary dysplasia with CC in PSC suggests use of dysplasia as a marker for current or developing malignancy. Some reports have suggested that biliary epithelial dysplasia on liver biopsy, even away from the site of the CC, is helpful, but these remain to be substantiated[14].

While all these markers may be associated with CC, it remains too early, in the view of the authors, to use such procedures for routine assessment or for timing of transplantation.

CC AND OUTCOME AFTER TRANSPLANTATION

CC remains a major risk facing the PSC patient, and develops in 15–30% of patients. To date the outcome following liver transplantation in PSC patients who have associated CC as a presenting feature has been poor. However, those patients who are found to have an incidental CC have an acceptable low incidence of recurrence of disease[15]. The results of liver transplantation for patients with clinically apparent CC are extremely poor; however, in patients in whom a microscopic tumour is detected in the explanted liver, survival is similar to those transplanted with PSC without CC[16].

For a small group of patients presenting with unresectable carcinoma above the cystic duct without intrahepatic or extrahepatic metastases, orthotopic liver transplantation, combined with preoperative irradiation and chemotherapy, may be available, and demonstrates improved survival on the basis of a recent study conducted at the Mayo Clinic. In the future, chemopreventive strategies aimed at blocking the links between inflammation (e.g. nitric oxide synthase and cyclooxygenase-2 inhibitors) and carcinogenesis may help prevent this often fatal disease[17].

Despite the overall advances in the ability to diagnose CC, some patients present with peri-hilar CC, and the prognosis for patients with this malignancy remains poor. Further improvements in the survival of patients with perihilar CC may come with the early diagnosis of these lesions. Complete surgical resection remains the only curative treatment for malignancies of the biliary tract. Aggressive surgical approaches are likely to continue, and the challenge remains to perform these procedures safely in jaundiced and sometimes septic patients. For those patients with unresectable lesions the optimal form of palliation, whether operative or non-operative, remains to be defined. Finally, advances in adjuvant chemotherapy and radiotherapy will be required to further improve the overall prognosis of patients with peri-hilar CC.

IBD

PSC is seen in association with IBD, with an incidence between 2.5% and 7.5%. Conversely, 50–75% of patients with PSC have IBD. This high degree of association suggests a common pathogenetic mechanism; however, no causal relationship has been established.

A recent meta-analysis of 11 studies showed that patients with ulcerative colitis (UC) and PSC have a significantly higher risk for the development of colorectal neoplasia, particularly in the proximal part of the colon, than do patients with UC but not PSC. More intensive colonoscopic surveillance should be considered for patients with UC and PSC[18].

A study from the Cleveland Clinic Foundation analysing the risk factors for colorectal cancer (CRC) and dysplasia in patients with PSC showed that 25% of 132 patients with UC and PSC developed CRC or dysplasia compared with 5.6% of 196 with UC alone, suggesting that those patients with UC and PSC are at increased risk of developing CRC or dysplasia. Chronically active disease may be a risk factor, whereas folate could have a protective effect. CRCs associated with PSC are more likely to be proximal, to be diagnosed at a more advanced stage, and to be fatal[19].

Patients with PSC are at greater risk of colonic cancer, but this risk may be reduced by ursodeoxycholic acid (UDCA)[20]. A study from the Mayo Clinic showed that UDCA significantly decreases the risk for developing colorectal dysplasia or cancer in patients with UC and PSC. UDCA has shown effectiveness as a colon cancer chemopreventive agent[21].

Patients with PSC and IBD have an increased risk of developing CRC after liver transplantation (LT). We evaluated patients with PSC after LT to identify risk factors for CRC and its impact on survival. A total of 152 patients with PSC who underwent 173 transplants between 1986 and 2000 were analysed in three groups: PSC without IBD, PSC with colectomy, and PSC with IBD and an intact colon. The incidence of CRC after LT was 5.3% compared with 0.6% in non-PSC cases. All CRCs in the PSC group were in patients with IBD and an intact colon. The cumulative risk of developing CRC in the 83 patients with an intact colon and IBD was 14% and 17% after 5 and 10 years, respectively. Multivariate analysis showed three significant variables related to the risk of developing CRC: colonic dysplasia after LT, duration of colitis more than 10 years, and pancolitis.

Patients with PSC undergoing orthotopic liver transplant (OLT) with a long history of UC and pancolitis have an increased risk of developing CRC with reduced survival, thus there should be aggressive colonic surveillance and colectomy in selected high-risk patients with long-standing severe colitis[22]; we also now recommend offering all patients with UC treatment with UDCA.

The Mayo Clinic experience with 150 consecutive PSC patients showed 78% of PSC patients had associated IBD, most commonly chronic UC, which did not adversely impact patient outcome post-transplantation. Of 150 patients who had LT for PSC, nine (13.5%) required proctocolectomy after LT; five because of intractable symptoms related to IBD and four due to the development of CRC/high-grade dysplasia[23]. It was also shown that the risk of carcinoma after LT compared with that expected for patients during a comparable (pre-transplantation) period was increased fourfold, but this difference was not statistically significant. However, the development of CRC had no overall impact on patient survival. Prophylactic proctocolectomy does not appear necessary, but annual surveillance colonoscopy was recommended[24].

OUTCOME OF PATIENTS WITH PSC AFTER LT

Over the past decade the outcome of LT in patients with PSC and end-stage liver disease has improved significantly, with many centres reporting 1-year patient and graft survival of 90–97% and 85–88%, respectively. Thus, LT has emerged as the treatment of choice for selected patients with end-stage disease[15]. Current data from the European Liver Transplant Registry show that the 1-, 5-, and 10-year patient survival for patients grafted for PSC is 83%, 75%, and 66%, respectively; for those with CC the 5- and 10-year survival is 29% and 25%, respectively.

Analysis from the Mayo Clinic on 150 consecutive PSC patients who received 174 liver allografts showed actuarial patient survival at 1, 2, 5, and 10 years was

94%, 92%, 86%, and 70%, respectively, whereas graft survival was 83%, 83%, 79%, and 61%, respectively. Mean follow-up was 55 months[23].

The outcome after LT for patients grafted for PSC was reported by the University of California in 127 consecutive patients grafted between 1984 and 1996 with a follow-up period of 3 years. Incidental cholangiocarcinoma (ICC) was defined as a tumour < 1 cm in size that was discovered at the time of pathological sectioning of the explanted liver. The 1-, 2-, and 5-year actuarial patient survival was 90%, 86%, and 85%, respectively, and graft survival was 82%, 77%, and 72%, respectively. Previous biliary surgery had no effect on patient survival. Eight per cent of patients had ICC and their survival was not significantly different from that of patients without ICC (100%, 83%, and 83% at 1, 2, and 5 years, respectively). Four patients were known to have CC at the time of OLT, tumour recurred in all within 6 months, and they had a significantly worse outcome. Recurrent sclerosing cholangitis developed in 9%. The patient and graft survival in this group was not different from those in whom recurrence did not develop (patient survival 100%, 90%, and 90%; graft survival 80%, 70%, and 52%); 23% underwent colectomy after LT for dysplasia–carcinoma or symptomatic colitis. It was concluded that LT provides excellent patient and graft survival rates for patients affected with PSC independent of pre-transplant biliary tract surgery, and ICC does not affect patient survival significantly. However, known CC or common duct frozen section biopsy specimen or both showing CC are associated with poor recipient survival, and OLT should be avoided in these cases. Post-transplant colectomy does not affect patient survival adversely[25].

PSC in children

PSC is increasingly diagnosed in children and adolescents, but its long-term prognosis remains uncertain. Therefore a longitudinal cohort study was conducted by the Mayo Clinic to determine the long-term outcome of children with PSC. Fifty-two children with cholangiography-proven PSC (34 boys and 18 girls), who were seen over a 20-year period, were followed up for up to 16.7 years. During follow-up, 11 children underwent LT for end-stage PSC and one child died. The median (50%) survival free of LT was 12.7 years. Compared with an age- and gender-matched US population, survival was significantly shorter in children with PSC. In a Cox regression model, lower platelet count, splenomegaly, and older age were associated with shorter survival. Presence of autoimmune hepatitis overlapping with PSC or medical therapy did not affect survival. Therefore PSC significantly decreases survival in this child population. Although pharmacological therapy may improve symptoms and liver test results initially, it does not seem to impact the long-term outcome[26].

RECURRENCE OF PSC AFTER LT

Recurrent PSC after LT may be difficult to diagnose because of the lack of a diagnostic gold standard. The diagnosis of recurrence is made primarily by imaging the biliary tree, using either percutaneous cholangiography or MRC.

ERCP is usually technically difficult because most patients grafted for PSC have a Roux loop. Histology of the graft may show the characteristic lesions of periductal fibrosis but, as in the native liver, such a finding is not always seen.

Causes of secondary biliary cirrhosis should be excluded; these include preservation injury, blood group type incompatibility between donor and recipient, chronic rejection, hepatic arterial occlusion, and viral infection.

The diagnosis of PSC is based on well-defined cholangiographic features combined with biochemical and histological findings. However, none of these features is specific for PSC, particularly after OLT, because biliary strictures in the liver allograft can occur from a variety of causes other than recurrence.

Some reports provide cholangiographic evidence that post-OLT biliary strictures occur more frequently in patients with PSC than in those who underwent OLT for other liver diseases (including patients with a Roux-en-Y biliary reconstruction). Because no other causes of biliary strictures could be invoked to explain the greater prevalence of these strictures, recurrent disease has been implicated.

There is also histological evidence suggesting that PSC recurs after OLT. Histological findings suggestive of PSC were found more often in PSC allografts compared with a control group. Furthermore, histological features typical for PSC (fibro-obliterative lesions) were seen exclusively in liver biopsy specimens from patients with PSC.

The Mayo Clinic investigated the recurrence of PSC using strict criteria in 150 patients who underwent LT between 1985 and 1996 for PSC; the mean follow-up was 55 months. The incidence of non-anastomotic biliary strictures and hepatic histological findings suggestive of PSC was compared between patients transplanted for PSC and a non-PSC transplant control group. The definition of recurrent PSC was based on characteristic cholangiographic and histological findings that occur in non-transplanted PSC patient (Table 8). Thirty patients with other known causes of post-transplant non-anastomotic biliary strictures were excluded, leaving 120 patients for analysis of recurrence of PSC.

Table 8   Definition of PSC recurrence following liver transplantation

---

Diagnosis
Confirmed diagnosis of PSC prior to liver transplantation

AND

Cholangiography
Intrahepatic and/or extrahepatic biliary structuring, beading, and irregularity >90 days

OR

Histology
Fibrous cholangitis and/or fibro-obliterative lesions with or without ductopenia, biliary fibrosis, or biliary cirrhosis

Exclusion criteria
Hepatic artery thrombosis/stenosis
Established ductopenic rejection
Anastomosis stricture alone
Non-anastomotic strictures before post-transplantation day 90
ABO incompatibility between donor and recipient

Evidence of PSC recurrence after LT was found in 24 patients (20%). Of these, 22 patients showed characteristic features of PSC on cholangiography and 11 had compatible hepatic histological abnormalities with a mean time to diagnosis of 360 and 1350 days, respectively. Both cholangiographic and hepatic histological findings suggestive of PSC recurrence were seen in nine patients. The higher incidence and later onset of non-anastomotic biliary strictures in patients with PSC compared with a non-PSC control group are supportive of the fact that PSC does recur following LT. No risk factor for PSC recurrence could be found, and recurrent disease did not influence patient or graft survival after a mean follow-up of 4.5 years.

The reported incidence of PSC recurrence varies between 5% and 20%. To date, patient and graft survival do not appear to be negatively affected by disease recurrence in the intermediate term of follow-up[27].

An association between PSC recurrence and colectomy was found in our patients. Recurrent PSC, defined by histology or imaging the biliary tree, occurred in 56 of 152 patients at a median of 36 months. Five of these patients developed graft failure as a consequence of end-stage recurrent PSC. Multivariate analysis showed that two factors were associated with the recurrence of disease: intact colon prior to LT and male gender. These findings suggest that colectomy may protect against recurrence of PSC[28].

It is not clear whether immunosuppression affects recurrence. Although recurrence of PSC was more often seen (but not statistically significantly so) in patients who received maintenance corticosteroids, the time to recurrence was not significantly different between those who were treated with maintenance, those who were not successfully weaned, and those who successfully weaned off corticosteroids within 3 months after LT. Orthoclone (OKT3) therapy was associated with a higher risk of PSC recurrence. Recurrence was not influenced by immunosuppression with either cyclosporin or tacrolimus. Coexistent IBD was a cause of failure to wean off corticosteroids, was associated with a shorter time to recurrence of PSC, and was responsible for significant co-morbidity (colon cancer). More immunosuppression seems to be detrimental to the outcome of our patients with PSC: use of OKT3 was associated with a greater incidence of recurrence. Length of corticosteroid use did not affect timing or risk of recurrence, and early corticosteroid withdrawal after LT is beneficial[29].

REJECTION OF THE LIVER ALLOGRAFT

Rejection of the liver allograft may be classified as massive haemorrhagic necrosis or acute and chronic rejection. Massive haemorrhagic necrosis is now rarely seen; it occurs within the first few days after transplantation and is associated with transplantation across the blood-type groups. Early acute rejection (within 28 days of transplantation) is usually of little clinical significance and responds well to additional immunosuppression, whereas later rejection is associated with a greater risk for progression to graft loss. The incidence of early, acute rejection is dependent on the immunosuppressive regimen used and will vary between 20% and 70%. Patients who undergo transplantation for hepatitis B viral infection and alcohol-related liver disease have a lower incidence of rejection compared with those who undergo transplantation for cholestatic diseases, such as PSC and primary biliary cirrhosis. Other factors that influence the incidence of acute rejection include age, race of recipient, and preservation injury. The incidence of chronic rejection is declining; most centres report current rates of 4% to 8%, whereas in earlier series rates of 15% to 20% were observed. The reasons for this decline are unknown, but may relate to better immunosuppression.

Chronic (or ductopenic) rejection usually presents within the first year post-transplantation. The greatest risk factor for chronic rejection is transplantation for chronic rejection; other factors include indication (especially PSC, primary biliary cirrhosis, and autoimmune hepatitis); cytomegalovirus infection, and low levels of immune suppression[30]. Patients with PSC had a higher incidence of acute cellular and chronic ductopenic rejection compared to a non-PSC control group. Chronic ductopenic rejection adversely affected patient and graft survival[23].

CONCLUSIONS

PSC is a chronic progressive destructive biliary disorder of unknown aetiology with a variable and fluctuating course. However, in the majority of patients the disease in the end progresses to liver failure. About 15% of the patients will develop CC. The majority of patients have associated IBD, mostly UC; only few have Crohn's disease. Until now no medical or surgical therapy has been shown effectively to stop the progression of the disease; therefore, LT remains the only effective therapy.

Over the past decade there have been significant advances in our understanding of the natural history of the disease. However, specific treatment still remains elusive and, despite several novel therapeutic approaches, treatment is largely supportive. Transplantation is the only effective therapy, but medium-term graft survival is affected by recurrence. Once the pathogenesis is defined it may be possible to develop logical approaches to treatment.

References

1. Devlin J, O'Grady J. Indications for referral and assessment in adult liver transplantation, BSG guidelines. Gut. 1999;45(Suppl. VI):VI1–VI22.
2. Neuberger J, Gunson B, Komolmit P, Davies MH, Christensen E. Pretransplant prediction of prognosis after liver transplantation on PSC using a Cox regression model. Hepatology. 1999; 29:1375–9.
3. Weisner RH, Grambsch PM, Dickson ER et al. Primary sclerosing cholangitis: natural history, prognostic factors and survival analysis. Hepatology. 1989;10:430–4.
4. Kim WR, Therneau TM, Weisner RH et al. A revised natural history model for primary sclerosing cholangitis. Mayo Clin Proc. 2000;75:688–94.
5. Ferrant JM, Hayllar KM, Wilkinson ML et al. Natural history and prognostic variables in PSC. Gastroenterology. 1991;100:1710–17.
6. Broome U, Olsson R, Loof L et al. Natural history and prognostic factors in 305 Swedish patients with PSC. Gut. 1996;38:610–15.
7. Okolicsanyi L, Fabris L, Viaggi S, Carulli N, Podda M, Ricci G. Primary sclerosing cholangitis: clinical presentation, natural history and prognostic variables: an Italian multicentre study, The Italian PSC Study Group. Eur J Gastroenterol Hepatol. 1996;8:685–91.

8. Shetty K, Rybicki L, Carey WD. The Child–Pugh classification as a prognostic indicators for survival in PSC. Hepatology. 1997;25:1049–53.
9. Boberg KM, Rocca G, Egeland T et al. Time-dependent Cox regression model is superior in prediction of prognosis in primary sclerosing cholangitis. Hepatology. 2002;35:652–7.
10. Boberg KM, Bergquist A, Mitchell S et al. Cholangiocarcinoma in PSC: risk factors and clinical presentation. Scand J Gastroenterol. 2002;37:1205–11.
11. Nashan B, Schlitt HJ, Tusch G et al. Biliary malignancies in PSC: timing for liver transplantation. Hepatology. 1996;23:1105–11.
12. Chalasani N, Baluyut A, Ismail A et al. Cholangiocarcinoma in patients with PSC: multicentre case–control study. Hepatology. 2000;31:7–11.
13. Kubicka S, Kuhnel F, Flemming P et al. K-ras mutations in the bile of patients with primary sclerosing cholangitis. Gut. 2001;48:403–8.
14. Fleming KA, Boberg KM, Glaumann H, Bergquist A, Smith D, Clausen OP. Biliary dysplasia as a marker of cholangiocarcinoma in PSC. J Hepatol. 2001;34:360–5.
15. Wiesner RH. Liver transplantation for PSC: timing, outcome, impact of inflammatory bowel disease and recurrence of disease. Best Pract Clin Gasteroenterol. 2001;15:667–80.
16. Gow PJ, Chapman RW. Liver transplantation for primary sclerosing cholangitis. Liver. 2000; 20:97–103.
17. Yoon JH, Gores GJ. Diagnosis, staging and treatment of cholangiocarcinoma. Curr Treat Options Gastroenterol. 2003;6:105–12.
18. Soetikno RM, Lin OS, Heidenreich PA, Young HS, Blackstone MO. Increased risk of colorectal neoplasia in patients with PSC and ulcerative colitis: a meta-analysis. Gastrointest Endosc. 2002; 56:48–54.
19. Shetty K, Rybicki L, Brzezinski A, Carey WD, Lashner BA. The risk for cancer or dysplasia in ulcerative colitis patients with primary sclerosing cholangitis. Am J Gasteroenterol. 1999;94: 1643–9.
20. Neuberger J. Liver transplantation for cholestatic liver disease. Curr Treat Options Gastroenterol. 2003;6:113–21.
21. Pardi DS, Loftus EV Jr, Kremers WK, Keach J, Lindor KD. Ursodeoxycholic acid as a chemopreventive agent in patients with ulcerative colitis and PSC. Gastroenterology. 2003;124:889–93.
22. Vera A, Gunson BK, Ussatoff V et al. Colorectal cancer in patients with inflammatory bowel disease after transplantation for primary sclerosing cholangitis. Transplantation. 2003;75:1983–8.
23. Graziadei IW, Weisner RH, Marotta PJ et al. Long-term results of patients undergoing liver transplantation for PSC. Hepatology. 1999;30:1121–7.
24. Loftus EV Jr, Aguliar HI, Sandborn WJ et al. Risk of colorectal neoplasia in patients with PSC and ulcerative colitis following orthotopic liver transplantation. Hepatology. 1998;27:685–90.
25. Goss JA, Shackleton CR, Farmer DG et al. Orthotopic liver transplantation for PSC. A 12-year single centre experience. Ann Surg. 1997;225:472–81.
26. Feldstein AE, Perrault J, El-Youssif M, Lindor KD, Freese DK, Angulo P. Primary sclerosing cholangitis in children: long-term follow up study. Hepatology. 2003;38:210–17.
27. Graziadei IW, Weisner RH, Batts KP et al. Recurrence of PSC following liver transplantation. Hepatology. 1999;29:1050–6.
28. Vera A, Moledina S, Gunson B et al. Risk factors for recurrence of PSC liver allograft. Lancet. 2002;360:1943–4.
29. Kugelmas M, Spiegelman P, Osgood MJ et al. Different immunosuppressive regimens and recurrence of PSC after liver transplantation. Liver Transplant. 2003;9:727–32.
30. Neuberger J. Incidence, timing, and risk factors for acute and chronic rejection. Liver Transplant Surg. 1999;5(4 Suppl. 1):S30–6.

Index

Falk Symposium Series

*These titles were published under the MTP Press imprint.

Falk Symposium Series

65. Hadziselimovic F, Herzog B, eds.: *Inflammatory Bowel Diseases and Morbus Hirschprung*. Falk Symposium No. 65. 1992   ISBN: 0-7923-8995-6

66. Martin F, McLeod RS, Sutherland LR, Williams CN, eds.: *Trends in Inflammatory Bowel Disease Therapy*. Falk Symposium No. 66. 1993   ISBN: 0-7923-8827-5

67. Schölmerich J, Kruis W, Goebell H, Hohenberger W, Gross V, eds.: *Inflammatory Bowel Diseases – Pathophysiology as Basis of Treatment*. Falk Symposium No. 67. 1993   ISBN: 0-7923-8996-4

68. Paumgartner G, Stiehl A, Gerok W, eds.: *Bile Acids and The Hepatobiliary System: From Basic Science to Clinical Practice*. Falk Symposium No. 68. 1993   ISBN: 0-7923-8829-1

69. Schmid R, Bianchi L, Gerok W, Maier K-P, eds.: *Extrahepatic Manifestations in Liver Diseases*. Falk Symposium No. 69. 1993   ISBN: 0-7923-8821-6

70. Meyer zum Büschenfelde K-H, Hoofnagle J, Manns M, eds.: *Immunology and Liver*. Falk Symposium No. 70. 1993   ISBN: 0-7923-8830-5

71. Surrenti C, Casini A, Milani S, Pinzani M , eds.: *Fat-Storing Cells and Liver Fibrosis*. Falk Symposium No. 71. 1994   ISBN: 0-7923-8842-9

72. Rachmilewitz D, ed.: *Inflammatory Bowel Diseases – 1994*. Falk Symposium No. 72. 1994   ISBN: 0-7923-8845-3

73. Binder HJ, Cummings J, Soergel KH, eds.: *Short Chain Fatty Acids*. Falk Symposium No. 73. 1994   ISBN: 0-7923-8849-6

73B. Möllmann HW, May B, eds.: *Glucocorticoid Therapy in Chronic Inflammatory Bowel Disease: from basic principles to rational therapy*. International Falk Workshop. 1996   ISBN 0-7923-8708-2

74. Keppler D, Jungermann K, eds.: *Transport in the Liver*. Falk Symposium No. 74. 1994   ISBN: 0-7923-8858-5

74B. Stange EF, ed.: *Chronic Inflammatory Bowel Disease*. Falk Symposium. 1995   ISBN: 0-7923-8876-3

75. van Berge Henegouwen GP, van Hoek B, De Groote J, Matern S, Stockbrügger RW, eds.: *Cholestatic Liver Diseases: New Strategies for Prevention and Treatment of Hepatobiliary and Cholestatic Liver Diseases*. Falk Symposium 75. 1994.   ISBN: 0-7923-8867-4

76. Monteiro E, Tavarela Veloso F, eds.: *Inflammatory Bowel Diseases: New Insights into Mechanisms of Inflammation and Challenges in Diagnosis and Treatment*. Falk Symposium 76. 1995.   ISBN 0-7923-8884-4

77. Singer MV, Ziegler R, Rohr G, eds.: *Gastrointestinal Tract and Endocrine System*. Falk Symposium 77. 1995.   ISBN 0-7923-8877-1

78. Decker K, Gerok W, Andus T, Gross V, eds.: *Cytokines and the Liver*. Falk Symposium 78. 1995.   ISBN 0-7923-8878-X

79. Holstege A, Schölmerich J, Hahn EG, eds.: *Portal Hypertension*. Falk Symposium 79. 1995.   ISBN 0-7923-8879-8

80. Hofmann AF, Paumgartner G, Stiehl A, eds.: *Bile Acids in Gastroenterology: Basic and Clinical Aspects*. Falk Symposium 80. 1995   ISBN 0-7923-8880-1

81. Riecken EO, Stallmach A, Zeitz M, Heise W, eds.: *Malignancy and Chronic Inflammation in the Gastrointestinal Tract – New Concepts*. Falk Symposium 81. 1995   ISBN 0-7923-8889-5

82. Fleig WE, ed.: *Inflammatory Bowel Diseases: New Developments and Standards*. Falk Symposium 82. 1995   ISBN 0-7923-8890-6

Falk Symposium Series

82B. Paumgartner G, Beuers U, eds.: *Bile Acids in Liver Diseases*. International Falk Workshop. 1995   ISBN 0-7923-8891-7

83. Dobrilla G, Felder M, de Pretis G, eds.: *Advances in Hepatobiliary and Pancreatic Diseases: Special Clinical Topics*. Falk Symposium 83. 1995.   ISBN 0-7923-8892-5

84. Fromm H, Leuschner U, eds.: *Bile Acids – Cholestasis – Gallstones: Advances in Basic and Clinical Bile Acid Research*. Falk Symposium 84. 1995   ISBN 0-7923-8893-3

85. Tytgat GNJ, Bartelsman JFWM, van Deventer SJH, eds.: *Inflammatory Bowel Diseases*. Falk Symposium 85. 1995   ISBN 0-7923-8894-1

86. Berg PA, Leuschner U, eds.: *Bile Acids and Immunology*. Falk Symposium 86. 1996
                                                                        ISBN 0-7923-8700-7

87. Schmid R, Bianchi L, Blum HE, Gerok W, Maier KP, Stalder GA, eds.: *Acute and Chronic Liver Diseases: Molecular Biology and Clinics*. Falk Symposium 87. 1996
                                                                        ISBN 0-7923-8701-5

88. Blum HE, Wu GY, Wu CH, eds.: *Molecular Diagnosis and Gene Therapy*. Falk Symposium 88. 1996   ISBN 0-7923-8702-3

88B. Poupon RE, Reichen J, eds.: *Surrogate Markers to Assess Efficacy of TReatment in Chronic Liver Diseases*. International Falk Workshop. 1996   ISBN 0-7923-8705-8

89. Reyes HB, Leuschner U, Arias IM, eds.: *Pregnancy, Sex Hormones and the Liver*. Falk Symposium 89. 1996   ISBN 0-7923-8704-X

89B. Broelsch CE, Burdelski M, Rogiers X, eds.: *Cholestatic Liver Diseases in Children and Adults*. International Falk Workshop. 1996   ISBN 0-7923-8710-4

90. Lam S-K, Paumgartner P, Wang B, eds.: *Update on Hepatobiliary Diseases 1996*. Falk Symposium 90. 1996   ISBN 0-7923-8715-5

91. Hadziselimovic F, Herzog B, eds.: *Inflammatory Bowel Diseases and Chronic Recurrent Abdominal Pain*. Falk Symposium 91. 1996   ISBN 0-7923-8722-8

91B. Alvaro D, Benedetti A, Strazzabosco M, eds.: *Vanishing Bile Duct Syndrome – Pathophysiology and Treatment*. International Falk Workshop. 1996
                                                                        ISBN 0-7923-8721-X

92. Gerok W, Loginov AS, Pokrowskij VI, eds.: *New Trends in Hepatology 1996*. Falk Symposium 92. 1997   ISBN 0-7923-8723-6

93. Paumgartner G, Stiehl A, Gerok W, eds.: *Bile Acids in Hepatobiliary Diseases – Basic Research and Clinical Application*. Falk Symposium 93. 1997   ISBN 0-7923-8725-2

94. Halter F, Winton D, Wright NA, eds.: *The Gut as a Model in Cell and Molecular Biology*. Falk Symposium 94. 1997   ISBN 0-7923-8726-0

94B. Kruse-Jarres JD, Schölmerich J, eds.: *Zinc and Diseases of the Digestive Tract*. International Falk Workshop. 1997   ISBN 0-7923-8724-4

95. Ewe K, Eckardt VF, Enck P, eds.: *Constipation and Anorectal Insufficiency*. Falk Symposium 95. 1997   ISBN 0-7923-8727-9

96. Andus T, Goebell H, Layer P, Schölmerich J, eds.: *Inflammatory Bowel Disease – from Bench to Bedside*. Falk Symposium 96. 1997   ISBN 0-7923-8728-7

97. Campieri M, Bianchi-Porro G, Fiocchi C, Schölmerich J, eds. *Clinical Challenges in Inflammatory Bowel Diseases: Diagnosis, Prognosis and Treatment*. Falk Symposium 97. 1998   ISBN 0-7923-8733-3

98. Lembcke B, Kruis W, Sartor RB, eds. *Systemic Manifestations of IBD: The Pending Challenge for Subtle Diagnosis and Treatment*. Falk Symposium 98. 1998
                                                                        ISBN 0-7923-8734-1

Falk Symposium Series

Falk Symposium Series

Falk Symposium Series

130. Holtmann G, Talley NJ, eds. *Gastrointestinal Inflammation and Disturbed Gut Function: The Challenge of New Concepts.* Falk Symposium 130. 2003
ISBN 0-7923-8783-X

131. Herfarth H, Feagan BJ, Folsch UR, Schölmerich J, Vatn MH, Zeitz M, eds. *Targets of Treatment in Chronic Inflammatory Bowel Diseases.* Falk Symposium 131. 2003
ISBN 0-7923-8784-8

132. Galle PR, Gerken G, Schmidt WE, Wiedenmann B, eds. *Disease Progression and Carcinogenesis in the Gastrointestinal Tract.* Falk Symposium 132. 2003
ISBN 0-7923-8785-6

132A. Staritz M, Adler G, Knuth A, Schmiegel W, Schmoll H-J, eds. *Side-effects of Chemotherapy on the Gastrointestinal Tract.* Falk Workshop. 2003
ISBN 0-7923-8791-0

132B. Reutter W, Schuppan D, Tauber R, Zeitz M, eds. *Cell Adhesion Molecules in Health and Disease.* Falk Workshop. 2003   ISBN 0-7923-8786-4

133. Duchmann R, Blumberg R, Neurath M, Schölmerich J, Strober W, Zeitz M. *Mechanisms of Intestinal Inflammation: Implications for Therapeutic Intervention in IBD.* Falk Symposium 133. 2004   ISBN 0-7923-8787-2

134. Dignass A, Lochs H, Stange E. *Trends and Controversies in IBD – Evidence-Based Approach or Individual Management?* Falk Symposium 134. 2004
ISBN 0-7923-8788-0

134A. Dignass A, Gross HJ, Buhr V, James OFW. *Topical Steroids in Gastroenterology and Hepatology.* Falk Workshop. 2004   ISBN 0-7923-8789-9

135. Lukáš M, Manns MP, Špičák J, Stange EF, eds. *Immunological Diseases of Liver and Gut.* Falk Symposium 135. 2004   ISBN 0-7923-8792-9

136. Leuschner U, Broomé U, Stiehl A, eds. *Cholestatic Liver Diseases: Therapeutic Options and Perspectives.* Falk Symposium 136. 2004   ISBN 0-7923-8793-7